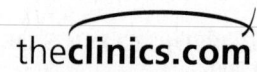

ORTHOPEDIC CLINICS OF NORTH AMERICA

Wrist Trauma

GUEST EDITOR
Steven Papp, MD, MSc, FRCS(C)

April 2007 • Volume 38 • Number 2

SAUNDERS

An Imprint of Elsevier, Inc.
PHILADELPHIA   LONDON   TORONTO   MONTREAL   SYDNEY   TOKYO

W.B. SAUNDERS COMPANY
A Division of Elsevier Inc.

Elsevier Inc., 1600 John F. Kennedy Blvd., Suite 1800, Philadelphia, PA 19103-2899.

http://www.orthopedic.theclinics.com

ORTHOPEDIC CLINICS OF NORTH AMERICA
April 2007
Editor: Debora Dellapena

Volume 38, Number 2
ISSN 0030-5898
ISBN-10: 1-4160-4348-9
ISBN-13: 978-1-4160-4348-5

Copyright © 2007 by Elsevier Inc. All rights reserved. No part of this publication may be reproduced or transmitted in any form or by any means, electronic or mechanical, including photocopy, recording, or any information retrieval system, without written permission from the Publisher.

Single photocopies of single articles may be made for personal use as allowed by national copyright laws. Permission of the Publisher and payment of a fee is required for all other photocopying, including multiple or systematic copying, copying for advertising or promotional purposes, resale, and all forms of document delivery. Special rates are available for educational institutions that wish to make photocopies for non-profit educational classroom use. Permissions may be sought directly from Elsevier's Rights Department in Philadelphia, PA, USA: phone (+1) 215 239 3804, fax (+1) 215 239 3805, e-mail healthpermissions@elsevier.com. Requests may also be completed on-line via the Elsevier homepage (http://www.elsevier.com/locate/permissions). In the USA, users may clear permissions and make payments through the Copyright Clearance Center, Inc., 222 Rosewood Drive, Danvers, MA 01923, USA; phone: (978) 750-8400, fax: (978) 750-4744, and in the UK through the copyright Licensing Agency Rapid Clearance Service (CLARCS), 90 Tottenham Court Road, London W1P 0LP, UK; phone (+44) 171 436 5931; fax: (+44) 171 436 3986. Other countries may have a local reprographic rights agency for payments.

The ideas and opinions expressed in *Orthopedic Clinics of North America* do not necessarily reflect those of the Publisher. The Publisher does not assume any responsibility for any injury and/or damage to persons or property arising out of or related to any use of the material contained in this periodical. The reader is advised to check the appropriate medical literature and the product information currently provided by the manufacturer of each drug to be administered to verify the dosage, the method and duration of administration, or contraindications. It is the responsibility of the treating physician or other health care professional, relying on independent experience and knowledge of the patient, to determine drug dosages and the best treatment for the patient. Mention of any product in this issue should not be construed as endorsement by the contributors, editors, or the Publisher of the product or manufacturers' claims.

Orthopedic Clinics of North America (ISSN 0030-5898) is published quarterly (For Post Office use only: Volume 38 issue 1 of 4) by Elsevier Inc., 360 Park Avenue South, New York, NY 10010-1710. Months of publication are January, April, July, and October. Business and Editorial Offices: 1600 John F. Kennedy Blvd., Suite 1800, Philadelphia, PA 19103-2899. Customer Service Office: 6277 Sea Harbor Drive, Orlando, FL 33887-4800. Periodicals postage paid at New York, NY and additional mailing offices. Subscription prices are $205.00 per year for (US individuals), $347.00 per year for (US institutions), $243.00 per year (Canadian individuals), $407.00 per year (Canadian institutions), $281.00 per year (international individuals), $407.00 per year (international institutions), $103.00 per year (US students), $140.00 per year (Canadian and international students). Foreign air speed delivery is included in all *Clinics* subscription prices. All prices are subject to change without notice. **POSTMASTER:** Send address changes to *Orthopedic Clinics of North America*, Elsevier Periodicals Customer Service, 6277 Sea Harbor Drive, Orlando, FL 32887-4800. **Customer Service: 1-800-654-2452 (US). From outside of the US, call 1-407-345-4000.** E-mail: elspcs@elsevier.com.

Reprints. For copies of 100 or more, of articles in this publication, please contact the Commercial Reprints Department, Elsevier Inc., 360 Park Avenue South, New York, New York 10010-1710. Tel. (212) 633-3813 Fax: (212) 462-1935 e-mail: reprints@elsevier.com.

Orthopedic Clinics of North America is covered in *Index Medicus, Cinahl, Excerpta Medica,* and *Cumulative Index to Nursing and Allied Health Literature.*

Printed in the United States of America.

WRIST TRAUMA

GUEST EDITOR

STEVEN PAPP, MD, MSc, FRCS(C), Assistant Professor, Ottawa Civic Hospital, Department of Orthopaedic Surgery, University of Ottawa, Ottawa, Ontario, Canada

CONTRIBUTORS

JULIE E. ADAMS, MD, Resident, Department of Orthopaedic Surgery, Mayo Clinic, Rochester, Minnesota

GEORGE S. ATHWAL, MD, FRCSC, Assistant Professor and Consultant, Hand and Upper Limb Centre, St. Joseph's Health Care, University of Western Ontario, London, Ontario, Canada

TERRY S. AXELROD, MD, MSc, FRCS(C), Consultant Orthopaedic Surgeon, Division of Orthopaedic Surgery, Sunnybrook Health Science Centre; Associate, Professor of Surgery, Department of Surgery, University of Toronto, Ontario, Canada

GREGORY K. BERRY, MD, FRCSC, Assistant Professor, McGill University Division of Orthopedic Surgery, Montreal, Quebec, Canada

ROY CARDOSO, MD, Department of Orthopaedic Surgery, University of California, Davis, School of Medicine, Sacramento, California

KENNETH J. FABER, MD, MHPE, FRCSC, Associate Professor and Consultant, Hand and Upper Limb Centre, St Joseph's Health Care, University of Western Ontario, London, Ontario, Canada

ALAN GIACHINO, MD, BPHE, FRCS(C), Professor, Department of Orthopaedics, University of Ottawa, Ottawa, Ontario, Canada

WADE GOFTON, MD, MEd, FRCSC, Department of Orthopaedic Surgery, University of Ottawa, The Ottawa Hospital, Civic Campus, Ottawa, Ontario, Canada

EDWARD J. HARVEY, MD, MSc, FRCSC, Associate Professor, McGill University Division of Orthopedic Surgery, Montreal, Quebec, Canada

ASIF M. ILYAS, MD, Fellow, Hand Surgery, Harvard Medical School, Massachusetts General Hospital; Orthopaedic Hand Service, Massachusetts General Hospital, Boston, Massachusetts

JESSE B. JUPITER, MD, Chief, Orthopaedic Hand Service, Massachusetts General Hospital; Professor, Department of Orthopaedic Surgery, Harvard Medical School; Orthopaedic Hand Service, Massachusetts General Hospital, Boston, Massachusetts

ALLAN LIEW, MD, FRCSC, Department of Orthopaedic Surgery, University of Ottawa, The Ottawa Hospital, Civic Campus, Ottawa, Ontario, Canada

SURIYA LUENAM, MD, Clinical Fellow, Division of Orthopaedic Surgery, Kingston General Hospital, Queen's University, Kingston, Ontario, Canada

JENNIFER MANUEL, MD, Hand Fellow, Division of Hand Surgery, Department of Orthopedics, Mayo Clinic, Rochester, Minnesota

PAUL A. MARTINEAU, MD, FRCSC, Fellow, Hand and Upper Extremity, University of Washington, Seattle, Washington

WREN V. McCALLISTER, MD, Fellow, Hand and Microvascular Surgery, Department of Orthopaedics and Sports Medicine, University of Washington, Seattle, Washington

MICHAEL D. McKEE, MD, FRCS(C), Associate Professor, Division of Orthopaedics, Department of Surgery, St. Michael's Hospital, University of Toronto, Toronto, Ontario, Canada

STEVEN L. MORAN, MD, Associate Professor of Plastic Surgery and Orthopedic Surgery, Division of Plastic Surgery, Mayo Clinic, Rochester, Minnesota

JONATHAN S. MULFORD, BMEDSC, MBBS, FRACS, Clinical Fellow, Division of Orthopaedic Surgery, Sunnybrook Health Science Centre, University of Toronto, Toronto, Ontario, Canada

NICHOLAS M. NEMECHEK, Research Assistant, Hand and Microvascular Surgery, Department of Orthopaedics and Sports Medicine, University of Washington, Seattle, Washington

STEVEN PAPP, MD, MSc, FRCS(C), Assistant Professor, Ottawa Civic Hospital, Department of Orthopaedic Surgery, University of Ottawa, Ottawa, Ontario, Canada

JUBIN B. PAYANDEH, MD, FRCS(C), Clinical Fellow, Division of Orthopaedics, Department of Surgery, St. Michael's Hospital, University of Toronto, Toronto, Ontario, Canada

H. JAMES PFAEFFLE, MD, PhD, Fellow, Hand and Microvascular Surgery, Department of Orthopaedics and Sports Medicine, University of Washington, Seattle, Washington

DAVID R. PICHORA, MD, FRCSC, Professor and Chair, Division of Orthopaedic Surgery, Kingston General Hospital, Queen's University, Kingston, Ontario, Canada

JAMES H. ROTH, MD, FRCSC, Professor of Surgery, Hand and Upper Limb Centre, St. Joseph's Health Care, University of Western Ontario, London, Ontario, Canada

DAVID J. SAUDER, MD, FRCSC, Clinical Fellow, Hand and Upper Limb Centre, St. Joseph's Health Care, University of Western Ontario, London, Ontario, Canada

BRADLEY E. SLAGEL, MD, Resident, Division of Orthopaedic Surgery, Kingston General Hospital, Queen's University, Kingston, Ontario, Canada

SCOTT P. STEINMANN, MD, Associate Professor of Orthopedics, Department of Orthopaedic Surgery, Mayo Clinic College of Medicine, Rochester, Minnesota

ROBERT M. SZABO, MD, MPH, Chief, Hand and Upper Extremity Service, Professor of Orthopaedics and Plastic Surgery, Department of Orthopaedic Surgery, University of California, Davis, School of Medicine, Sacramento, California

THOMAS E. TRUMBLE, MD, Professor and Chief, Hand and Microvascular Surgery, Department of Orthopaedics and Sports Medicine, University of Washington Hand Surgery Institute, Seattle, Washington

ROBERT G. TURNER, MB, BCh, FRCS, Clinical Fellow, Hand and Upper Limb Centre, St. Joseph's Health Care, University of Western Ontario, London, Ontario, Canada

THANAPONG WAITAYAWINYU, MD, Research Fellow, Hand and Microvascular Surgery, Department of Orthopaedics and Sports Medicine, University of Washington School of Medicine, Seattle, Washington

DARRYL YOUNG, MD, BSc(H), Resident, University of Ottawa, Ottawa, Ontario, Canada

WRIST TRAUMA

CONTENTS

Preface ix
Steven Papp

Wrist Anatomy and Surgical Approaches 127
Roy Cardoso and Robert M. Szabo

> Appreciation and knowledge of anatomy as it relates to surgical approaches is critical for planning treatment of traumatic wrist injuries. This article discusses the pertinent anatomy and some of the more commonly used approaches to wrist trauma.

Physical Examination of the Wrist 149
Darryl Young, Steven Papp and Alan Giachino

> Physical examination of the wrist requires knowledge of wrist anatomy and pathology to make a diagnosis or narrow the differential diagnosis. Symptoms are provoked by palpation and signs are produced by manipulation. Negative findings elsewhere in the wrist are important. Final diagnosis may require diagnostic imaging. By having all three methods of assessment agree one is assured of correct diagnosis. The physical examination of the wrist is not unlike that of other joints, in that a systematic approach includes observation, range of motion, palpation, and special tests.

Distal Radius Fractures—Classification of Treatment and Indications for Surgery 167
Asif M. Ilyas and Jesse B. Jupiter

> Distal radius fractures are common injuries. Multiple classification systems have highlighted the evolution of the understanding of distal radius fractures. Understanding the classifications of distal radius fractures is important in identifying the important aspects that affect their outcome. Surgical indications of distal radius fractures can be divided into the following categories: patient factors, fracture reduction, fracture stability, and the presence of associated injuries.

Distal Radius Fractures: Nonoperative and Percutaneous Pinning Treatment Options 175
Wade Gofton and Allan Liew

> Nonoperative treatment of distal radial fractures by reduction and immobilization remains the most common treatment, based on the incidence of appropriate fracture types, as seen in many epidemiological studies in the literature. In this article, the indications, technique, predictors of failure, outcomes, and complications are reviewed. A variety of

treatment options have been proposed for distal radial fractures that are predicted, or subsequently identified, to be too unstable for nonoperative management. Percutaneous pinning is an effective option for select fractures. The authors also review the indications, described techniques, complications and outcomes associated with this treatment option.

External Fixation of Distal Radius Fractures 187
Jubin B. Payandeh and Michael D. McKee

Fractures of the distal radius are the most common fractures that occur in patients between ages 15 and 75 years. Many methods for treating displaced distal radius fractures are available. All forms of treatment involve obtaining fracture reduction, which may then be maintained by casting, functional bracing, external fixation, percutaneous pinning, internal fixation, or a combination of these methods. This article discusses the indications and technique of fracture treatment with external fixation and, when required, adjuvant percutaneous pins.

Plating for Distal Radius Fractures 193
Paul A. Martineau, Gregory K. Berry and Edward J. Harvey

No area of fracture management has had such a recent explosion of new treatment modalities as distal radius plating. This explosion has largely been implant- and industry-driven, with little evidence-based research guiding the way. A perceived difficulty with commonly used modalities by the orthopedic community has been enough to drive an entire new set of options for distal radius fixation. A drift from dorsal to volar plating has occurred that has been unexamined by randomized research. Segment specific fixation has been a new mindset that has resulted in a novel plate line and has caused other manufacturers to redesign their product lines. Other novel approaches for proposed problems include locking plates, nail-plate combinations, and others. This article outlines some of these options with a literature opinion and a clarification from the authors. A treatment plan for common fractures of the distal radius is also outlined.

Management of Post-Traumatic Malunion of Fractures of the Distal Radius 203
Bradley E. Slagel, Suriya Luenam and David R. Pichora

Distal radius malunions are a common cause of patient morbidity. This review of the literature surrounding distal radius malunion covers the demographics, pathologic anatomy, and indications for surgery, surgical techniques, and salvage options. Particular emphasis is placed on subject areas that have not been reviewed as extensively in previous articles, including: intra-articular malunion, computer-assisted techniques, bone graft alternatives, and volar fixed-angle plate osteosynthesis.

Complications of Distal Radius Fractures 217
Robert G. Turner, Kenneth J. Faber and George S. Athwal

Fractures occur at the distal end of the radius more frequently than at any other location. The reported complication rates of distal radius fractures in the literature vary from 6% to 80%. Complications may occur from the fracture or its treatment. This article reviews complications caused by distal radius fractures and their treatment. Complications are divided chronologically in to immediate, early (less than 6 weeks), and late (greater than 6 weeks).

Acute Scaphoid Fractures 229
Julie E. Adams and Scott P. Steinmann

Scaphoid fractures are a common problem encountered in clinical practice. This manuscript provides an algorithm for the diagnosis, evaluation, and treatment of acute scaphoid fractures.

Management of Scaphoid Nonunions 237
Thanapong Waitayawinyu, H. James Pfaeffle, Wren V. McCallister,
Nicholas M. Nemechek, and Thomas E. Trumble

> Scaphoid nonunions can exist with or without avascular necrosis of the proximal pole, and waist fractures may have an associated humpback deformity. CT best shows the deformity and bone loss, whereas MRI will show avascular necrosis. Operative treatment should be directed at correcting the deformity with open reduction and internal fixation and bone grafting. Vascularized bone grafts should be used in cases of avascular necrosis.

Carpal Bone Fractures 251
Steven Papp

> Carpal bone fractures make up a significant proportion of injuries to the wrist. The complex bone shape and articulations make diagnosis more difficult and missed injuries more common. This article reviews carpal bone fractures excluding the scaphoid.

The Diagnosis and Treatment of Scapholunate Instability 261
Jennifer Manuel and Steven L. Moran

> Scapholunate instability is the most common form of carpal instability. Pain produced by this condition is caused by the wrist's inability to sustain physiologic loads because of an injury to the linkage between the scaphoid and lunate. The term scapholunate instability may describe a wide spectrum of clinical conditions ranging from mild wrist dysfunction and partial ligamentous tear to debilitating pain with associated rupture of the scapholunate interosseus ligament complex. This article reviews the pathophysiology of scapholunate instability and its identification and treatment.

Perilunate Injuries 279
David J. Sauder, George S. Athwal, Kenneth J. Faber, and James H. Roth

> Perilunate injuries are complex injuries of the bony and ligamentous structures of the wrist. They require operative management with careful restoration of carpal alignment and open reduction and internal fixation of associated fractures. Even with optimal treatment, mild to moderate dysfunction affects most patients.

Traumatic Problems of the Distal Radioulnar Joint 289
Jonathan S. Mulford and Terry S. Axelrod

> Traumatic injuries of the distal radioulnar joint (DRUJ) may give rise to complex wrist pathologies. Substantial ongoing disability can arise should these injuries go unrecognized resulting in sub-optimal treatment and lack of appropriate rehabilitation. Injuries of the DRUJ may occur in isolation but more commonly are found with a fracture of the radius. These challenging DRUJ injuries may be simple or complex (irreducible or severe instability), acute or chronic. An adequate knowledge of the stabilizers of the DRUJ is essential in understanding treatment options. Traumatic instability of the DRUJ is reviewed and the anatomy and stabilizing factors are discussed. An algorithm to guide selection of treatment options in complex cases is presented.

Index 299

FORTHCOMING ISSUES

July 2007

Minimally Invasive Spine Surgery
Dino Samartzis, DSc, MSc, DipEBHC
Francis H. Shen, MD
D. Greg Anderson, MD, *Guest Editors*

October 2007

Scoliosis
Anthony A. Stans, MD, *Guest Editor*

RECENT ISSUES

January 2007

Vascularized Bone Grafting in Orthopedic Surgery
Alexander Y. Shin, MD
Steven L. Moran, MD, *Guest Editors*

October 2006

Sexual Dimorphism in Musculoskeletal Health
Laura L. Tosi, MD
Letha Y. Griffin, MD
Mary I. O'Connor, MD, *Guest Editors*

July 2006

Advances in Musculoskeletal Imaging
Peter L. Munk, MD, CM, FRCPC
Bassam Masri, MD, FRCSC, *Guest Editors*

The Clinics are now available online!

Access your subscription at:
http://www.theclinics.com

Preface

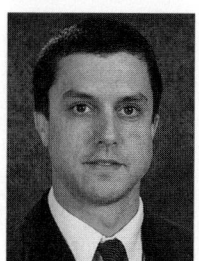

Steven Papp, MD, MSc, FRCS(C)
Guest Editor

It is an honor to act as guest editor for this edition of *Orthopedic Clinics of North America*. I currently practice in Ottawa, Ontario—home to the largest skating rink in the world. For the months of January to March, the Rideau Canal is transformed into an 8-kilometer skating rink for people to enjoy or even skate to work! Unfortunately, experienced and beginner skaters alike commonly have falls on this amazing but sometimes treacherous rink. Our volume of radius fractures, scaphoid fractures, and other wrist injuries dramatically goes up during these months. As I am sure many other orthopedic surgeons have experienced, the increased population, increased life expectancy, and increased general activity level have all translated into a great demand on physicians that deal with these problems. In Canada, the shortage of orthopedic specialists can compound this problem. Correct treatment can have a great impact on the patient and on society in terms of health care costs.

In this issue, leading authors and researchers from around North America have contributed articles on various topics in wrist trauma. The authors have vast experience with many research publications in this field, many of whom I look up to greatly.

In the first two articles, the anatomy and physical examination of the wrist serve as the building blocks for making a diagnosis in a patient who has a wrist injury. The next six articles cover various topics and treatment options related to distal radius fractures, as this is probably the most common problem a treating physician will encounter. There has been an explosion of literature and implants available to deal with this common problem. The remaining articles cover scaphoid fractures, carpal bone fractures, distal radio-ulnar joint injuries, and ligament injuries common to the wrist. My hope is the orthopedic surgeon or training resident can use this issue as a reference for injuries to the wrist.

I have enjoyed the experience of putting this issue together immensely. Asking some of my senior colleagues to contribute was daunting, but luckily all of the authors were happy to contribute. I would like to thank them for their hard work and excellent and thoughtful articles. I would like to thank Deb Dellapena, the editor of this issue, for her diligent work on this project. I dedicate this issue to my wife Brenda and my children—Rosemary, Ryan, and Renée for their great support.

Steven Papp, MD, MSc, FRCS(C)
Ottawa Civic Hospital
Department of Orthopaedic Surgery
University of Ottawa
1053 Carling Avenue
Ottawa, Ontario
Canada K1Y 4E9

E-mail address: spapp@ottawahospital.on.ca

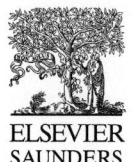

Wrist Anatomy and Surgical Approaches
Roy Cardoso, MD, Robert M. Szabo, MD, MPH*

Department of Orthopaedic Surgery, University of California, Davis, School of Medicine, 4860 Y Street, Suite 3800, Sacramento, CA 95817, USA

Appreciation and knowledge of anatomy as it relates to surgical approaches is critical for planning treatment of traumatic wrist injuries. This article discusses the pertinent anatomy and some of the more commonly used approaches to wrist trauma.

Surface landmarks

Important dorsal landmarks include the styloid process of the long-finger metacarpal, anatomic snuffbox, Lister's tubercle, lunate fossa, the radial styloid, and the head of the ulna (Fig. 1).

The anatomic snuffbox is formed by the third dorsal compartment (extensor pollicis longus) ulnarly, the first dorsal compartment (abductor pollicis longus, extensor pollicis brevis) radially, and the extensor retinaculum proximally. Its contents include the dorsal continuation of the radial artery and branches of the radial sensory nerve.

Lister's tubercle, a dorsal prominence over the distal aspect of the radius, redirects the extensor pollicis longus, which lies just ulnar to it, approximately 0.5 cm proximal to the radiocarpal joint [1]. The lunate fossa is a palpable depression found in line with the third metacarpal. The lunate bone lies directly below this depression.

Important landmarks on the palm and volar aspect of the wrist are illustrated in Fig. 2. Kaplan described his *cardinal line* in 1953 [2]. As a surface marker, this line helps localize deeper structures in the hand and wrist. Although experts disagree on the exact manner in which the line is drawn and its relationship to deeper structures, it continues to be an important and widely used tool [3].

Kaplan's line is made by extending a transverse line across the palm, in line with the distal aspect of the thumb metacarpal. Additionally, longitudinal lines are drawn perpendicular to Kaplan's line, along the radial aspect of long finger and the ulnar aspect of the ring finger. The intersecting lines form a grid whose points demarcate underlying neurovascular structures (Fig. 3).

Osteology and joint anatomy

The skeletal components of the wrist include the distal radius and ulna, eight carpal bones, and the proximal ends of the five metacarpals (Fig. 4). The articular surface of the distal radius is typically tilted with 22° of radial inclination, 11° of volar tilt, and 12 mm of radial height (Fig. 5). Its articulation is composed of two fossae—the ovoid-shaped lunate fossa and triangular scaphoid fossa—which articulate with the lunate and scaphoid bones, respectively (Fig. 6). The radiocarpal joint allows multiple axes of motion, including flexion, extension, radial deviation, and ulnar deviation [4]. On the ulnar aspect of the distal radius, the sigmoid notch articulates with the distal ulna to form the distal radioulnar joint (DRUJ). The DRUJ, a pivot joint, permits pronation and supination of the wrist. Although the arc of curvature of the sigmoid notch varies, it is typically greater than that of the ulnar head. This incongruity permits both translation and rotation of the DRUJ. Consequently, the ulna translates dorsally in pronation and volarly

---

* Corresponding author.
 E-mail address: rmszabo@ucdavis.edu (R.M. Szabo).

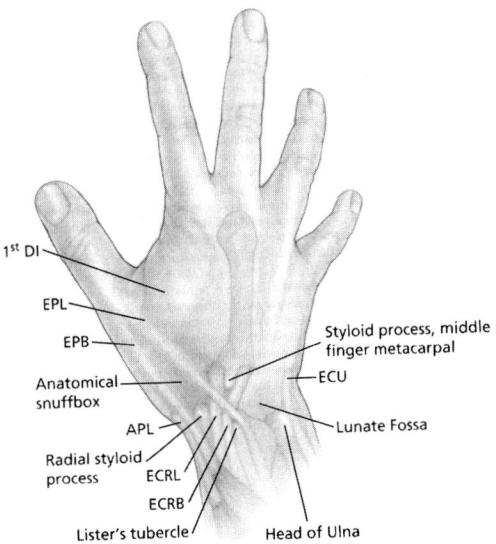

Fig. 1. Dorsal wrist landmarks. (*Reproduced from* Doyle JR, Botte MJ. Surgical anatomy of the hand and upper extremity. Philadelphia: Lippincott Williams and Wilkins; 2003. p. 486–529; with permission.)

in supination. Although the joint is primarily stabilized by the triangular fibrocartilage complex (TFCC), additional stability is imparted by the joint capsule, interosseous membrane, pronator quadratus, and extensor carpi ulnaris [5].

The distal ulna does not typically articulate with the carpus. Its distal surface, covered by the triangular fibrocartilage (TFC), is composed of the head, seat, styloid, and fovea. The carpal bones are arranged into a proximal and distal row. The midcarpal joint is the articulation between the rows. The proximal row, formed by the scaphoid, lunate, and triquetrum, has no muscular attachments; it articulates with the trapezium, trapezoid, capitate, and hamate. The scaphoid occupies both rows. The eighth carpal bone, the pisiform, is a sesamoid bone of the flexor carpi ulnaris and does not contribute to midcarpal joint motion.

Ligament anatomy

The ligaments of the wrist have been described and named differently by several investigators. Taleisnik [6] groups wrist ligaments into extrinsic and intrinsic, palmar, and dorsal. The extrinsic ligaments span the radiocarpal and midcarpal joints, whereas the intrinsic ligaments connect the carpal bones.

The palmar radiocarpal ligaments are extrinsic, originating from the palmar edge of the distal radius and traveling toward to the scaphoid, lunate, and capitate (Fig. 7). The radial-most

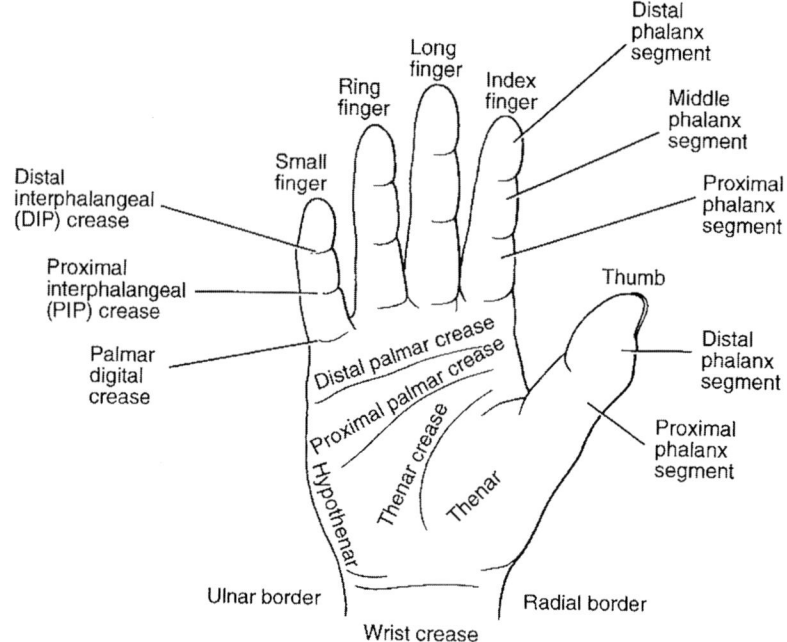

Fig. 2. Palmar wrist landmarks. (*From* Trumble TE. Principles of hand surgery and therapy. Philadelphia: W.B. Saunders; 2000. p. 1–18; with permission.)

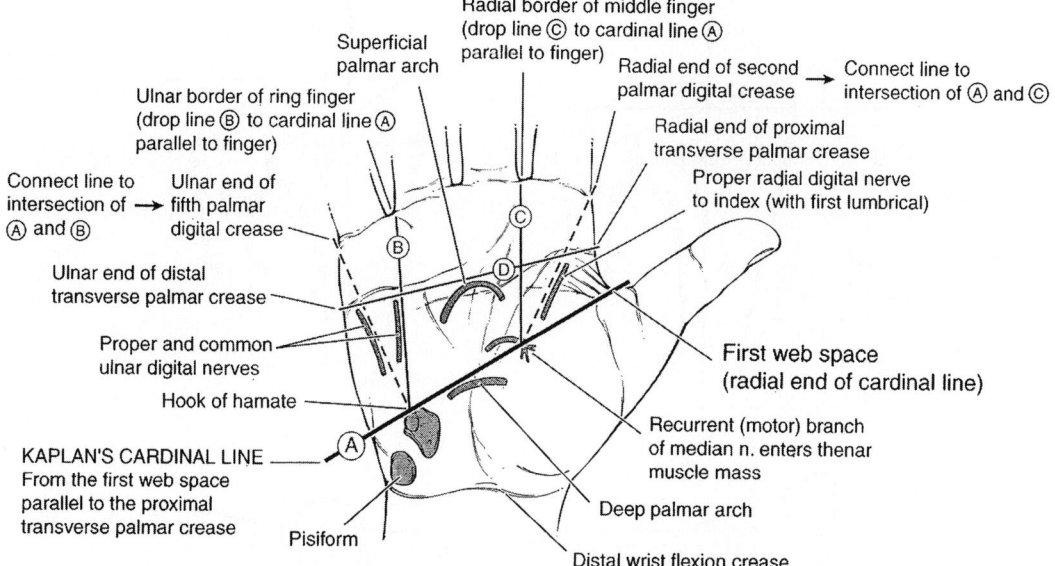

Fig. 3. Kaplan's cardinal line and associated structures. (*Reproduced from* Carlson GC. Surgical approaches to the hand and wrist. In: Chapman MW, editor. Chapman's orthopaedic surgery. 3rd edition. Philadelphia: Lippincott Williams & Wilkins; 2001. p. 1239–46; with permission.)

extrinsic ligament, the radioscaphocapitate ligament (RSC), originates from the radial styloid, travels across the waist and distal pole of the scaphoid, crosses the capitate, and coalesces with the ulnocapitate ligament (Fig. 8). The RSC is typically divided when performing a volar approach to the scaphoid and should be repaired because it is an important stabilizer of the radial wrist. The long radiolunate ligament lies just ulnar to the RSC and may also be encountered during a volar approach to the scaphoid. Along with the short radiolunate, the long radiolunate ligament functions as a primary restraint to lunate displacement with perilunate dislocations [6]. The radioscapholunate ligament, also known as the ligament of Testut, is actually a neurovascular bundle and contributes nothing to carpal stability.

The ulnocarpal ligaments (see Figs. 8 and 9) arise from the distal ulna and, in conjunction with the TFC and the sheath of the extensor carpi ulnaris, form the TFCC. The TFCC serves as the primary stabilizer of the DRUJ [7,8]. The TFC originates from the lunate and sigmoid fossae of the distal radius and inserts into the base of the ulnar styloid. Its peripheral layer is composed of thick, well-vascularized volar and dorsal ligamentous bands: the dorsal and palmar radioulnar ligaments. Between these bands, a central area of fibrocartilage is avascular, load-bearing, and often likened to the meniscus of the knee. It articulates with the distal ulna and triquetrum (Fig. 9) [5].

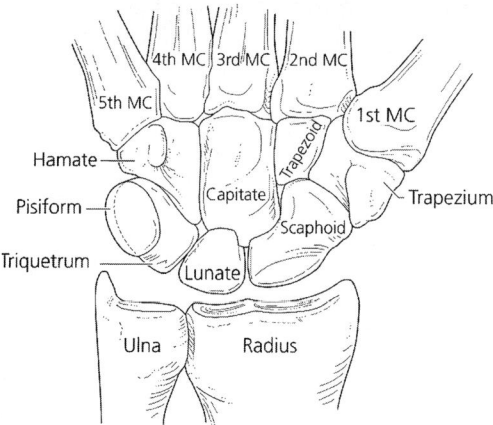

Fig. 4. Osseous Anatomy of the wrist. (*From* Steinburg BD, Plancher KD. Clinical anatomy of the wrist and elbow. Clin Sports Med 1995;14(2):299–313; with permission.)

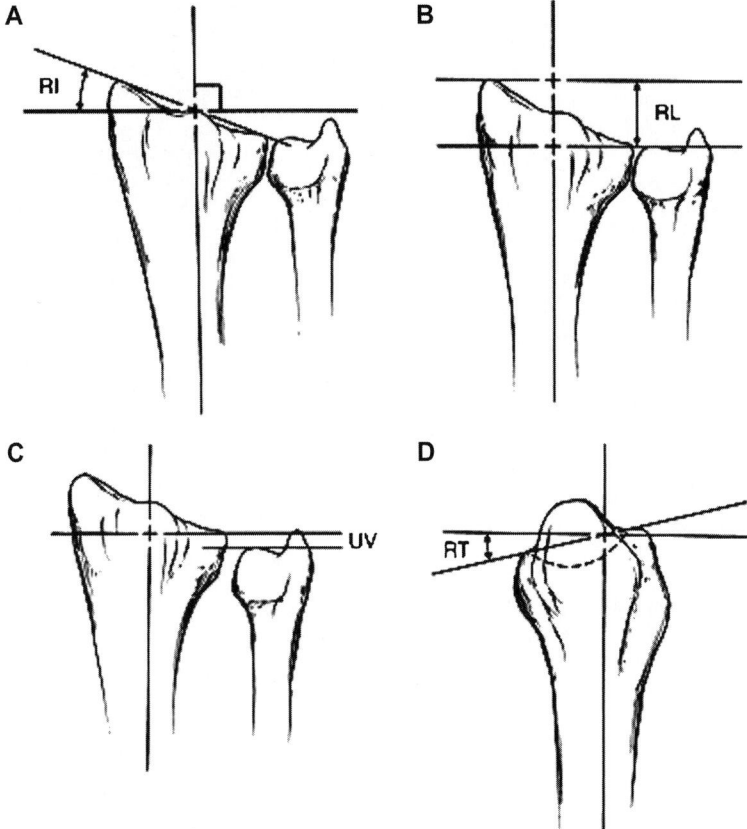

Fig. 5. The various angles to assess in distal radius fractures. (*A*) Radial inclination (RI), normal, 22°. (*B*) Radial length (RL), normal, 12 mm. (*C*) Ulnar variance (UV), normal, 0–2 mm. (*D*) Radial tilt (RT), normal, 11° volar. (*Reproduced from* Graham TJ. Surgical correction of malunited fractures of the distal radius. J Am Acad Orthop Surg 1997;5:270–81; with permission.)

Dorsally, the dorsal radiotriquetral (radiocarpal) ligament and the dorsal intercarpal ligament help stabilize the wrist. The former helps stabilize the lunotriquetral joint, preventing volar intercalated segment instability (Fig. 10). The latter is an

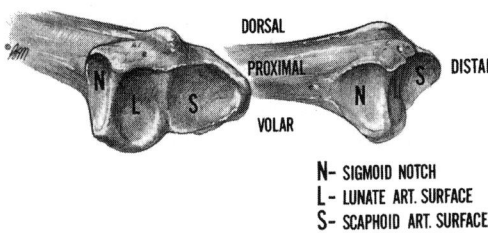

Fig. 6. Articular surface of the distal radius. (*From* Bowers WH. The distal radioulnar joint. In: Green DP, Hotchkiss RN, Pederson WC, editors. Operative hand surgery. 3rd edition. New York: Churchill Livingstone; 1993. p. 976; with permission.)

important stabilizer of the proximal pole of the scaphoid. Frequently injured intercarpal ligaments include the scapholunate interosseous ligament and the lunotriquetral interosseous ligament. The scapholunate ligament has proximal, dorsal, and volar components, with the dorsal the strongest and therefore most critical joint stabilizer. When torn, dorsal intercalated segment instability can result. In contrast, the lunotriquetral ligament is strongest at its volar aspect. Injury to this ligament may result in volar intercalated segment instability [9].

Retinacular anatomy

Two distinct fascial layers encompass the volar wrist. The superficial layer consists of the volar carpal ligament and palmar fascia. A deeper layer, the flexor retinaculum, is divided into three

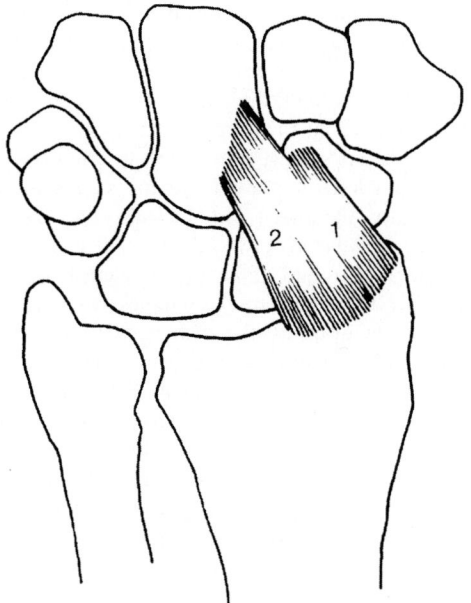

Fig. 7. Components of the radioscaphocapitate ligament. 1, radioscaphoid component; 2, radiocapitate component. (*From* Weber ER. Physiologic bases for wrist function. In: Lichtman DM, Alexander AH, editors. The wrist and its disorders. Philadelphia: W.B. Saunders; 1997; with permission.)

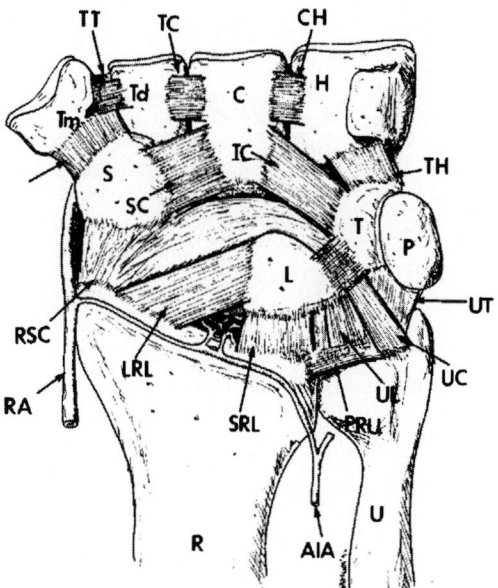

Fig. 8. The anatomy of the palmar wrist ligaments. AIA, anterior interosseous artery; C, capitate; CH, palmar capitohamate ligament; H, hamate; L, lunate; LRL, long radiolunate ligament; P, pisiform; PRU, palmar radioulnar ligament; PTC, palmar trapezocapitate ligament; R, radius; RA, radial artery; RSC, radioscaphocapitate ligament; S, scaphoid; SC, scaphocapitate ligament; SRL, short and radiolunate ligament; STT, scaphotrapziotrapezoid ligament; T, triquetrum; TC, triquetrocapitate ligament; Td, trapezoid; TH, triquetrohamate ligament; Tm, trapezium; TT, palmar trapeziotrapezoid ligament; U, ulna; UC, ulnocapitate ligament; UL, ulnolunate ligament; UT, ulnotriquetral ligament. (*From* Berger RA. Arthroscopic anatomy of the wrist and distal radioulnar joint. Hand Clin 1999;15:393–413; with permission.)

anatomic zones from proximal to distal (Fig. 11). The proximal portion is largely contiguous with the antebrachial fascia. The middle portion, the transverse carpal ligament (TCL), attaches ulnarly to the hook of the hamate and the pisiform, and radially to the scaphoid tubercle and trapezial tuberosity. The TCL serves as the roof of the carpal canal. The distal portion is the aponeurosis between the thenar and hypothenar muscles.

The carpal canal lies directly under the TCL and contains the flexor pollicis longus radially, the median nerve volarly, and the eight tendons of the flexor digitorum superficialis and the flexor digitorum profundus. Guyon's canal is ulnar to the carpal canal and contains the ulnar nerve and artery. Guyon's canal lies above the transverse carpal ligament, between the pisiform and hook of the hamate. Its floor is formed by the TCL and its roof by the volar carpal ligament and palmaris brevis. It is bordered radially by the hook of the hamate and the digital flexor tendons and ulnarly by the pisiform, flexor carpi ulnaris, and abductor digiti minimi (Fig. 12).

The extensor retinaculum lies across the dorsum of the wrist and prevents bowstringing of the extensor tendons. The extensor tendons of the wrist and digits pass under the extensor retinaculum through six discrete tunnels, or dorsal compartments (Fig. 13). In addition to their intended function, the dorsal compartments are excellent landmarks for surgical approaches.

Vascular anatomy

The radial artery enters the wrist just radial to the flexor carpi radialis. It is the most consistent arterial supply and has seven major carpal branches. The ulnar artery has several branches,

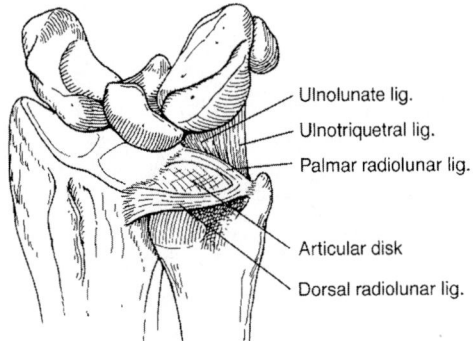

Fig. 9. The components of the triangular fibrocartilage complex. (*From* Loftus JB, Palmer AK. Disorders of the DRUJ and TFCC. In: Lichtman DM, Alexander AH, editors. The wrist and its disorders. Philadelphia; W.B. Saunders: 1997; with permission.)

both volar and dorsal, at the level of the wrist. The artery travels across the radiocarpal joint just radial to the ulnar nerve. As the nerve enters Guyon's canal, the ulnar artery travels distally and radially to form the superficial palmar arch. The anterior interosseous artery bifurcates at the proximal border of the pronator quadratus into dorsal and palmar branches. The dorsal branch travels along the interosseous membrane to anastomose with the three dorsal carpal arches. The palmar branch travels deep to the pronator quadratus to supply the palmar radiocarpal arch and terminates at the deep palmar arch.

The radial, ulnar, and anterior interosseous arteries coalesce to form the extraosseous blood supply to the wrist and hand. The extraosseous vascular supply to the wrist is composed of three volar and three dorsal carpal arches. Dorsally, the radiocarpal arch lies deep in the extensor tendons at the radiocarpal joint and supplies the lunate and triquetrum. The intercarpal arch, the largest and most consistent arch, tends to supply the distal carpal row before anastomosing with the radiocarpal arch. Finally, the basal metacarpal arch, the smallest and least consistently present arch, helps supply the distal carpal row (Fig. 14) [10]. Volarly, the palmar radiocarpal arch runs within the wrist capsule and supplies the volar portions of the lunate and triquetrum. The most important of the three arches, the deep palmar arch, is located at the metacarpal bases. It is a continuation of the radial artery and supplies the distal carpal row through the radial and ulnar recurrent branches (Fig. 15) [10].

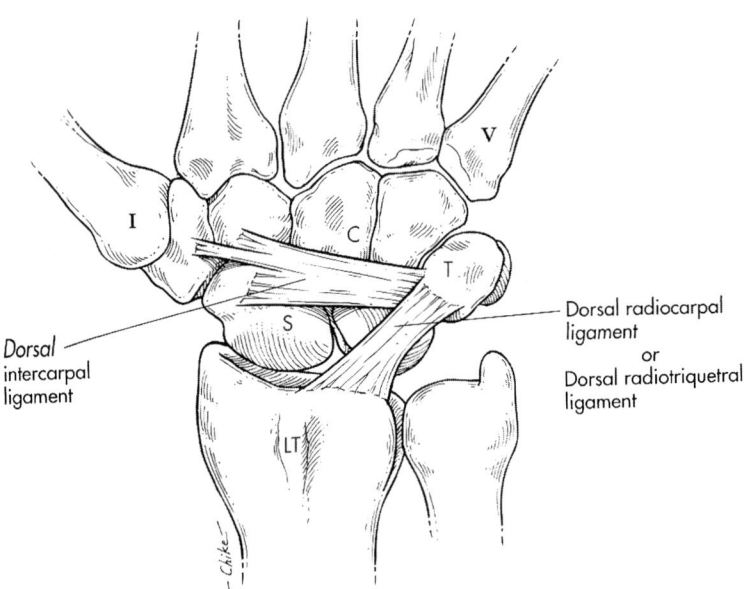

Fig. 10. The dorsal Intercarpal ligament and dorsal radiotriquetral ligament. (*From* Berger RA. Ligament anatomy. In: Cooney WP, Linscheid RL, Dobyns JH, editors. The wrist: diagnosis and operative treatment. St. Louis (MO): Mosby; 1997; with permission.)

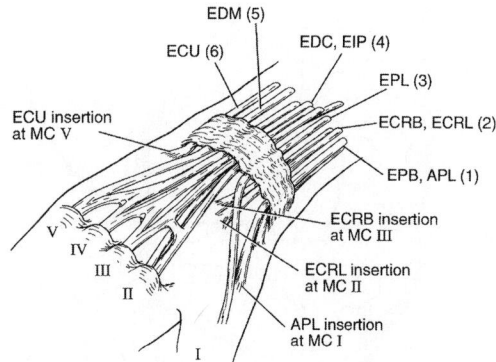

Fig. 13. The extensor retinaculum and six dorsal compartments. (*From* Trumble TE. Principles of hand surgery and therapy. Philadelphia: W.B. Saunders; 2000. p. 1–18; with permission.)

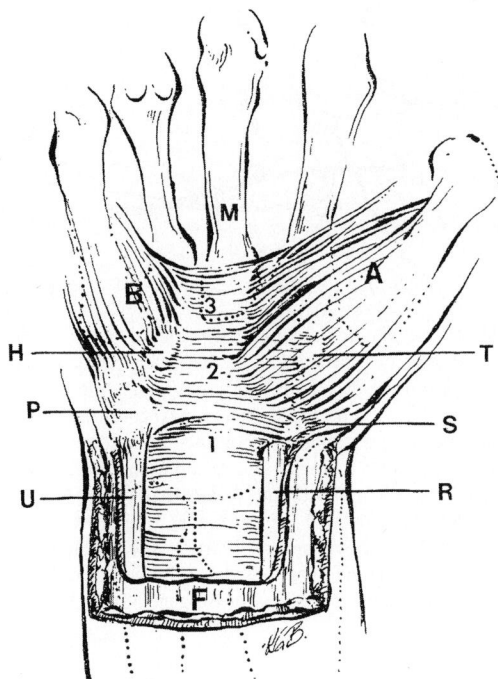

Fig. 11. The three portions of the flexor retinaculum. A, thenar muscles; B, hypothenar muscles; H, hamate; P, pisiform; R, flexor carpi radialis; S, scaphoid; T, trapezium; U, flexor carpi ulnaris. (*From* Cobb TK, Dalley BK, Posteraro RH, et al. Anatomy of the flexor retinaculum. J Hand Surg [Am] 1993;18:91–9; with permission from The American Society for Surgery of the Hand.)

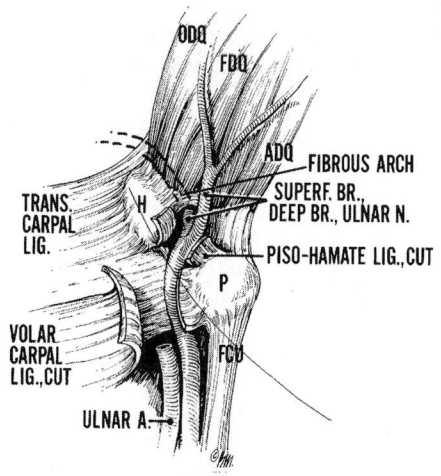

Fig. 12. Guyon's canal. Note that the ulnar artery travels radial to the canal. (*From* Szabo RM. Compression neuropathies. In: Green DP, Hotchkiss RN, Pederson WC, editors. Operative hand surgery. 4th edition. New York: Churchill Livingstone; 1999; with permission.)

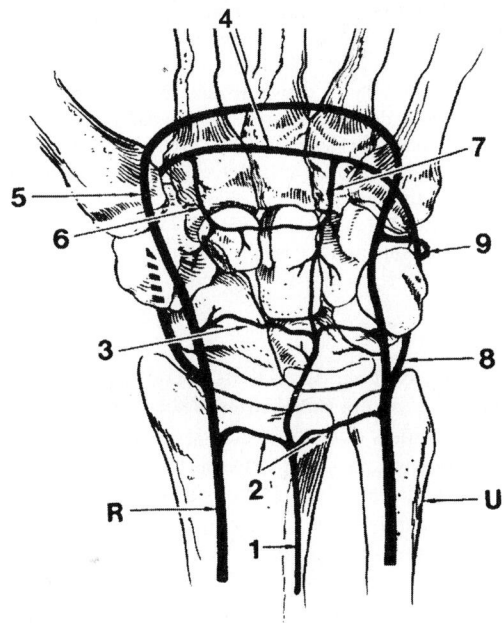

Fig. 14. Schematic drawing of the arterial supply of the palmar aspect of the wrist. R, radial artery; U, ulnar artery; 1, palmar branch, anterior interosseous artery; 2, palmar radiocarpal arch; 3, palmar intercarpal arch; 4, deep palmar arch; 5, superficial palmar arch; 6, radial recurrent artery; 7, ulnar recurrent artery; 8, medial branch, ulnar artery; 9, branch off ulnar artery contributing to dorsal intercarpal arch. (*From* Gelberman RH, Panagis JS, Taleisnik J, et al. The arterial anatomy of the human carpus. Part I: the extraosseous vascularity. J Hand Surg 1983;8:367–75; with permission from The American Society for Surgery of the Hand.)

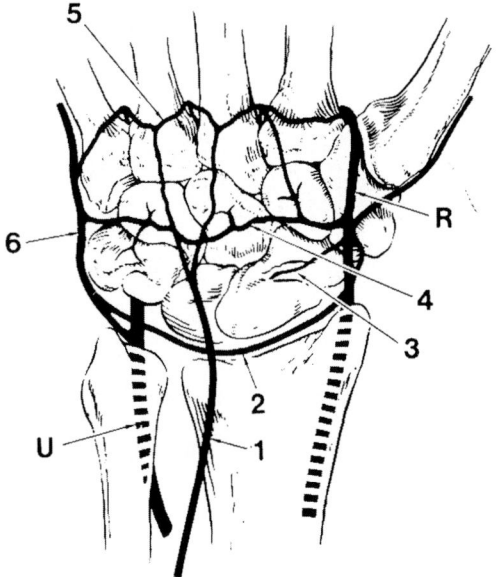

Fig. 15. Schematic drawing of the arterial supply of the dorsal aspect of the wrist. R, radial artery; U, ulnar artery; 1, dorsal branch, anterior interosseous artery; 2, dorsal radiocarpal arch; 3, branch to the dorsal ridge of the scaphoid; 4, dorsal intercarpal arch; 5, basal metacarpal arch; 6, medial branch of the ulnar artery. (*From* Gelberman RH, Panagis JS, Taleisnik J, et al. The arterial anatomy of the human carpus. Part I: the extraosseous vascularity. J Hand Surg 1983;8:367–75; with permission from The American Society for Surgery of the Hand.)

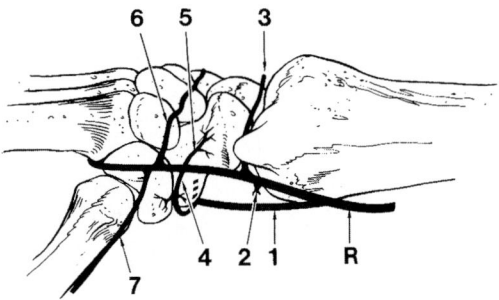

Fig. 16. Schematic drawing of the arterial supply of the lateral aspect of the wrist. R, radial artery; U, ulnar artery; 1, superficial palmar artery; 2, palmar radiocarpal arch; 3, dorsal radiocarpal arch; 4, branch to the scaphoid tubercle and trapezium; 5, branch to the dorsal ridge of the scaphoid; 6, dorsal intercarpal arch; 7, branch to lateral trapezium and thumb metacarpal. (*From* Gelberman RH, Panagis JS, Taleisnik J, et al. The arterial anatomy of the human carpus. Part I: the extraosseous vascularity. J Hand Surg 1983;8:367–75; with permission from The American Society for Surgery of the Hand.)

The scaphoid receives its blood supply from branches of the radial artery; 80% of its blood supply enters dorsally. A dorsal ridge at the level of the scaphoid waist, between the radius, trapezoid, and trapezium, is the site of vessel entry. Consequently, this vessel must be preserved during a dorsal approach to the scaphoid. Furthermore, blood supply to the proximal pole is supplied by a single intraosseous vessel, making fractures to this region prone to nonunion (Fig. 16) [10].

Surgical approaches

Volar radial approach

Indications and landmarks

The standard volar radial approach allows the volar surface of the distal radius to be accessed through the interval between the flexor carpi radialis (FCR) tendon and radial artery. Landmarks include the FCR tendon, radial artery, and distal wrist crease (Fig. 17).

Technique

A skin incision is made along the forearm, starting from the distal wrist crease longitudinally or in a zigzag fashion, overlying the FCR tendon. After dissection through subcutaneous tissue, the FCR tendon sheath is readily visualized. The radial artery and its venae comitantes, which lie immediately radial to the FCR tendon, should be identified and tagged.

Care is taken to incise the sheath directly over the tendon, avoiding the palmar cutaneous branch of the median nerve (PCBMN), just ulnar to the FCR and radial artery. The tendon is then mobilized ulnarly to reveal the floor of the tendon sheath and protect the median nerve and its palmar cutaneous branch. The floor of the sheath is incised longitudinally to expose the pronator quadratus. More proximally, the flexor digitorum superficialis to the index finger and the flexor pollicus longus are encountered overlying the pronator quadratus. The flexor digitorum superficialis can be swept ulnarly and the flexor pollicis longus is mobilized radially to better visualize the pronator quadratus. The space between the flexor pollicis longus and radial septum can be developed to further improve visualization. As this space is developed, branches from the radial

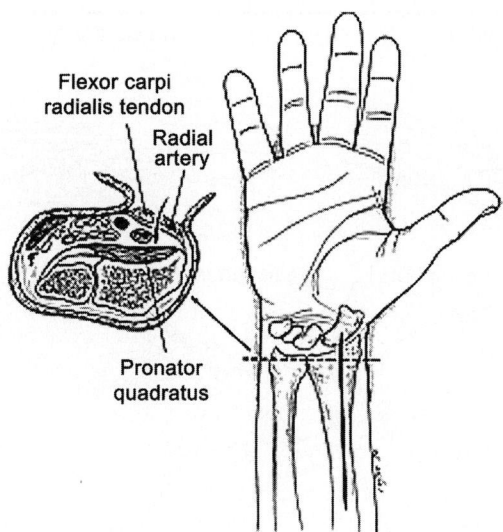

Fig. 17. The volar radial approach uses the interval between the flexor carpi radialis tendon and the radial artery. The pronator quadratus is elevated sharply, starting at its insertion on the distal radius. (*Reproduced from* Fernandez DL, Jupiter JB. Fractures of the distal radius. New York: Springer; 1996. p. 67–102; with permission.)

artery are sometimes encountered and must be cauterized to facilitate exposure. When the pronator quadratus is well visualized, its radial and distal borders are sharply released in an L-shaped fashion. The pronator quadratus is then reflected ulnarly to expose the volar surface of the radius. The brachioradialis is often released from its insertion to facilitate manipulation of fracture fragments (Fig. 18).

Extended flexor carpi radialis approach

The extended FCR approach, popularized by Orbay et al. [11], allows access to dorsally comminuted and displaced distal radius fractures from a volar approach. Pronating the proximal fragment of the radius out of the way allows the dorsal aspect of the distal radius to be visualized (Fig. 19).

Technique

The FCR approach is extended by first releasing the brachioradialis from its insertion. The brachioradialis insertion is found on the floor of the first dorsal compartment within the radial septum (Fig. 20). After incising the compartment sheath, the abductor pollicis longus is retracted radially to expose the brachioradialis insertion. Some experts advocate releasing the brachioradialis in a step-cut fashion to later facilitate its repair. The repaired brachioradialis can subsequently be used as an anchor-point to reattach the pronator quadratus after hardware placement. Releasing the brachioradialis also alleviates its deforming force on distal radial fracture fragments, permitting better fracture reduction. Next, the first dorsal compartment is lifted off the proximal fragment, followed by the dorsal periosteal attachments. Finally, the proximal radial fragment is pronated out of the way to better visualize the dorsal aspect of the fracture (Fig. 19) [11].

Volar approach to the scaphoid (Russe)

Indications and landmarks

The Russe or volar approach to the scaphoid is ideal for screw fixation of acute, scaphoid waist fractures and treating scaphoid nonunions with bone grafting. Like the volar approach to the wrist, this approach uses the FCR tendon as a landmark. The scaphoid waist lies at the intersection of the FCR tendon and the proximal palmar wrist crease, at the level of the radial styloid.

Technique

A longitudinal 5-cm incision is started over the FCR tendon centered on the proximal wrist crease. The incision crosses the wrist crease at a 45° angle to follow the ulnar border of the thumb metacarpal (Fig. 21). After incising the skin and subcutaneous tissues, care is taken to avoid the palmar cutaneous branch of the median

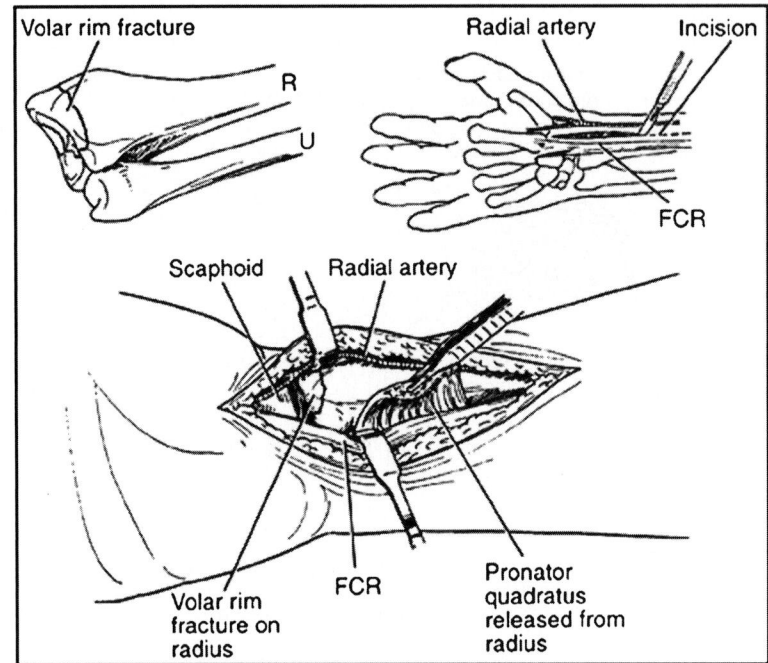

Fig. 18. The volar radial approach is through the interval between the flexor carpi radialis (FCR) and the radial artery. R, radius; U, ulna. (*Reproduced from* Trumble TE, Culp R, Hanel DP, et al. Intra-articular fractures of the distal aspect of the radius. J Bone Joint Surg Am 1998;80:582–600; reprinted with permission from The Journal of Bone and Joint Surgery, Inc.)

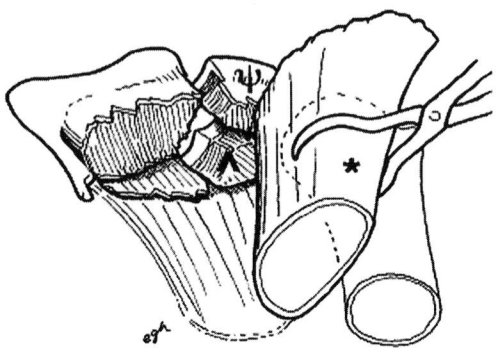

Fig. 19. The extended FCR approach allows dorsal access to intra-articular fragments from a volar approach. The pronated proximal radius fragment (*), dorsal die-punch fragment (Λ), and volar die punch fragment (Ψ) are shown. (*From* Orbay JL. Fernandez DL. Volar fixation for dorsally displaced fractures of the distal radius: a preliminary report. J Hand Surg [Am] 2002;27(2):205–15; with permission from The American Society for Surgery of the Hand.)

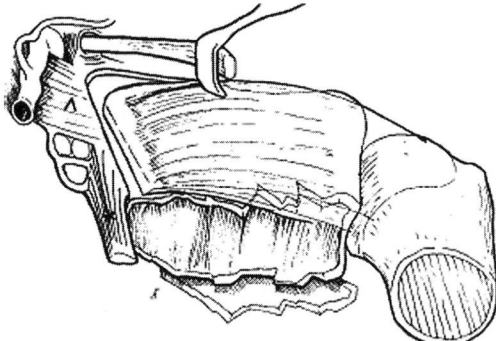

Fig. 20. The radial septum is a complex fascial structure consisting of the intramuscular membrane, brachioradialis insertion (*), and first extensor compartment (Λ). (*From* Orbay JL. Fernandez DL. Volar fixation for dorsally displaced fractures of the distal radius: a preliminary report. J Hand Surg [Am] 2002;27(2):205–15; with permission from The American Society for Surgery of the Hand.)

nerve, ulnar to the FCR. The radial artery and its venae comitantes, which lie immediately radial to the FCR tendon, should be identified and tagged. The FCR tendon sheath is incised distally and the tendon retracted ulnarly to reveal the RSC and long radiolunate ligaments. The RSC is incised longitudinally with the intention to repair later. The palmar branch of the radial artery is typically found at this level and may be ligated for better exposure, if necessary. The capsule is then visualized and incised in a longitudinal fashion. Further exposure can also be gained by mobilizing the thenar muscles radially. To visualize the joint surface of the distal pole, a capsulotomy is performed at the scaphotrapezial joint. The wrist is then flexed and ulnarly deviated to better view the scaphoid (Fig. 22).

Carpal tunnel approach

Indications and landmarks

The carpal tunnel approach provides access to the carpal canal and its contents and limited access to the mid-carpus and the hook of the hamate. Landmarks include Kaplan's line, the pisiform, the hook of the hamate, the thenar and hypothenar eminences, the distal wrist crease, the FCR, and the palmaris longus (when present). Although no true neurovascular plane exists, small palmar cutaneous branches of the median nerve and branches of the ulnar cutaneous nerves should be avoided if possible.

Nonunions of the hook of the hamate may be approached through the carpal tunnel or Guyon's canal. However, the carpal tunnel approach has the disadvantage of requiring release of the transverse carpal ligament, which may prolong recovery.

Technique

A longitudinal or slightly curvilinear 3- to 4-cm incision is started at Kaplan's line and is carried to the level of the distal wrist crease. The incision travels in the depression between the thenar and hypothenar eminences, in line with the central axis of the ring finger. The incision can be extended proximally by coursing at a 45° angle to the distal wrist crease, after which it can be extended more proximally along the course of the ulnar artery or by curving back radially (Fig. 23). After incising the skin and subcutaneous fat and palmar fascia, the transverse fibers of the flexor retinaculum should become apparent. The palmaris longus (if present) is moved radially to better expose the flexor retinaculum and protect the palmar cutaneous branch of the median nerve. Gentle dissection is then performed to identify the proximal and distal extent of the flexor retinaculum. The distal border can be identified by looking for a fat pad, which also demarcates the position of the superficial palmar arch.

Proximally, the antebrachial fascia is recognized as being very thin compared with the TCL. This proximal fascia should be incised first, and then the median nerve immediately identified. The flexor retinaculum is then incised longitudinally from proximal to distal, aiming at the long finger along the ulnar border of the median nerve. Care is taken not to encroach on the hook of the hamate, which lies near the ulnar artery and nerve. The median nerve and digital flexor tendons lie immediately dorsal to the TCL and may be retracted radially to gain limited access to the carpus. The recurrent motor branch of the median nerve should be identified before closure and, if an extended radial incision is used, the palmar cutaneous branch of the median nerve should also be identified [12].

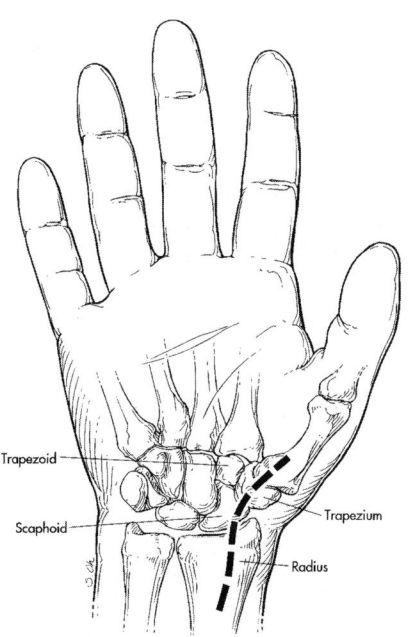

Fig. 21. Skin incision for volar approach to the scaphoid. (*From* Ruby LK. Arthrotomy. In: Cooney WP, Linscheid RL, Dobyns JH, editors. The wrist: diagnosis and operative treatment. St. Louis (MO): Mosby; 1997; with permission.)

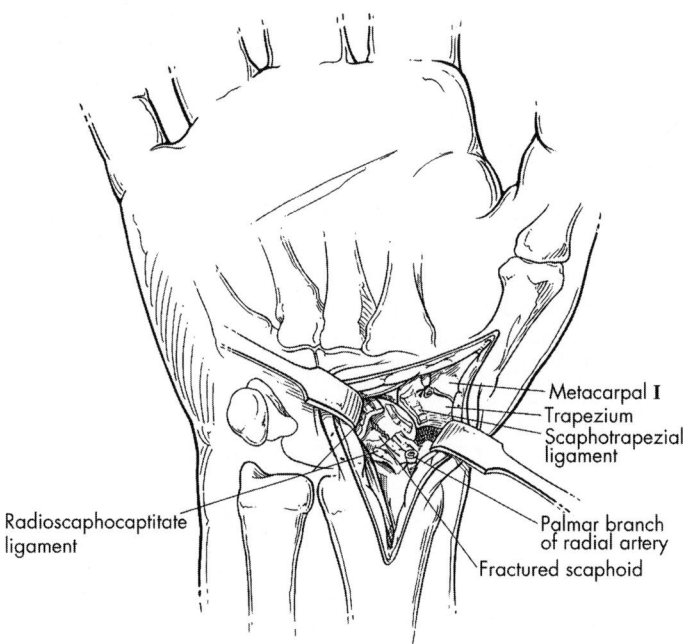

Fig. 22. Visualization of the volar scaphoid after incising radioscaphocapitate and trapezium scaphotrapezial ligaments. (*From* Ruby LK. Arthrotomy. In: Cooney WP, Linscheid RL, Dobyns JH, editors. The wrist: diagnosis and operative treatment. St. Louis (MO): Mosby; 1997; with permission.)

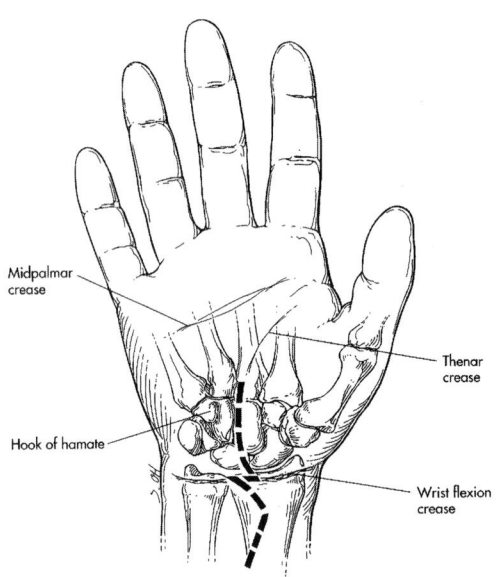

Fig. 23. Midpalmar approach. The incision stops at the distal wrist crease for carpal tunnel approach. (*From* Ruby LK. Arthrotomy. In: Cooney WP, Linscheid RL, Dobyns JH, editors. The wrist: diagnosis and operative treatment. St. Louis (MO): Mosby; 1997; with permission.)

To access the hook of the hamate, the median nerve and finger flexors are gently retracted radially while the TLC is lifted ulnarly. The entire hook of the hamate is accessible without excessive dissection of the ulnar nerve or artery (Fig. 24).

Central palmar approach

This approach is an extension of the carpal tunnel approach and provides access to the ulnar aspect of the distal radius and the palmar portion of the DRUJ, and better exposure to the volar carpus (Fig. 25).

Technique

The incision, starting at Kaplan's line, is an extension of the incision to expose the carpal canal. The incision is carried proximally, crossing the wrist crease in a curvilinear or oblique fashion. The incision is continued longitudinally along the ulnar border of the palmaris longus to avoid the palmar cutaneous branch of the median nerve, which lies just radial to it. The median nerve should be identified as it travels beneath the muscle belly of the middle-finger flexor digitorum superficialis. The palmar cutaneous branch of the median nerve should also be identified as it

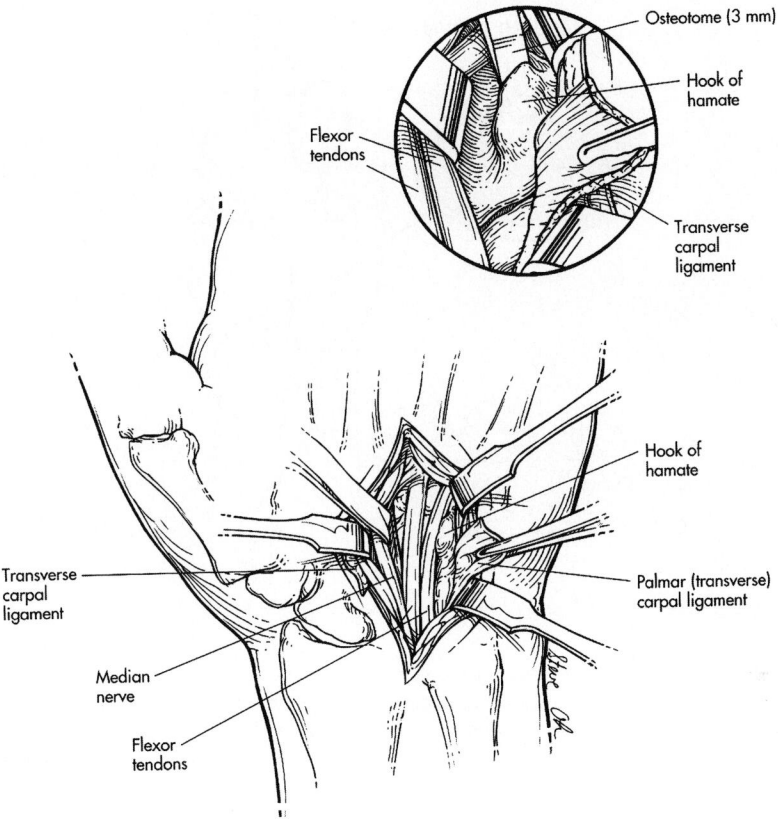

Fig. 24. Carpal tunnel approach with access to the hook of the hamate. (*From* Ruby LK. Arthrotomy. In: Cooney WP, Linscheid RL, Dobyns JH, editors. The wrist: diagnosis and operative treatment. St. Louis (MO): Mosby; 1997; with permission.)

branches radially off the median between 4 and 8 cm proximal to the distal wrist crease. The palmaris longus tendon is then freed from the flexor retinaculum and moved radially. The flexor retinaculum should be incised as discussed in the carpal tunnel approach section. The median nerve along with the digital flexors can then be retracted ulnarly or radially to gain access to deeper structures in the wrist (Fig. 26). Immediately below the digital flexors lies the pronator quadratus. Just proximally, the anterior interosseous artery and nerve are identified traveling along the interosseous membrane before supplying the pronator quadratus. Care is taken to visualize the ulnar artery, which lies between the flexor carpi ulnaris and the flexor digitorum superficialis to the ring and small fingers. The pronator quadratus may be released either radially or ulnarly to access the radius and the volar portion of the distal radioulnar joint (Figs. 27 and 28).

Approach to Guyon's canal

Indications and landmarks

Fractures and nonunions of the pisiform and hook of the hamate and injuries to the ulnar nerve and artery may be addressed through this incision. Landmarks include the flexor carpi ulnaris tendon, pisiform, and hook of the hamate.

Technique

An incision started just proximal to the wrist crease is carried in a zigzag fashion distally between the pisiform and hook of the hamate. Blunt dissection through the subcutaneous tissues is recommended to avoid injuring the palmar cutaneous branches of the ulnar nerve that may be encountered. Proximally, the flexor carpi ulnaris is identified and retracted ulnarly to expose the ulnar artery and nerve. The ulnar nerve is traced from the palmar crease to the level

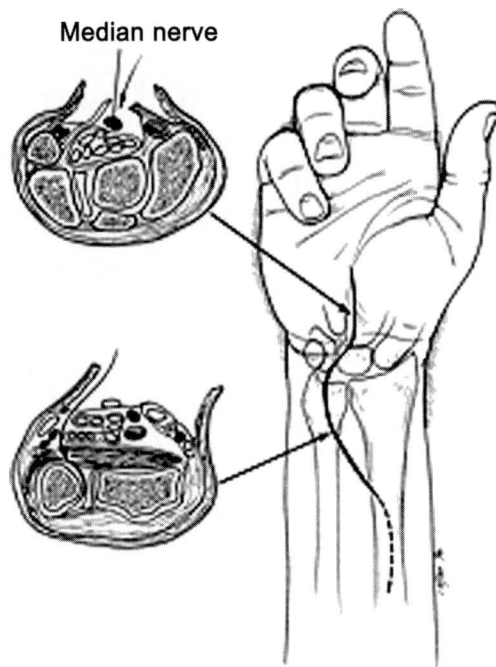

Fig. 25. The mid-palmar approach can be extended distally to release the median nerve from the carpal tunnel. Bottom detail, at the level of the distal radius, the flexor tendons and the median nerve are retracted radially to expose the volar medial distal radius. (*From* Fernandez DL, Jupiter JB. Fractures of the distal radius. New York: Springer; 1996. p. 67–102; with permission.)

of Guyon's canal. The palmaris brevis muscle is seen and moved ulnarly. The volar carpal and pisohamate ligaments are identified and divided. The fibrous arch of the origin of the hypothenar muscles is then encountered and incised to unroof the ulnar nerve and artery. The pisiform and hook of the hamate are easily palpable and can be further exposed with subperiosteal elevation (Fig. 29) [12].

Radial approach to the scaphoid

Indications

The radial approach to the scaphoid allows excellent visualization of the proximal pole of the scaphoid and dorsal exposure for placing bone graft. The incision may be extended proximally to address fractures of the radial styloid. Landmarks include the anatomic snuffbox formed by the tendons of the first and third dorsal compartments, and the tip of the radial styloid.

Technique

A curvilinear incision is made overlying the anatomic snuffbox between the first and third dorsal compartments (Fig. 30). Further dissection is performed carefully as the superficial branches of the radial nerve lie subcutaneous to the incision. Volar retraction of the extensor pollicis brevis reveals the radial artery, which should be gently swept volarly. The capsule may then be incised longitudinally to expose the scaphoid (see Fig. 30). Care should be taken to avoid stripping the blood supply to the proximal pole of the scaphoid, found at its dorsal ridge [13].

Longitudinal dorsal approach

Indications

The longitudinal dorsal approach has several uses, including access to the dorsal aspect of the distal radius, the radiocarpal and radioulnar joints, the carpal bones, and the extensor tendons. Landmarks include Lister's tubercle, the lunate fossa, the long-finger metacarpal, and the radial and ulnar styloid. The extensor retinaculum may be incised at different levels depending on the required exposure. Access to the digital extensors is through the fourth dorsal compartment, whereas the DRUJ is visualized through the fifth dorsal compartment. Access to most dorsal structures of the dorsal wrist, including the distal

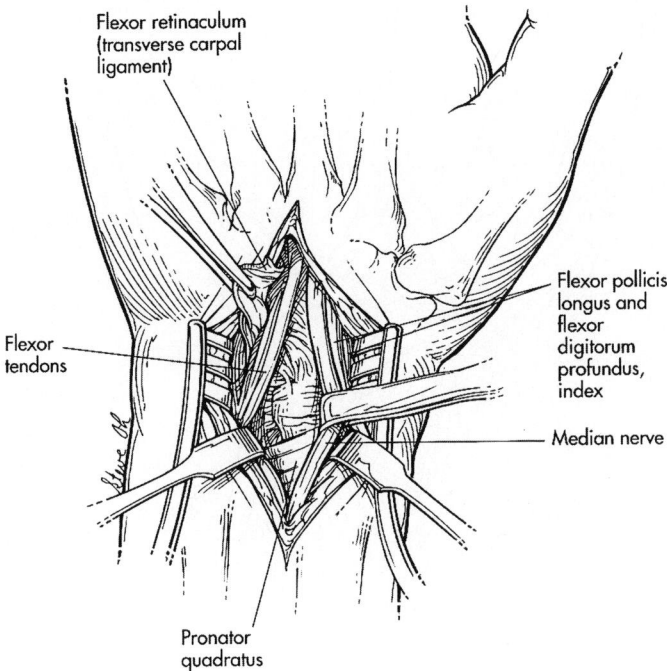

Fig. 26. Midpalmar approach. The medial nerve, flexor pollicis longus, and index profundus are retracted radially, and the rest of the digital flexors are retracted ulnarly. (*From* Ruby LK. Arthrotomy. In: Cooney WP, Linscheid RL, Dobyns JH, editors. The wrist: diagnosis and operative treatment. St. Louis (MO): Mosby; 1997; with permission.)

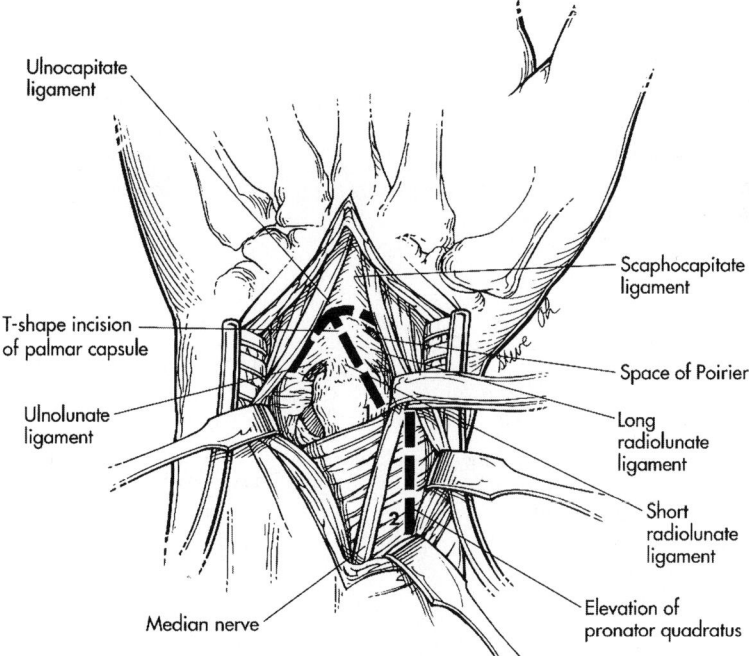

Fig. 27. Palmar capsule incisions: through the space of Poirier and between palmar radiocarpal ligaments. The pronator quadratus is also elevated for further exposure. (*From* Ruby LK. Arthrotomy. In: Cooney WP, Linscheid RL, Dobyns JH, editors. The wrist: diagnosis and operative treatment. St. Louis (MO): Mosby; 1997; with permission.)

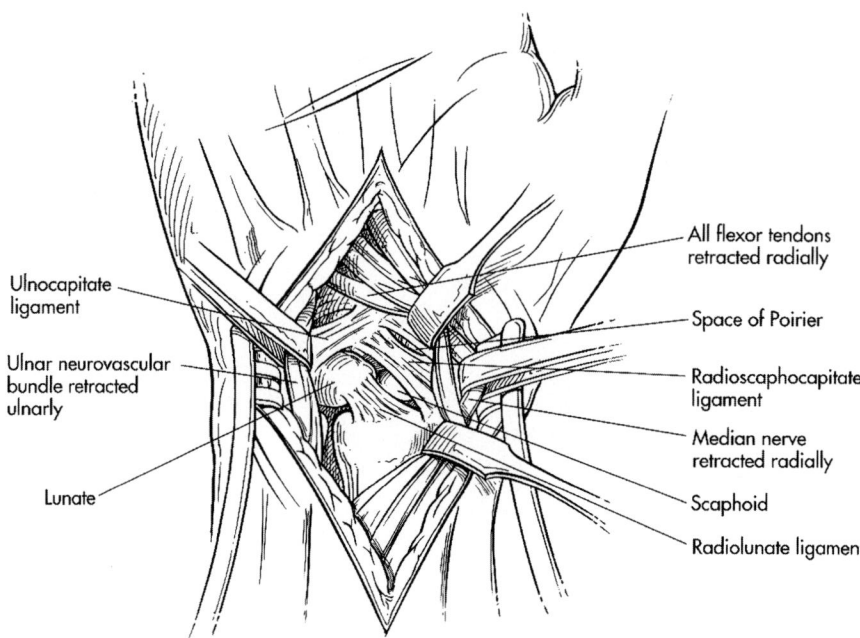

Fig. 28. Radial retraction of the flexor tendons allows visualization of the ulnar aspect of the radius and the palmar aspect of the DRUJ. (*From* Ruby LK. Arthrotomy. In: Cooney WP, Linscheid RL, Dobyns JH, editors. The wrist: diagnosis and operative treatment. St. Louis (MO): Mosby; 1997; with permission.)

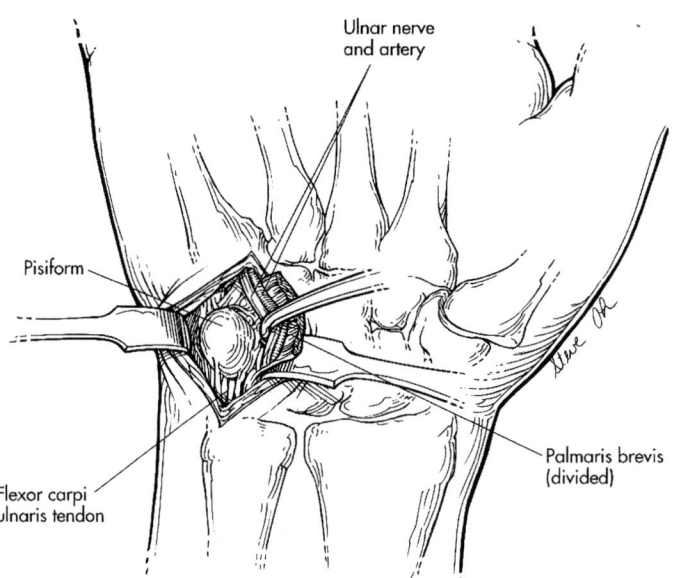

Fig. 29. Approach to Guyon's canal allows access to the pisiform and hook of the hamate. (*From* Ruby LK. Arthrotomy. In: Cooney WP, Linscheid RL, Dobyns JH, editors. The wrist: diagnosis and operative treatment. St. Louis (MO): Mosby; 1997; with permission.)

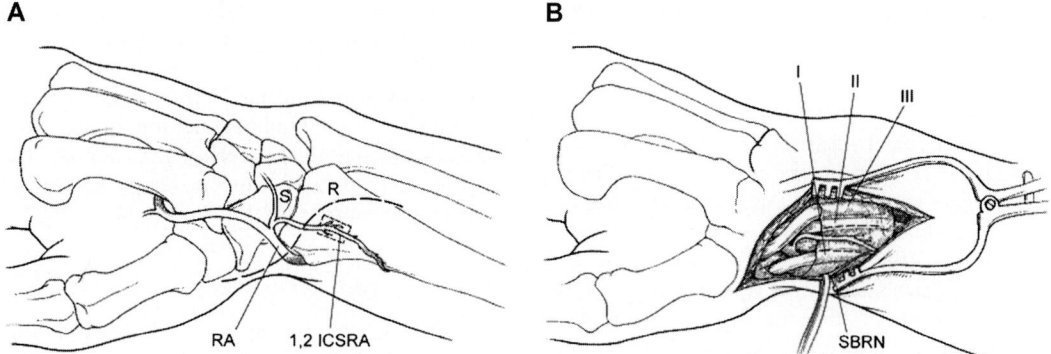

Fig. 30. Dorsoradial approach to the scaphoid. (*A*) The incision (*dashed line*) exposes the scaphoid and bone graft donor site. Subcutaneous tissues are raised from the extensor retinaculum, and the 1,2 ICSRA is identified. RA, radial artery; S, scaphoid; R, radius. (*B*) Branches (I, II, III) of the superficial branch of the radial nerve (SBRN) are identified and protected. Dashed lines indicate incisions of the first and second extensor compartments. (*From* Shin AY, Bishop AT, Berger RA. Vascularized pedicled bone graft for disorders of the carpus. Tech Hand Up Extrem Surg 1998;2(2):100; with permission.)

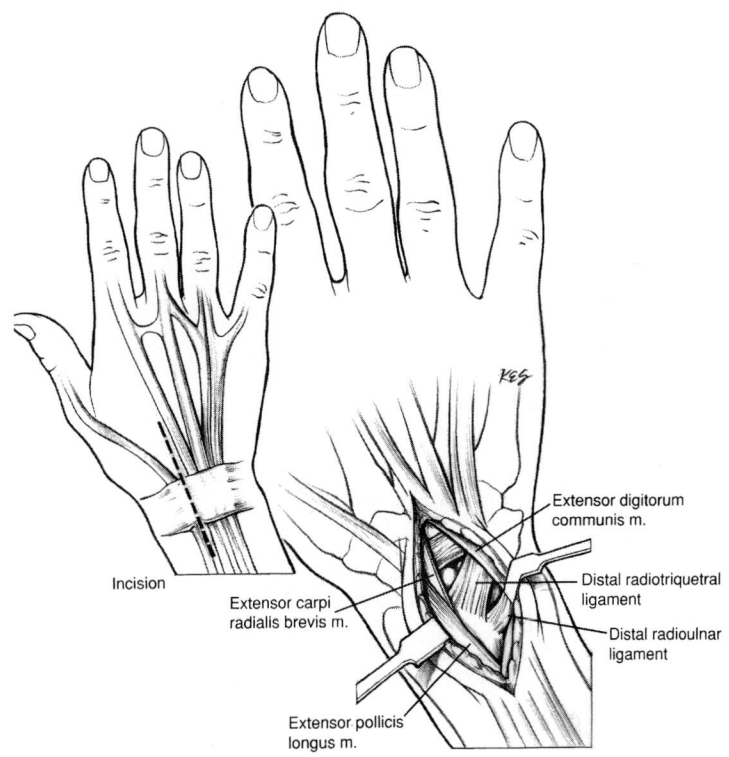

Fig. 31. Standard dorsal approach. An incision is made inline with the index finger metacarpal. The capsule is approached between the third and fourth dorsal compartments. (*From* Szabo RM, Newland CC. Open reduction and ligamentous repair for acute lunate and perilunate dislocations. In: Gelberman RH, editor. Masters techniques in orthopaedic surgery, the wrist. New York: Raven Press; 1994. p. 172; with permission.)

radius and mid-carpus, can be accessed between the third and fourth dorsal compartments.

Technique

A longitudinal incision is made over the dorsum of the wrist in line with the index-finger metacarpal. Alternatively, a more centralized incision in line with the long-finger metacarpal may be used (Fig. 31). The incision starts at the base of the carpometacarpal ligament and travels just ulnar to Lister's tubercle. The incision is carried down to the level of the extensor retinaculum, taking care to avoid injury to sensory nerves and large dorsal veins. Skin flaps are made as thick as possible because of the delicate nature of the dorsal skin.

The extensor retinaculum is then visualized and incised between the third and fourth dorsal compartments. The extensor pollicis longus is radially retracted from the groove formed by Lister's tubercle. The fourth compartment is then elevated ulnarly, taking care to remain subperiosteal to avoid tendon adhesions. Subperiosteal dissection is continued to expose the distal radius and carpal capsule. The capsule is entered by making a longitudinal incision in line with Lister's tubercle to the level of the capitate. The capsule may then be subperiostially elevated to visualize the carpus [14,15].

Dorsal approach to the distal radioulnar joint

This less-extensile approach is used if only access to the DRUJ is required.

Technique

A longitudinal or zigzag skin incision is made directly over the dorsal ulna in line with the ulnar aspect of the ring-finger metacarpal (Fig. 32). After skin flaps are raised, the fifth dorsal compartment is identified. The dorsal cutaneous branch of the ulnar nerve should be identified

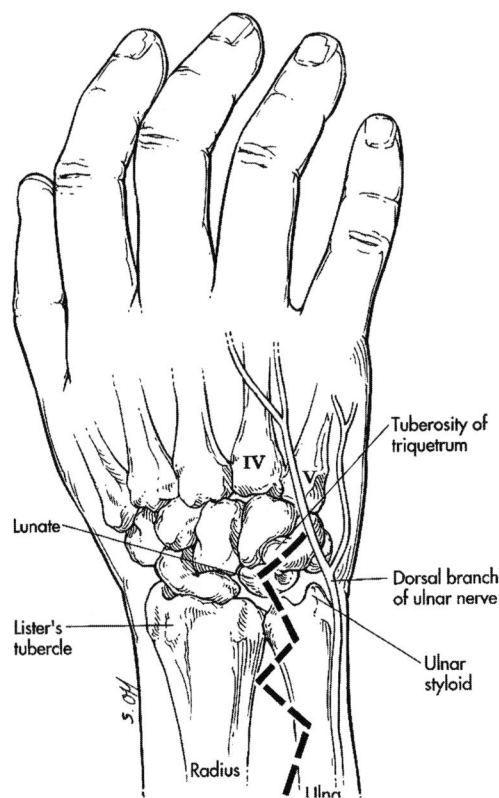

Fig. 32. Limited dorsal approach to the DRUJ. (*From* Ruby LK. Arthrotomy. In: Cooney WP, Linscheid RL, Dobyns JH, editors. The wrist: diagnosis and operative treatment. St. Louis (MO): Mosby; 1997; with permission.)

and protected in the distal aspect of the incision. A longitudinal incision through the extensor retinaculum permits ulnar reflection of the extensor carpi ulnaris and radial reflection of the extensor digiti minimi (Fig. 33). The capsule of the distal radioulnar joint, directly below the compartment, can be entered through a longitudinal incision. The ulnocarpal joint is visualized by continuing the capsular incision distally to the lunotriquetral joint. Care must be taken to avoid cutting the dorsal radioulnar ligament or TFC (Fig. 34).

Direct ulnar approach

Indications and landmarks

The direct ulnar approach is useful for treatment of distal ulnar styloid fractures, excision of the distal ulna, exposure of the extensor carpi ulnaris, and limited exposure of the TFCC. Landmarks include the subcutaneous border of the ulna, the extensor carpi ulnaris tendon, and the ulnar styloid (if not displaced).

Technique

A longitudinal incision is made over the ulnar aspect of the distal ulna. The incision is centered just volar to the extensor carpi ulnaris tendon and carried distally across the carpus. The dorsal cutaneous branch of the ulnar nerve should be localized as is crosses the ulna from volar to dorsal. The nerve should be gently freed from the subcutaneous tissue and retracted volarly. The extensor retinaculum should be incised over the extensor carpi ulnaris and the tendon retracted dorsally. The ulnar styloid and ulnocarpal joint should now be apparent. To access the TFCC, a longitudinal incision should be made through the capsule, taking care not to injure the underlying TFCC. Wound closure should include a careful repair of

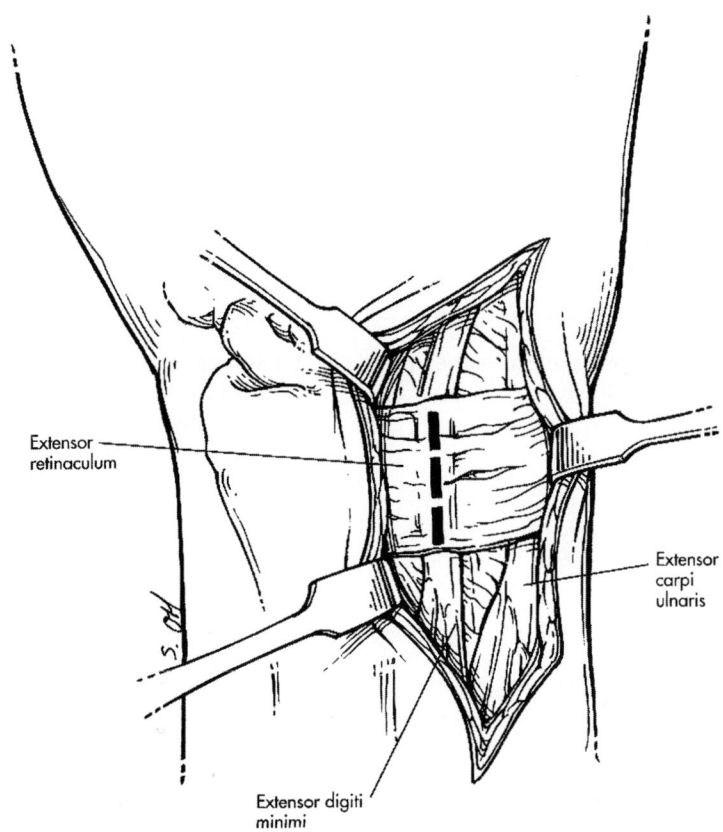

Fig. 33. The extensor retinaculum is incised over the fifth dorsal compartment. (*From* Ruby LK. Arthrotomy. In: Cooney WP, Linscheid RL, Dobyns JH, editors. The wrist: diagnosis and operative treatment. St. Louis (MO): Mosby; 1997; with permission.)

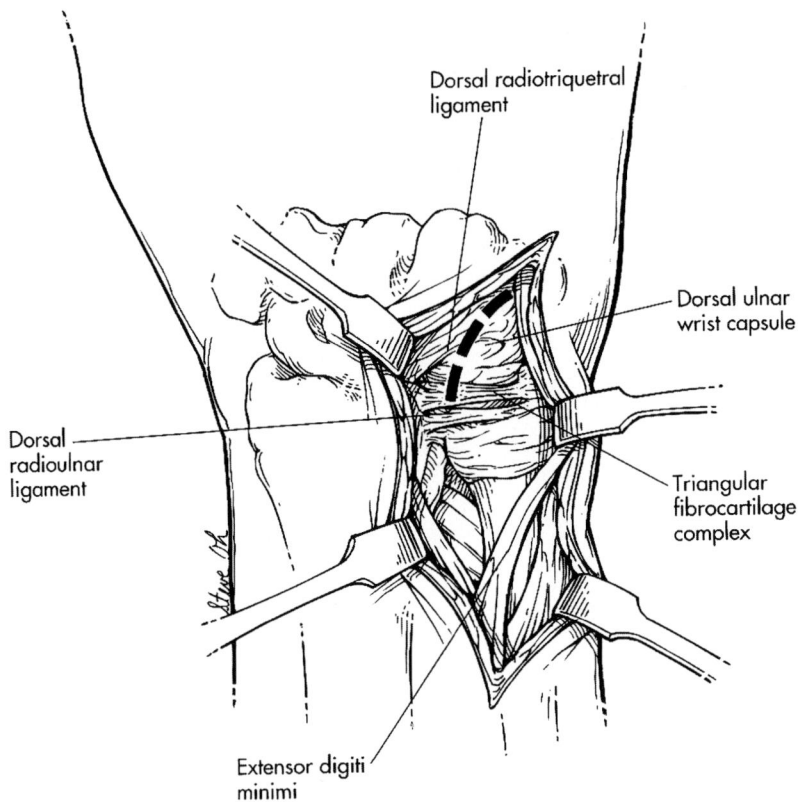

Fig. 34. The DRUJ can be visualized by ulnar retraction of the extensor digiti minimi. Care is taken to avoid incising the TFCC. The TFC and dorsal radiotriquetral ligament may be visualized by incision of the dorsal ulnar wrist capsule. (*From* Ruby LK. Arthrotomy. In: Cooney WP, Linscheid RL, Dobyns JH, editors. The wrist: diagnosis and operative treatment. St. Louis (MO): Mosby; 1997; with permission.)

the extensor retinaculum over the extensor carpi ulnaris to prevent tendon subluxation [13].

Application of an external fixator

Indications

An external fixator is indicated for stabilizing distal radius fractures, radiocarpal dislocations, and carpal injuries.

Technique

Typically two pins are applied to the dorsoradial aspect of the index finger metacarpal, followed by two pins to the dorsoradial aspect of the radial shaft. Percutaneous placement is not recommended because of the proximity of the superficial branch of the radial nerve and lateral antibrachial cutaneous nerve. The metacarpal incisions are made first to ensure adequate fixator length.

Either one or two incisions are made over the dorsoradial aspect of the index finger metacarpal. If two incisions are used, the distal one overlies the midshaft of the metacarpal, whereas the proximal one lies at its base. Subcutaneously, sensory branches of the radial nerve may be encountered and retracted away. The dissection is then carried to bone. The metacarpophalangeal joint should be held in flexion to slide the lateral band and first dorsal interosseous aponeurosis distally and away from the site of pin insertion.

For the proximal pins, a reduction should be attempted before the site of incision is planned to decrease the chance of excessive skin tension when the external fixator is finally applied. A longitudinal incision is conventionally made on the dorsoradial aspect of the radial shaft, approximately 10 cm proximal to the radial styloid. Alternatively, the incision may be planned 5 cm proximal to the fracture. Subcutaneously,

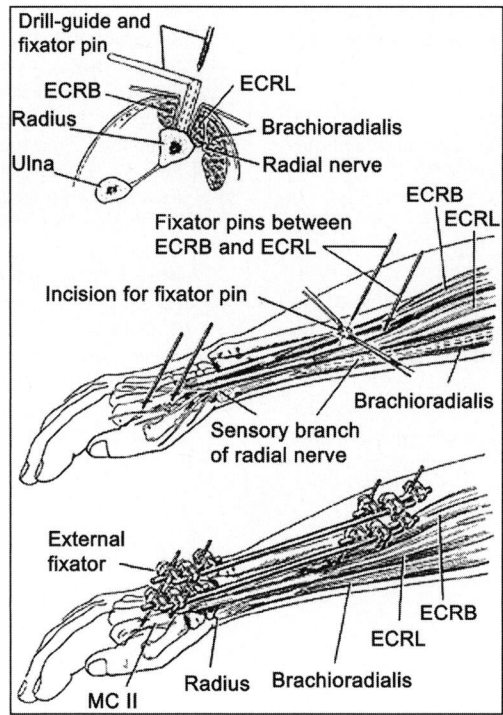

Fig. 35. The partially threaded pins for the external fixation device are inserted in the interval between the extensor carpi radialis longus (ECRL) and the extensor carpi radialis brevis (ECRB) to protect the sensory branch of the radial nerve. MC II, second metacarpal. (*From* Trumble TE, Culp R, Hanel DP, et al. Intra-articular fractures of the distal aspect of the radius. Bone Joint Surg Am 1998;80:582–600; reprinted with permission from The Journal of Bone and Joint Surgery, Inc.)

branches of the lateral antebrachial cutaneous nerve may be identified and protected. The brachioradialis tendon and extensor carpi radialis longus are next encountered. The latter is distinguished by noting tendon excursion with wrist flexion and extension. The space between the brachioradialis and extensor carpi radialis longus is developed by first opening the overlying fascial sheath. As the dissection is carried deeper, the radial sensory nerve should be identified and protected as it exits between the brachioradialis tendon and the extensor carpi radialis longus. The interval is carried down to the level of the radius, where the half pins are placed under direct visualization.

Some authors advocate placing pins in the interval between the extensor carpi radialis longus and brevis. Placement in this interval reduces contact with the radial sensory nerve. Furthermore, with the wrist immobilized, excursion between the extensor carpi radialis longus and brevis tendons is eliminated, thus alleviating soft tissue motion about the pins (Fig. 35) [4].

References

[1] Doyle JR, Botte MJ. Surgical anatomy of the hand and upper extremity. Philadelphia: Lippincott Williams and Wilkins; 2003. p. 486–529.
[2] Vella JC, Hartigan BJ, Stern PJ. Kaplan's cardinal line. J Hand Surg [Am] 2006;31(6):912–8.
[3] Kaplan EB. Guide lines to deep structures and dynamics of intrinsic muscles of the hand. Surg Clin North Am 1968;48:993–1002.
[4] Trumble TE, Culp R, Hanel DP, et al. Instructional course lectures, The American Academy of Orthopaedic Surgeons–intra-articular fractures of the distal aspect of the radius. J Bone Joint Surg Am 1998; 80:582–600.
[5] Szabo RM. Distal radioulnar joint instability. J Bone Joint Surg [Am] 2006;88(4):884–94.
[6] Taleisnik J. The ligaments of the wrist. J Hand Surg [Am] 1976;1(2):110–8.

[7] Gofton WT, Gordon KD, Dunning CE, et al. Soft-tissue stabilizers of the distal radioulnar joint: an in vitro kinematic study. J Hand Surg [Am] 2004;29: 423–31.

[8] Kihara H, Short WH, Werner FW, et al. The stabilizing mechanism of the distal radioulnar joint during pronation and supination. J Hand Surg [Am] 1995;20:930–6.

[9] Gelberman RH, Cooney WP, Szabo RM. Carpal instability. J Bone Joint Surg [Am] 2000;82: 578–94.

[10] Gelberman RH, Panagis JS, Taleisnik J, et al. The arterial anatomy of the human carpus. Part I: the extraosseous vascularity. J Hand Surg [Am] 1983; 8:367–75.

[11] Orbay JL, Badia A, Indriago IR, et al. The extended flexor carpi radialis approach: a new perspective for the distal radius fracture. Tech Hand Up Extrem Surg 2001;5(4):204–11.

[12] Szabo RM. Compression neuropathies. In: Green DP, Hotchkiss RN, Pederson WC, editors. Operative hand surgery. 4th edition. New York: Churchill Livingstone; 1999. p. 1404–47.

[13] Shin AY, Bishop AT, Berger RA. Vascularized pedicled bone graft for disorders of carpus. Tech Hand Up Extrem Surg 1998;2(2):100.

[14] Carlson GC. Surgical approaches to the hand and wrist. In: Chapman MW, editor. Chapman's orthopaedic surgery. 3rd edition. Philadelphia: Lippincott Williams & Wilkins; 2001. p. 1239–46.

[15] Ruby LK. Arthrotomy. In: Cooney WP, Linscheid RL, Dobyns JH, editors. The wrist: diagnosis and operative treatment. St. Louis (MO): Mosby; 1997. p. 128–68.

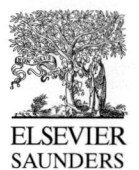

Physical Examination of the Wrist

Darryl Young, MD, BSc (H)[a], Steven Papp, MD, MSc, FRCS(C)[b,*], Alan Giachino, MD, BPHE, FRCS(C)[c]

[a]Department of Orthopaedics, University of Ottawa, The Ottawa Hospital, 501 Smyth Road, Room 3041, Ottawa, Ontario, Canada K1H 8L6
[b]Department of Orthopaedics, University of Ottawa, Ottawa Civic Hospital, 1053 Carling Ave, Ottawa, Ontario, Canada K1Y 4E9
[c]University of Ottawa, Suite 206, 1929 Russell Road, Ottawa, Ontario, Canada K1G 4G3

As with many joints, a focused history and well-performed physical examination of the wrist requires knowledge of anatomy and pathology of this area. Based on physical examination, one should be able to make a diagnosis or narrow the differential diagnosis dramatically. This examination is a summation of anatomical locations where symptoms are provoked by palpation and where signs, often with symptoms, are produced by manipulation. Negative findings elsewhere in the wrist are important. A final diagnosis may require diagnostic imaging (radiographs, bone scan, MRI, and the like) for confirmation. But only by having all three methods of assessment point to the same diagnosis is one assured of the correct diagnosis. A history of dorsoradial wrist pain with a physical examination indicating tenderness over the lunate and a triangular fibrocartilage complex (TFCC) tear seen with MRI does not lead to a secure diagnosis. The physical examination of the wrist is not unlike other joints, in that a systematic approach includes observation, range of motion, palpation and special tests.

Observation and range of motion

How the patient uses and holds the hand and wrist will give important clues as to the degree of pain and disability. Wasting of muscles and a shiny skin with discoloration may suggest reflex sympathetic dystrophy. Scars and other skin changes should be noted. All range of motion, both active and passive, should be documented Fig. 1. For example, if the past history indicates an old distal radial fracture, a lateral view may show a "dinner-fork" deformity. A pronation malunion can be assessed comparing both forearms (Fig. 2A, B). Usually, the patient holds both arms with a similar amount of proximal rotation. If one side pronates more distally, then the "peak at the palm sign" is present. CT scan confirms the pronation deformity in (Fig. 2C, D). Shortening of the radius can be assessed by a clinical test for ulnar variance (Fig. 3). Look for swellings and malalignment.

Palpation

Feeling for the exact localization of tenderness and structural abnormalities is the mainstay of the physical examination. It is essential to recognize three main principles:

1. The exact point of local tenderness is the location of the pathology.
2. If one knows the exact location, that is, the anatomical structure, one likely knows the diagnosis.
3. The diagnosis is arrived at by a summation of the positive and negative physical findings.

Special tests

Dynamic tests for instability, for articular and fibrous cartilage assessment, and for painful sensory feedback provide valuable information that may be missed with simple palpation alone.

* Corresponding author.
  E-mail address: spapp@Ottawahospital.on.ca (S. Papp).

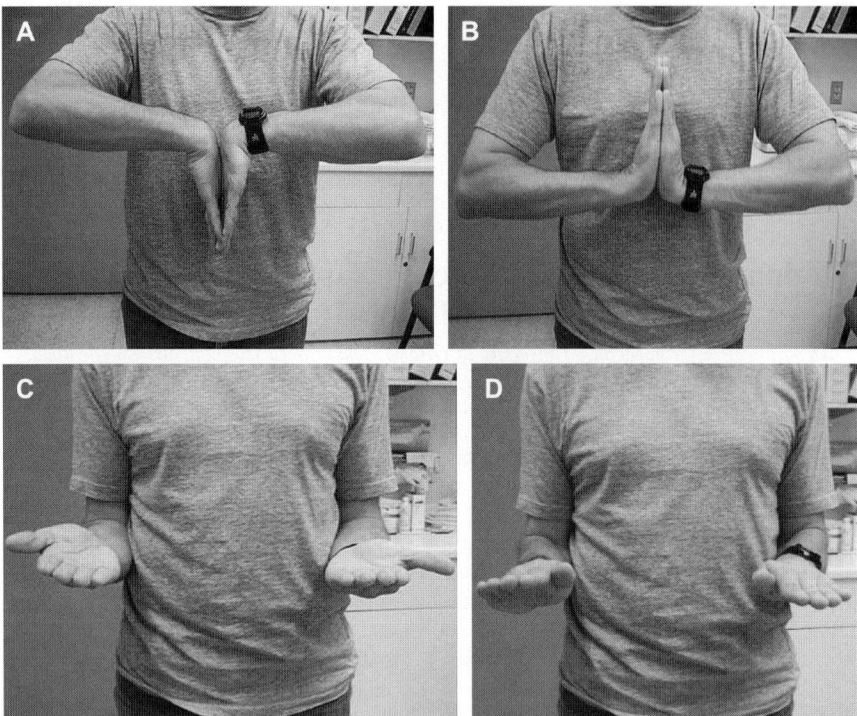

Fig. 1. Examining the range of motion of the wrist. (*A*) Flexion. (*B*) Extension. (*C*) Supination. (*D*) Pronation. Radial and ulnar deviation not shown.

Understanding the special tests of the wrist examination is complicated by the fact that there are often numerous descriptions of similar tests by different authors, sometimes even given the same name. Furthermore, as with other joints, the tests and interpretations of findings are often modified by clinicians over time to be different than in the original author's description. In this section, the authors attempt to provide a comprehensive review of the original authors' descriptions of special tests and how they define and interpret positive or negative findings. The senior author (AG) also provides his personal approach.

The approach to the wrist examination can be simplified by dividing it into four regions: radial, dorsal, ulnar, and palmar. The description of the wrist examination that follows uses this regional approach, starting radially and progressing around the wrist. For each region the authors describe a systematic approach of observation, palpation, and special tests. Provocative tests of instability are described separately at the end.

Radial wrist examination

Palmar scaphoid

To begin, start at the palmar radial aspect of the wrist. Sit comfortably with the elbows flexed and use the right hand as the dominant examining action hand for the patient's right wrist and the left for the patient's left. Curl one's fingers about the radial aspect to the dorsum of the patient's wrist while the thumb is palmar and points distally (Fig. 4A). Palpate the distal palmar tuberosity of the scaphoid. This is located immediately proximal to the thenar eminence and immediately radial to the flexor carpi radialis tendon (Fig. 4B). Use the opposite hand to move the patient's hand/wrist unit into flexion-extension and radioulnar deviation. If one is palpating the distal pole of the scaphoid, this small bony lump will move, demonstrating that it is part of the carpus and not the radius. More importantly, the distal pole will become prominent palmarly with wrist flexion and with radial deviation as the scaphoid rotates into flexion. Alternatively, it will be less

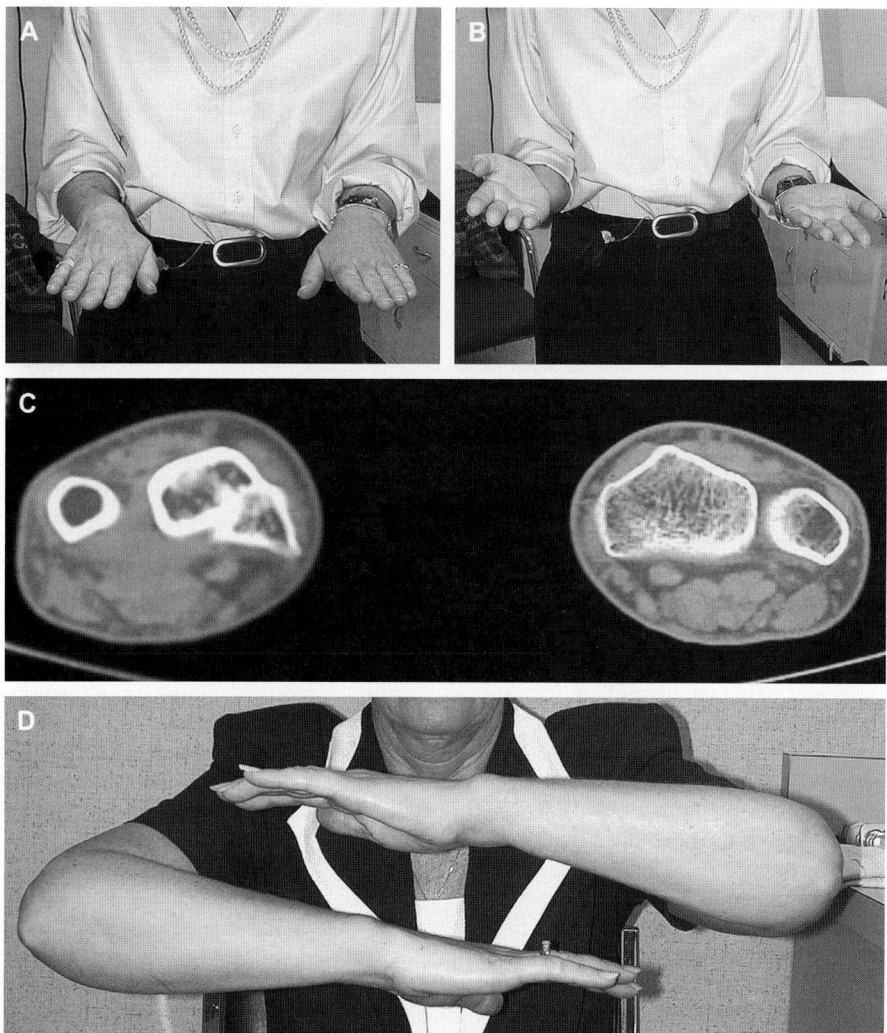

Fig. 2. Pronation malunion of distal radius fractures. (*A*) Full active pronation. (*B*) Limited supination on side of malunion (*right*). (*C*) CT scan revealing pronation malunion on right side. (*D*) Different patient who had pronation malunion demonstrating "peak at palm sign," whereby the increased pronation results in more of the palm being visible on the affected side (*left side*).

prominent with dorsiflexion and ulnar deviation as the scaphoid rotates into extension to line up with the long axis of the forearm. Find this bony landmark. Move the wrist through the ranges of motion to be convinced that the bony structure felt is indeed the tuberosity of the scaphoid. Tighten and loosen your grip on the patient so that the tip of the thumb forces the scaphoid tuberosity dorsally. The counterpressure is applied by the fingers of the same hand resting on the dorsum of the distal radius.

Rotate the patient's forearm so that you can view the radial aspect of the wrist. Assuming you are examining the right wrist, continue to hold the patient's hand with your left hand (to prevent dorsiflexion) and observe the dorsal translation of the patient's wrist that occurs when pressure is exerted by the examining thumb with dorsal counter pressure. Once this has been mastered, move to the next step, which secures the anatomical localization of the examining thumb and introduces relevant carpal kinematics. With your left hand, hold the patient's right hand dorsiflexed and ulnarly deviated. With the right hand and thumb in the above position, forcefully apply pressure to the scaphoid tuberosity, remove your

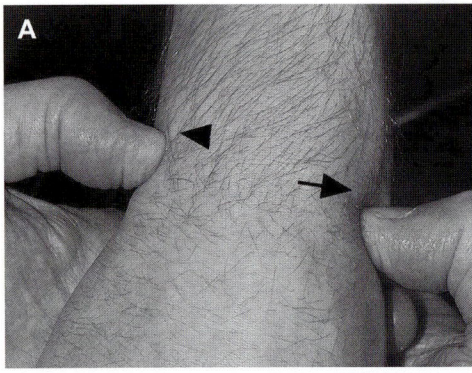
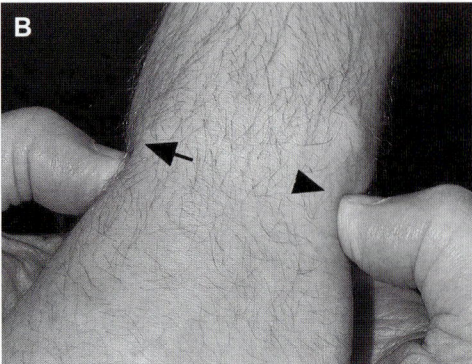

Fig. 3. Clinical examination of ulnar variance. Put the nail beds of the thumbs at 90° to the long axis of the forearm, one at the radial styloid (*arrow*) and the other at the ulnar styloid (*arrowhead*). Comparing the respective levels of these landmarks gives a measure of "clinical ulnar variance" (referenced from ulnar styloid) as opposed to "true ulnar variance" (referenced from ulnar head). (*A*) Right wrist with normal ulnar variance. (*B*) Left wrist with increased ulnar variance after distal radius malunion.

left hand, and request the patient to radially deviate. Feel the tuberosity attempting to rotate volarly, but if sufficient pressure is applied, the tuberosity will not be able to rotate volarly, and thus the wrist will be unable to radially deviate. The patient will feel this restriction and may experience pain as a result of the increased forces that are generated at the radioscaphoid articular surface and in the scapholunate (SL) ligament. This aspect of the examination illustrates that if the scaphoid is prevented from flexing, the carpus cannot move into radial deviation.

To further illustrate this point, ease the pressure exerted by the thumb and allow the wrist to move into radial deviation. The thumb should feel the distal pole of scaphoid become more prominent as scaphoid flexion occurs. The same sensation should be felt with wrist flexion. Practice these maneuvers, because they constitute the basis for understanding the tests for scapholunate instability, assessment of chondromalacia of the scaphoid facet of radius, occult scaphoid fractures, and ganglions in the SL ligament. In addition, the feedback insures that one is definitely palpating the scaphoid tuberosity, thus securing the anatomical landmark.

Flexor carpi radialis

Adjacent and immediately ulnar to the scaphoid tuberosity is the tendon of the flexor carpi radialis (FCR). This can often be visualized proximally, and if not, it can be palpated. Follow it proximally by laying three fingers on it while

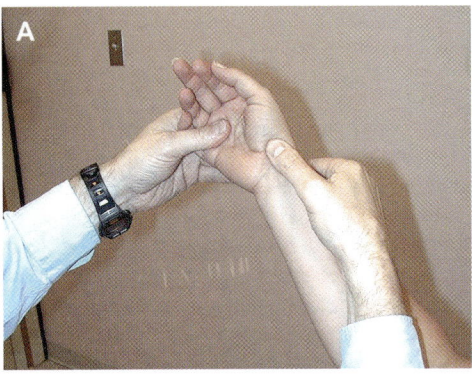
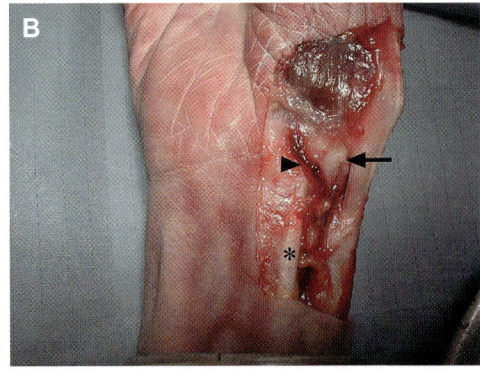

Fig. 4. The palmar scaphoid examination. (*A*) Position of the hands when palpating the scaphoid tuberosity or performing provocative tests of scaphoid instability (eg, scaphoid shift test). (*B*) Gross anatomy demonstrating the location of the scaphoid tuberosity (*arrow*) immediately radial to flexor carpi radialis tendon (*). Superficial palmar branch of radial artery (*arrowhead*).

palmar and dorsiflexing a clenched fist. As one palpates distally, the distinct nature of the tendon becomes obscured as it passes by the scaphoid tubercle. Palpate this area carefully and feel the bony roof of the fibro-osseous canal that the tendon enters in the trapezium as it dives to insert into the base of the second metacarpal. FCR tendonitis can manifest as tenderness upon palpation distally near the fibro-osseus tunnel in the trapezium. There is usually localized pain with hyperextension of the wrist caused by tendon stretch and with resisted wrist flexion and radial deviation.

Scaphotrapezial joint

Immediately radial to this point and distal to the scaphoid tuberosity is the scaphotrapezial (ST) joint. At this location, place your thumb nail transversely and at 90° to the long axis of the forearm. Ask the patient to move his thumb. There will be an appreciation of movement distally while the scaphoid tuberosity remains still. This will be useful for localizing pain related to ST arthritis, a common cause of radial palmar wrist pain, and to localize the entry point for an injection into that joint. Localized swelling or tenderness may indicate synovitis or arthritis in this joint (Fig. 5). Likewise, stress loading can elicit pain in an arthritic ST joint. This can be performed by combining radial deviation of the wrist and dorsally directed force on the scaphoid tuberosity [1].

Radial artery

Just proximal to the scaphoid tuberosity and coursing obliquely across the palmar-radial aspect of the wrist is the superficial palmar branch of the radial artery (see Fig. 4). This small artery is variable in size. The pulse can be palpated. Lay two finger pulps on this area and feel the pulse. If small, this artery is often sacrificed in the Russe approach. Follow the pulse proximally to identify the pulse of the radial artery, then trace this radial artery pulse distally to discover that it disappears about a finger's breadth proximal to the scaphoid tubercle. It is at this point where it courses deep to the first dorsal wrist compartment and is surrounded by fat in the snuffbox.

First dorsal compartment

Move the thumb into abduction and adduction and observe the prominent tendons of the first dorsal compartment, abductor pollicis longus (APL) and extensor pollicis brevis (EPB). These form the radial-palmar limit of the snuffbox. Palpate them with the thumb and index fingers and trace them proximally to determine that they are firmly secured to bone in a fibro-osseous tunnel on the distal radial surface. This is the first dorsal compartment. The tendons will not move medially or laterally here because they are firmly held in the sheath. It is this fibro-osseous sheath that is the source of symptoms in de Quervain's disease

Next determine where the two tendons insert. Palpate both the palmar and dorsal edge of these tendons while you firstly abduct then adduct the thumb metacarpal, while holding the metacarpophalangeal (MCP) joint stationary and slightly flexed. Determine which side of this tendon mass is most active during this maneuver and where the active motion tendon inserts. Then, keep the

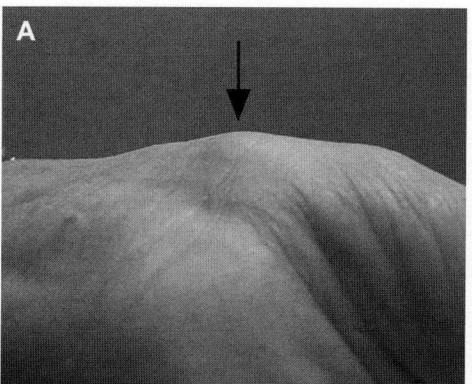
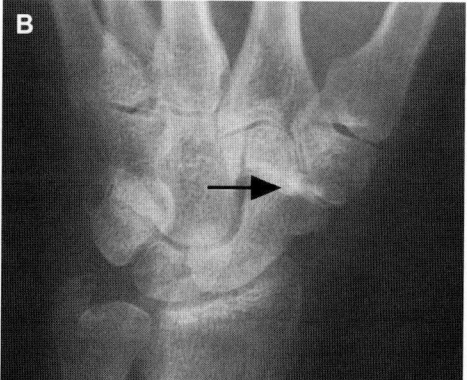

Fig. 5. Scaphotrapezial (ST) joint arthritis. (*A*) Swelling localized to the ST joint (*arrow*). (*B*) Radiographic evidence of ST arthritis (*arrow*).

thumb metacarpal still at the carpometacarpal (CMC) joint and extend and flex the MCP joint while feeling these tendons. Again determine which side of the tendon mass is moving and where it inserts. This exercise clearly demonstrates that the palmar tendon inserts into the proximal radial base of thumb metacarpal, and that the dorsal tendon moves the thumb MCP joint.

Deep to this first compartment, just distal to where the fibro-osseous sheath ends, is the radial styloid process. Palpate this with the thumb and index finger and determine the level of the distal tip by using your thumbnail. Learn what the dorsal ridge of the radial styloid feels like. In many wrist pathologies, this area will develop osteophytes, which will be palpable, tender, and occasionally visible as a lump. Pain localized over the radial styloid can be caused by intrinsic radiocarpal joint pathology, undisplaced fracture, or radiocarpal ligamentous sprain. Extrinsic soft-tissue pathology, such as de Quervain's tenosynovitis, intersection syndrome, and radial neuritis, are nearby but easily differentiated with a competent examination.

de Quervain's tenosynovitis

Tenosynovitis of the first dorsal compartment manifests as pain, swelling and tenderness of the APL and EPB tendons directly over the fibro-osseous tunnel, located just proximal to the radial styloid. Localized pain may be elicited with resisted thumb extension and abduction. Finklestein's test helps confirm the diagnosis [2]. This is performed by having the patient grasp his or her own thumb into the palm. A positive test is when pain is elicited near the fibro-osseous tunnel as the patient's wrist is brought from radial deviation into full ulnar deviation. This maneuver may be mildly painful in normal wrists.

Intersection syndrome

Intersection syndrome, also known as peritendonitis crepitans, is an overuse condition resulting in inflammation in the area where the muscle bellies of the APL and EPB cross the underlying extensor carpi radialis longus (ECRL) and brevis (ECRB) tendons [3,4]. The underlying pathologic abnormalities include stenosing tenosynovitis of the tendon sheath of ECRL and ECRB tendons [4] or APL bursitis [3]. It presents as pain, swelling, tenderness, and crepitus in the radiodorsal forearm about 4 cm proximal to the tip of the radial styloid, corresponding to the intersection of the first and second extensor compartments. Finklestein's test is often painful with APL bursitis, although the pain is usually more proximal in the radiodorsal forearm [3].

Superficial branch of the radial nerve

Back to the area of the sheath of the first dorsal compartment, one can usually see the cephalic vein just dorsal to this sheath. Deep to this vein is the superficial branch of the radial nerve. Deviate the wrist ulnarly to put the nerve under a mild degree of tension, and with the tip of your thumb, a thumb's breadth proximal to the snuffbox, drag the thumb transversely across the dorsolateral aspect of the radius. Apply mild to moderate pressure and do not move the thumb back and forth—drag it only in one direction. Feel the firm dorsal tissue on the radius, and as this is done, the superficial nerve will be bowstrung and snap back into its normal position. Proximally it will be singular, but close to the radiocarpal joint one should feel two or three small nerves as they snap back. In thin patients, you should be able to visualize the nerve as it relocates to its normal anatomical position (Fig. 6). Realize that it is not tender. Pathology in the nerve will produce symptoms. Radial neuritis (Wartenberg's cheiralgia or cheiralgia paresthetica) is an inflammation of the radial nerve secondary to injury such as stretch, compression, or direct blow. It manifests as pain and tenderness 1 to 2 cm proximal to the radial styloid, and radicular pain distally along the course of the superficial radial nerve elicited by percussion. Pain in this structure is much more likely related to a traumatic neuroma.

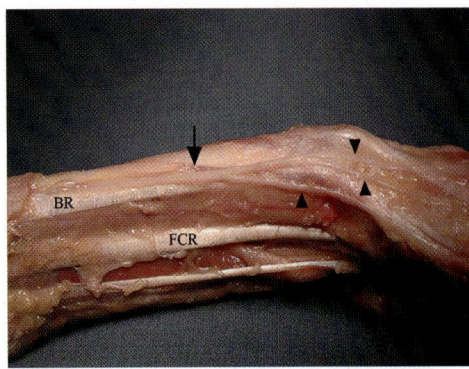

Fig. 6. Anatomy of the radial side of the wrist. Superficial branch of radial nerve (*arrow*) and its branches distally (*arrowheads*). BR, brachioradialis tendon.

First carpometacarpal joint

In line with the first compartment tendons, and just proximal to where the APL inserts, is the first CMC joint. It is between the distal aspect of the trapezium and the metacarpal. It is easier to localize radially, whereas the ST joint is localized volarly. When pathology is present in the first CMC joint, subluxation may be present, and slight longitudinal traction on the thumb with gentle pressure directed ulnarly on the base of the first metacarpal will reduce the subluxation. Usually this is accompanied by palpable crepitus and a painful sensation. If the subluxation is more than 2 or 3 mm, the outline of the thumb will form a slight step, called the "shoulder sign" (Fig. 7). Also, an axial load on the thumb may reproduce symptoms in the setting of degenerative disease of the first CMC joint. The grind test is a variation of this, in which an axial load is applied through the first metacarpal while the examiner's other hand is placed at the CMC joint and shifts the metacarpal base medially and laterally [5]. Exacerbation of the patient's pain and palpable crepitus indicate degenerative disease. Symptoms may be increased with rotation of the metacarpal effected by flexing the MCP joint and using the proximal phalanx as the lever for rotation. Try to establish by history which end (articular surface) of the trapezium is most painful. Flexion/extension of the wrist with the thumb immobilized will cause motion at the ST joint. Motion of the thumb with the wrist immobilized will mainly cause motion at the CMC joint.

The snuffbox

Distally in the snuffbox, the palmar border is formed by the first dorsal compartment tendons. The dorsal border is formed by the combined second and third compartments. The proximal border is the distal radius and the distal border the base of the first and second metacarpals. Spend a moment and find these limits. The snuffbox contains fat, the radial artery traversing obliquely, and the wrist joint capsule. Through this capsule the waist of the scaphoid can be readily felt when the wrist is ulnarly deviated (Fig. 8). The junctional point along the radial border of the scaphoid, where the proximal articular surface changes to nonarticular surface, is referred to as the scaphoid articular-nonarticular (ANA) junction. With the wrist in ulnar deviation, the ANA junction can be palpated with the examiner's index finger placed just distal to the radial styloid. Whereas mild tenderness is present there in normal wrists, scaphoid instability or synovitis is said to result in more severe pain [5,6]. Asymmetry on bilateral examination is important.

Move to the dorsal border of the snuffbox and realize that this border consists of both superficial and deep components. The extensor pollicis longus (EPL) forms the superficial border and heads toward the thumb. Deep to this is the ECRL tendon. Extend the interphalangeal (IP) joint of the thumb and feel the EPL. Dorsiflex the wrist and feel the ECRL. Follow the ECRL distally to its insertion in bone. Make a clenched fist and put the tip of the index finger into the V that forms

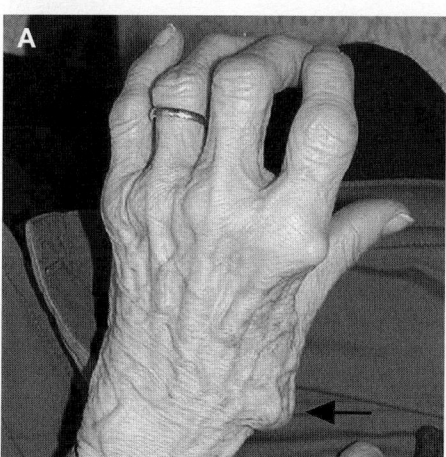 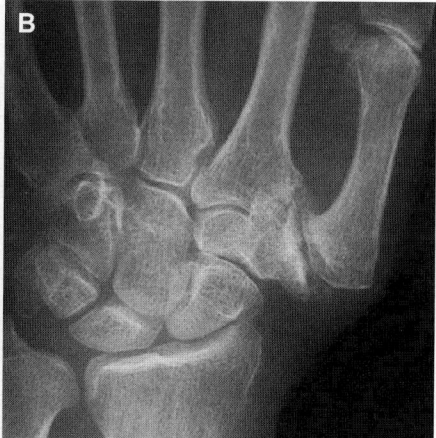

Fig. 7. First carpometacarpal arthritis. (*A*) Radial subluxation of the base of the first metacarpal giving the "shoulder sign" (*arrow*). (*B*) Anteroposterior (AP) radiograph of the same hand.

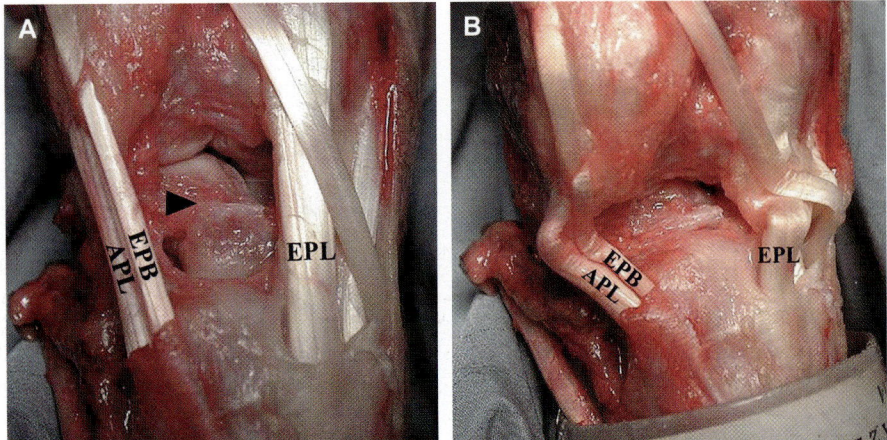

Fig. 8. Anatomy of the snuffbox. (*A*) With ulnar deviation, the waist of the scaphoid (*arrowhead*) is exposed and easily palpable. (*B*) With radial deviation, the waist of the scaphoid is no longer palpable. EPL, extensor pollicis longus.

distally between the ECRL and ECRB. Determine the exact insertion of these tendons. The ECRL inserts into the base of the second metacarpal, but does it insert into the center, the radial border, or the ulnar border? The ECRB inserts into the base of the third metacarpal, but again, exactly where? Feel for the answer, and be sure you agree that it is clearly the radial aspect of the base for both (Fig. 9A).

Extend the IP joint and abduct the thumb. The EPL should stand out visibly and be easily palpable through its course to the mid-dorsal radius, where it courses about the ulnar aspect of Lister's tubercle. Feel this definite short oblong bump with the tendon moving next to it. Feel the beginning of the radiocarpal joint just 2 to 3 mm distal to this tubercle. Move the wrist into dorsi- and palmar flexion and be certain that the "lump" remains stationary.

Next, hold the hand and apply thumb pressure in the interval between the two arms of the V made by the ECRL and ECRB. Flex and extend the wrist. In flexion, appreciate a smooth firm bump becoming prominent in this interval. This is the dorsal proximal pole of the scaphoid covered by capsule (Fig. 9B). It should be firm and not

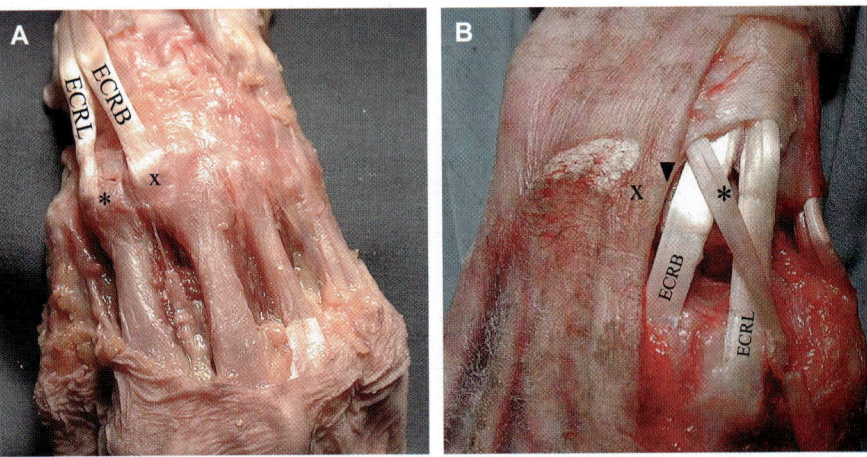

Fig. 9. Anatomy of the dorsum of the wrist. (*A*) ECRL tendon inserting into the base of second metatarsal (*). ECRB tendon inserting into the base of the third metatarsal (*x*). (*B*) The proximal pole of the scaphoid (*) can be palpated in the apex of the V formed by the ECRL and ECRB tendons. Ulnar to this, in line with the third metacarpal and covered by EDC tendons, one can palpate the dorsal pole of the lunate (*x*). Both bones become prominent when the wrist is flexed. The palpable gap between the two is the SL interval (*arrowhead*).

painful to press on. Scaphoid impaction is a condition in which repetitive hyperextension of the wrist causes impingement of the scaphoid onto the dorsal lip of the radius. A tender dorsal osteophyte or spur on the dorsal radial lip or dorsal scaphoid rim may be palpable, and extension of the wrist may be limited or painful [7].

Dorsal wrist examination

Scapholunate interval

Move ulnarly and place your thumb just distal to the dorsal lip of radius in line with the long metacarpal. Flex and extend the wrist and feel a poorly defined hard lump becoming prominent in flexion. This is the dorsal pole of lunate (see Fig. 9B). It is covered by capsule, extensor digitorum longus, tenosynovium, and retinaculum, and is not felt very distinctly—but it is felt. Pressure on this area is generally not painful unless a fracture or Kienbock's disease is present. Appreciate the hard fullness felt with palmar flexion, and move back and forth between the dorsal pole of the lunate and proximal pole of the scaphoid. Palpate the intervening SL area. Appreciate the slight valley that exists. This area should not be painful unless there is a recent SL ligament tear or a chronic occult ganglion. This is usually the area where the dorsal ganglion becomes obvious.

Fourth and fifth extensor compartment

The extensor digitorum communis (EDC) tendons (fourth compartment) and their tenosynovium is easily appreciated by flexing and extending the fingers at the MCP joints. This can be done as a unit, but is better appreciated if done in rhythmical consecutive fashion. Similarly, place the fingers in a "piccolo" fashion longitudinally between the EDC and head of ulna, and flex and extend the little digit. The tendon of the extensor digiti minimi (EDM) can be felt moving. Tenosynovitis is a common source of pain, swelling, and tenderness in the dorsum of the wrist. Ganglion cysts and vestigial wrist extensor muscles (extensor digitorum brevis manus) are less common but may have a similar presentation.

Carpometacarpal joints

Sprains of the second through fifth CMC joints can be associated with localized tenderness and swelling. Stressing the joint by flexion, extension, and rotational forces may add additional information [8]. A bony prominence at the base of second or third metacarpal, often involving the CMC joints, is called a carpal boss. The cause and significance of this prominence is unknown, and caution is suggested when considering any surgical treatment.

Ulnar wrist examination

Dorsal ulnar structures

Palpate the ulnocarpal space with pressure directed toward the proximal ulnar aspect of the lunate, best done with the wrist is in flexion. If this is painful, it may indicate chondromalacia on the ulnar aspect of lunate, and suggests the diagnosis of ulnocarpal impaction (UCI) or a TFCC tear. To test this diagnosis, a "grind test" is done [1,9]. Hold the dorsal and palmar aspect of the patient's metacarpal region in one hand (Fig. 10) and use the supporting hand to stabilize the distal forearm. The wrist is deviated ulnarly and put through a series of repetitive maneuvers that combine ulnar deviation and a proximally directed force with alternating pronation and supination. A positive test will produce a click or feeling of crepitus or be subjectively painful. Such a positive test may indicate a TFCC tear or UCI.

With the forearm pronated, palpate ulnar and distal to the ulnar head. Deviate the wrist radial

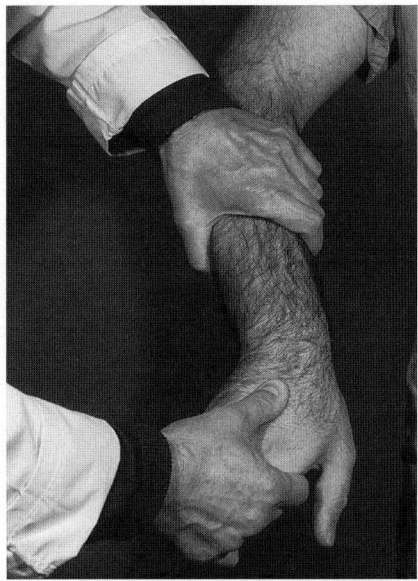

Fig. 10. The "grind test" for ulnocarpal impaction or TFCC tears. The wrist is ulnarly deviated and axially loaded with alternating pronation and supination.

and ulnar, and feel the tendon of the extensor carpi ulnaris (ECU) become prominent on ulnar deviation. Trace this tendon distally to its insertion into the dorso-ulnar base of the fifth metacarpal. Trace the tendon proximally to the sheath of the ECU, which begins at the distal aspect of the ulnar head. Feel that the ECU is ulnar when the forearm is pronated, but is relatively central when supinated. The ECU has not actually changed its position relative to the ulna, but rather the hand and radius has changed. Dorsiflex the wrist while the forearm is supinated, and appreciate that the ECU is more prominent than when the forearm is pronated. Tenderness along the tendon sheath or pain and weakness with resisted wrist extension and ulnar deviation suggest tendonitis.

The ulnar styloid (US) is best felt when the forearm is pronated. It is distal to the ulnar head and palmar to the ECU. It is slightly obscured by the ECU when the forearm is supinated. It should not be tender to palpate unless there has been a recent fracture or ulnar styloid-triquetral impaction (USTI) is present. To search for clinical support for this diagnosis, a USTI provocative test [10] is performed. This USTI test is based on the fact that the US is ulnar in pronation, and is more central and dorsal in supination (Fig. 11). Because the ECU is held firmly to the ulnar head by its subsheath, the US has the same relationship to the wrist as we have just appreciated for the ECU. Thus it is evident that to approximate the US to the triquetrum, one needs to bring the US closer to the carpus by supinating the forearm, and bring the carpus closer to the US by dorsiflexing the wrist. Therefore, begin the test with the wrist dorsiflexed and the forearm pronated, and simply add one motion, supination, while maintaining dorsiflexion (Fig. 12). A typical positive test will produce pain at the US when one approaches full supination. In a small series of patients with USTI, Topper and colleagues [10] reported that the USTI provocative test was positive in all patients preoperatively, and negative in all following partial ulnar styloidectomy. To support the diagnosis, the US should also be tender exactly over its tip. This is tested in pronation and neutral wrist flexion. The patient may indicate from the history that this test produces pain. The pain with the hand in the back pocket, repetitive page turning, or the distal supinated hand on the ice hockey stick may be historical evidence of a positive USTI provocative test.

The lunotriquetral (LT) joint can be localized as a depression just distal to the radial side of the ulnar styloid, because the head of the ulna articulates with one half of the lunate and one half of the triquetrum. Direct palpation of the LT joint may be tender when LT pathology is present; however, more information can often be obtained by the numerous LT stress maneuvers discussed later.

In the same general area, but located ulnarly and midway between the pisiform and US, palpate deeply with the tip of one's finger. This test may be slightly uncomfortable, but if there is more discomfort than expected, it may indicate pathology in the ulnotriquetral ligaments. Berger calls this the foveal sign [11]. The dorsal superficial branch of the ulnar nerve obliquely traverses this same area (Fig. 13). It can be bowstrung and palpated in the same fashion as one does

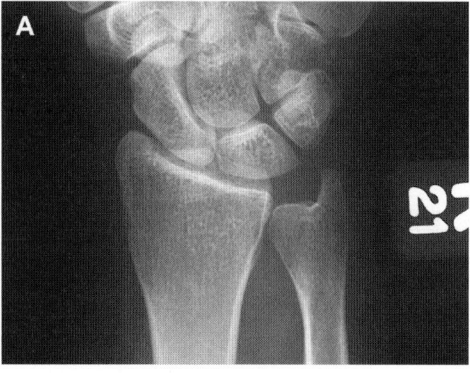 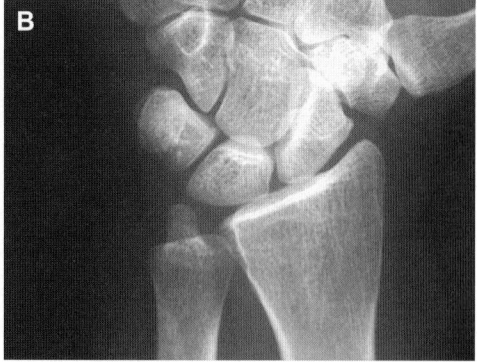

Fig. 11. The position of the US in relation to forearm rotation. (*A*) AP radiograph with the forearm in pronation, demonstrating that the US is located ulnarly. (*B*) AP radiograph with the forearm in supination, demonstating that the US is located dorsally and centrally.

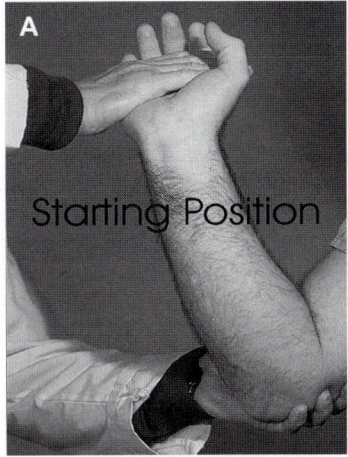 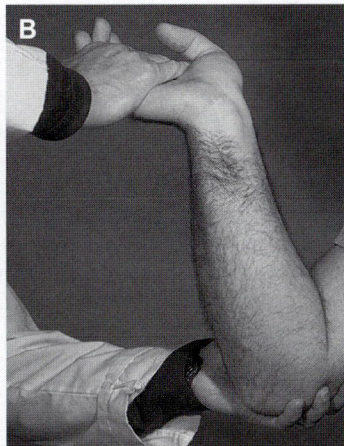 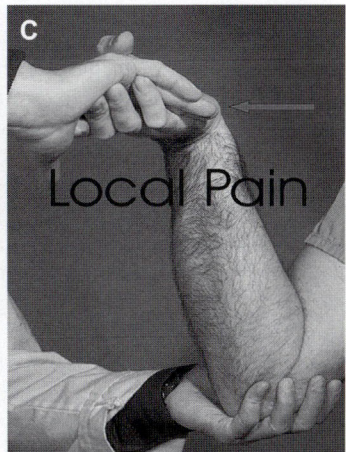

Fig. 12. The UST provocative test. (*A*) Starting position of pronation and wrist extension. (*B*) While maintaining wrist extension, the examiner moves the forearm into supination. (*C*) The final position of full supination produces localized pain at the ulnar styloid in USTI.

for the superficial branch of the radial nerve. Develop the ability to palpate and move these superficial nerves, and by patient feedback determine if symptoms are related to it. To facilitate the palpation of this nerve, radially deviate the wrist. This will place the branches under tension. Then drag one's thumb across the nerves perpendicular to its course. It is usually easy to palpate as it crosses the ECU near the insertion into fifth metacarpal. In addition, realize that a pathological process, such as neuroma, will likely show signs of decreased sensation over the appropriate area served by that nerve.

Distal radioulnar joint

Instability or degenerative disease of the distal radioulnar joint (DRUJ) is often associated with diminished or painful pronosupination. Instability can occasionally be appreciated on inspection, looking laterally at the wrist in full pronation and supination. A dimple sign may be appreciated. The piano key test for DRUJ instability could be done with one hand or two. With this test, the examiner depresses the ulnar head palmarly while the pisiform is stabilized with a dorsally directed force. A positive piano key sign is when the ulnar head springs back into position like a piano key when the forces are released [12]. Additional information can be obtained from testing both the palmar and dorsal displacement of the ulnar head in pronation, neutral, and supination, and comparing it with the opposite side. This is referred to as the distal ulna ballottement test [13]. In addition, press the ulnar head against the sigmoid notch as it translates, to appreciate the status of the articular cartilage as well as the ligamentous stability. This is referred to as the ulnar compression test [1].

Palmar ulnar structures

Hold the pisiform between the index finger and thumb. Flex and extend the wrist and move the pisiform medially and laterally while applying dorsally directed pressure, compressing the pisiform on the triquetrum, to search for articular cartilage crepitus or pain associated with pisotriquetral degenerative joint disease. This is referred to as the pisotriquetral grind test [1].

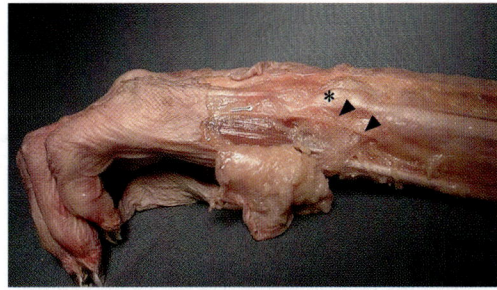

Fig. 13. Anatomy of the ulnar side of the wrist. Dorsal superficial branch of the ulnar nerve (*arrowheads*) in relation to the ulnar styloid (*).

Palpate the hook of the hamate just distal and radial from the pisiform. It is localized by placing the IP joint of the examiner's thumb over the more superficial pisiform, with the tip of the thumb directed toward the metacarpal head of the long finger. Deep palpation with the tip of the examiner's thumb reveals the hook of the hamate. This can be tender in the setting of fracture or nonunion of the hook of the hamate. Remember that this is the area of the ulnar nerve, and deep palpation onto this nerve is usually painful.

Palpate the flexor carpi ulnaris (FCU) proximally from the pisiform. It is most prominent by having the patient make a clenched fist during mild wrist flexion. Tenderness along the tendon sheath or pain and weakness with resisted wrist flexion and ulnar deviation suggest tendonitis.

With the tip of the thumb on the radial palmar side of the pisiform, add deep pressure. The uncomfortable sensation is related to pressure on the ulnar nerve. Although one cannot objectively feel this nerve, this means of localization will be of value for assessing symptoms or injecting local anesthetic.

The palmar wrist examination

The palmaris longus (PL) tendon is central and superficial in the palmar distal forearm. It stands out with a flexed grip, and can be visualized and palpated. It may be absent. At the wrist crease between the PL and FCR, an astute examiner can often palpate a fine snapping of the palmar cutaneous branch of the median nerve. This subtle finding is aided by tensioning the nerve with dorsiflexion of the wrist and then drawing the tip of the examining digit across the interval with slight deep pressure. Finally, circumferential wrist compression with the thumb and index will produce pain when a synovitis and effusion is present.

Provocative tests of carpal instability

Scapholunate instability

Watson [14] described the first test of SL instability, called the scaphoid shift maneuver, in 1978; however, it was not until 1988 that Watson and colleagues [15] first published a detailed description and interpretation of the maneuver. They stressed the point that the scaphoid shift is a provocative maneuver rather than a test, because it does not offer a simple positive or negative result, but rather a variety of findings, with emphasis being on asymmetry on bilateral examination [5,15]. The maneuver is performed starting with the wrist in slight extension and ulnar deviation. The examiner grasps the wrist from the radial side, placing a thumb on the palmar prominence of the scaphoid while wrapping fingers around the distal radius for counterpressure. The wrist is then passively moved into radial deviation and slight flexion by the examiner's other hand. The examiner's thumb resists the attempt of the scaphoid tuberosity to rotate volarly, creating a dorsally directed subluxation stress. This subluxation stress causes the proximal pole of the scaphoid to "shift" dorsally in relation to other bones of the carpus and the distal radius, even in normal wrists. The degree of the shift is related to the amount of examiner pressure, the degree of scaphoid flexion, the amount of ligamentous laxity, and the status of the SL ligament. A ruptured SL ligament allows the proximal pole to move more dorsally and frequently rest on the dorsal lip of the radius. The maneuver is best done with the patient's wrist flexed, because this causes the scaphoid to be angled to such a degree that the proximal pole may be only partially constrained by the bony architecture of the dorsal lip of the radius (Fig. 14). As the thumb pressure is withdrawn, there may be a palpable "clunk" as the scaphoid returns to its normal position. Pain that replicates the patient's symptoms or asymmetrical laxity when comparing with the contralateral wrist are considered significant findings.

The scaphoid shift is perhaps the most studied provocative test of the wrist examination. Radiographic displacement of the scaphoid has been shown to correlate with clinical grade of subluxation [16]. Likewise, objective evaluation of displacement using a customized instrument has been shown to correlate with clinical grade of subluxation [17]; however, Watson and other authors agree that it is a subjective test, and that experience is required to determine the clinical significance of the degree of scaphoid mobility elicited [5,15–17]. There are many reports of "positive" scaphoid shifts in normal patients who have no symptoms or history of wrist trauma [6,17–19]. This calls into question the positive predictive value of the test. Watson and colleagues [6] examined 1000 random individuals who had no prior wrist complaints, and found that 21% had unilateral increased scaphoid mobility on the scaphoid shift test. Only 37% of these had associated symptoms. Similarly, Easterling and Wolfe [19] examined 100 uninjured asymptomatic patients, and found that

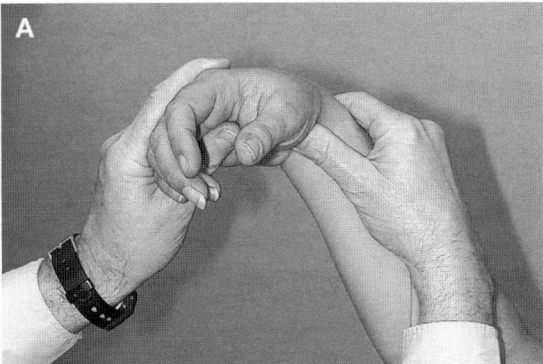
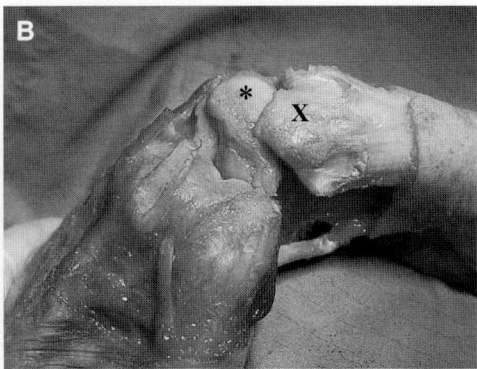

Fig. 14. The scaphoid shift test. (*A*) Starting with the wrist in ulnar deviation and slight extension, the wrist is passively moved into radial deviation and slight flexion while the examiner's thumb resists the attempt of the scaphoid tuberosity to rotate volarly. (*B*) The resulting dorsally directed subluxation stress causes the proximal pole of the scaphoid (*) to "shift" dorsally in relation to the distal radius (*x*).

32% had bilateral and 14% had unilateral increased scaphoid mobility on the scaphoid shift test, with a palpable "clunk" on release of the pressure on the scaphoid tubercle. There was an association between positive tests and generalized ligamentous laxity. None of the patients had a painful shift, thus supporting Watson and colleagues' [15] emphasis on the clinical significance of reproducing the patient's symptoms. The importance of a pain associated with the scaphoid shift is also supported by radiographic evidence of greater displacement of the scaphoid correlating with painful shifts compared with painless shifts [16].

The scaphoid shift maneuver is usually considered a test for SL rupture and scaphoid instability; however, this test is also important for assessing the articular cartilage status of the proximal pole of scaphoid and radial facet, with a gritty sensation or clicking suggesting condromalacia or loss of articular cartilage [15]. It will also produce symptoms when an occult dorsal ganglion or an occult scaphoid fracture is present. Because the test produces a dorsal displacement of the scaphoid and traction on the SL ligament, if an occult dorsal ganglion is present, the test will generally be painful [20]. Likewise, thumb pressure produces a force that begins on the tuberosity of the scaphoid and travels up the longitudinal axis of the scaphoid. This test will produce a painful stimulus if any fracture exists, and should be considered a mandatory test for all cases diagnosed as "clinical scaphoid fracture."

The scaphoid thrust [21,22] and the scaphoid lift [1] are additional tests of scapholunate instability that have been described. They involve slight variations in the technique of loading the distal pole of the scaphoid, and are not as well-studied as Watson's original scaphoid shift test.

Lunotriquetral instability

The LT compression test [1,23] loads the LT joint in an ulnar-to-radial direction, eliciting pain with LT instability or degenerative joint disease. The examiner's thumb applies a radially directed pressure on the triquetrum just distal to the US at the "ulnar snuffbox," the space between the tendons of FCU and ECU. This maneuver is similar to the radiocarpal glide test described later for radiocarpal instability (Fig. 15).

LT ballottement tests and LT shear tests demonstrate instability by exerting pressure in opposite directions upon the adjacent carpal bones. The LT ballottement test, as described by Reagan and colleagues [24], is performed by grasping the lunate between the thumb and index finger of one hand while applying alternating dorsal and palmar loads at the pisotriquetral unit with the thumb and index finger of the other hand (Fig. 16). The test is considered positive if the maneuver elicits pain, crepitus, and increased anteroposterior laxity at the LT joint. A variation of this ballottement test was also described by Masquelet [25]. The LT shear test, as described by Kleinman [26], is performed by applying a dorsally directed load on the pisotriquetral unit with the examiner's thumb to create a shear force at the LT joint.

Triquetral lift maneuver [27] is similar to the scaphoid sift maneuver in that the examiner resists

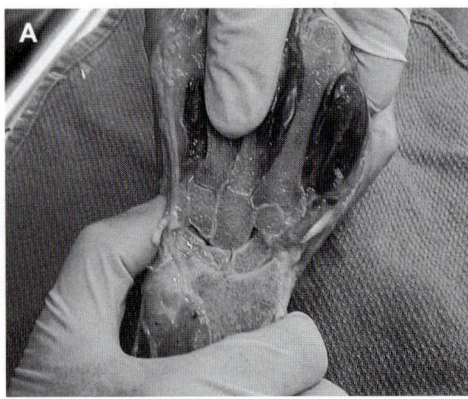 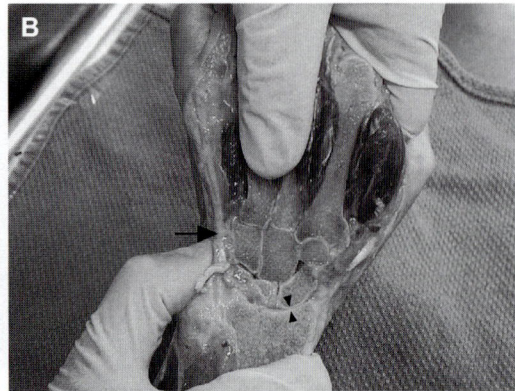

Fig. 15. Gross anatomy of the radiocarpal glide test. (*A*) Starting position. (*B*) The examiner's thumb exerts a radially directed force on the triquetrum (*arrow*). This results in a radial shift of the proximal carpal row relative to the distal radius in the setting of radiocarpal instability. The articular surface of the radiocarpal joint can also be assessed by noting crepitus caused by degenerative disease (*arrowheads*).

the normal dorsal translocation of the triquetrum as the wrist moves from ulnar deviation into radial deviation. The patient's hand is placed in full pronation, and the examiner places his or her thumb over the dorsal aspect of the triquetrum, resisting the dorsal lift of the triquetrum as the wrist is brought from ulnar deviation into radial deviation. Resisting the lift stresses both the LT joint and the triquetrohamate joint, eliciting pain if instability is present.

Radiocarpal instability

The anteroposterior drawer test [28] can be used to assess for instability of either the radiocarpal or midcarpal joints. The examiner stabilizes distal forearm with one hand while the other hand grips the metacarpals, applying longitudinal traction and an anteroposterior force. A "drawer" is elicited though the radiocarpal or midcarpal joint, and compared with the contralateral side.

The radiocarpal glide will test the articular surface of the proximal carpal row and the extrinsic ligaments (see Fig. 15). The examiner's thumb exerts a radially directed force on the triquetrum. A radial shift of the proximal carpal row relative to the distal radius may be appreciated in the setting of radiocarpal instability. Crepitus may be felt in the setting of articular pathology of the radiocarpal joint.

Midcarpal instability

The catch-up clunk test was first described Lichtman and colleagues [29]. With the forearm in pronation, the patient actively moves the wrist back and forth from radial deviation to ulnar deviation. Normally as the wrist moves from radial to ulnar deviation, the proximal carpal row rotates smoothly from flexion to extension while the distal row translates from palmar to dorsal. With midcarpal instability, the proximal row remains flexed and the distal row remains volarly translated longer than normal during ulnar deviation. As ulnar deviation progresses, the soft-tissue and bony restraints cause a sudden "catch-up" of the proximal row into extension and the distal row into dorsal translation, which is often an audible or palpable "clunk" [30]. This abnormal carpal motion has been confirmed using videoflouroscopy [31]. The catch-up clunk test is not specific for midcarpal instability because a similar clunk may be present in radiocarpal instability [27,32],

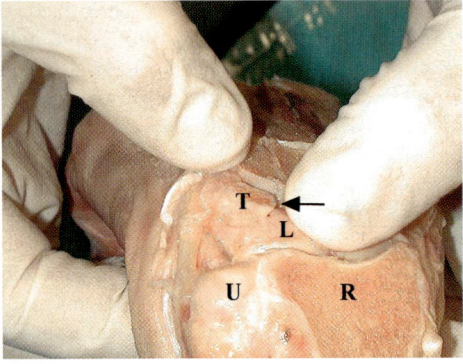

Fig. 16. Gross anatomy of the LT ballottement test. Note the step (*arrow*) between the lunate (L) and triquetrum (T). U, ulnar head; R, distal radius.

in which the proximal row may suddenly sublux dorsally with ulnar deviation [32].

Lichtman and colleagues [31,32] later added a provocative maneuver referred to as the midcarpal shift test (Fig. 17). With the wrist in neutral ulnoradial deviation, the examiner stabilizes the forearm in pronation with one hand, and with the other hand applies a palmarly directed pressure at the level of the distal capitate, noting the ease and extent of palmar translation. The wrist is then axially loaded and passively ulnar deviated. The test is positive if a painful catch-up clunk occurs with ulnar deviation that reproduces the patient's symptoms. The presence of palmar translation or a clunk alone without the reproduced symptoms are not considered positive, because they can occur in normal asymptomatic patients [30,32]. The test is very subjective; however, Lichtman and colleagues [32] later developed a grading system (Grades I–IV) to help quantify the severity of the palmar translation and catch-up clunk. The validity of the test is supported by studies showing the correlation between clinical grading and objective mechanical measurements of displacement [30,32].

The anteroposterior drawer test [28], as previously described for radiocarpal instability, can also be used to assess for instability of the midcarpal joint. Additionally, a pivot shift test [33] of the midcarpal instability has been described, but is not as well studied as the midcarpal shift test.

Capitolunate instability

Capitolunate instability is rare and can be tested with a dorsally directed force to the hand. The dorsal capitate-displacement apprehension test to demonstrate capitolunate instability was described by Johnson and Carrera [34]. The examiner stabilizes the distal forearm with one hand, while exerting a dorsally directed force on the capitate with the thumb of the other hand. Apprehension and discomfort with dorsal subluxation of the capitate are considered a positive test. Johnson and Carrera's original description of the test includes fluoroscopy to directly visualize the degree of dorsal subluxation of the capitate. Other authors have described similar dorsal capitolunate displacement tests that load the capitate at different locations, such as through the scaphoid tuberosity [35] or the metacarpals (Fig. 18) [33]. Apergis [36] described a positive wrist hanging test, in which hanging the wrist over the end of the table with the forearm supinated causes

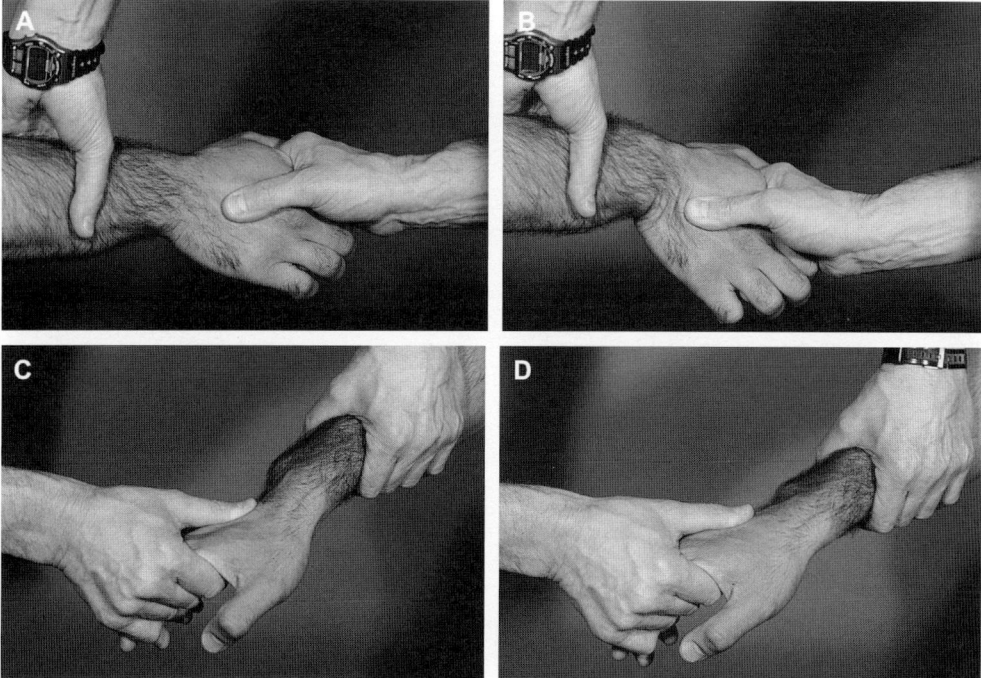

Fig. 17. (*A–D*) The midcarpal shift test.

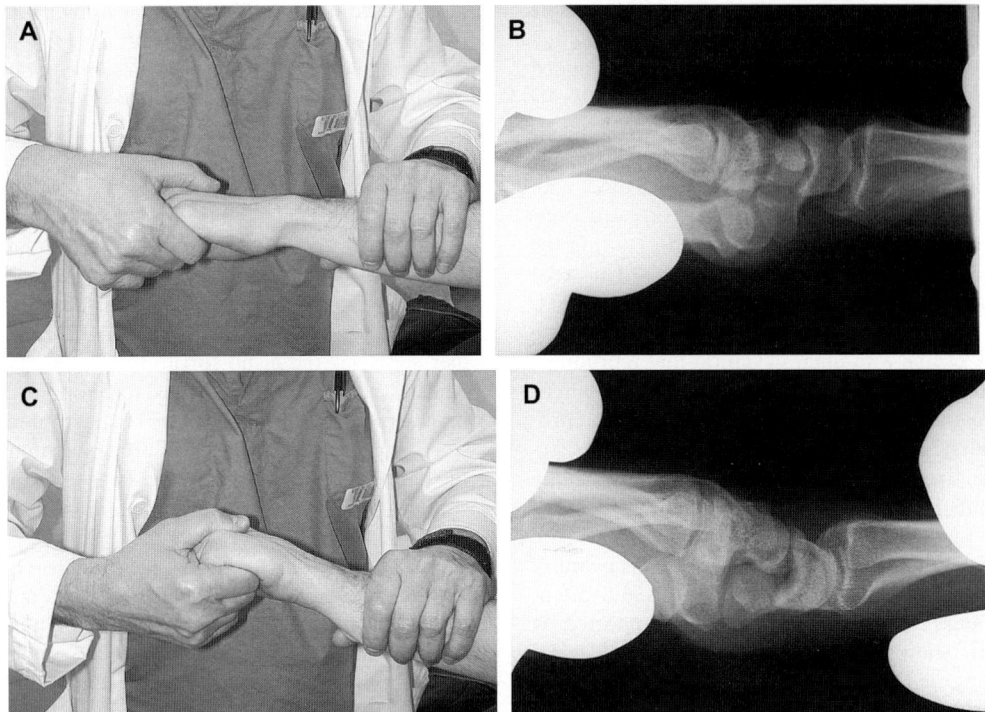

Fig. 18. Dorsal capitolunate displacement test. (*A*) Starting position before dorsally loading the wrist. (*B*) Corresponding lateral radiograph (before load) showing reduced capitolunate joint. (*C*) Dorsal load applied through the metacarpals with resulting dorsal midcarpal subluxation. (*D*) Corresponding lateral radiograph (during dorsal load) demonstrating dorsal subluxation of the capitate on the lunate.

discomfort. This was positive in two thirds of patients who had capitolunate instability. All of the wrists in that same series had a palmar sag appearance [36].

The finger extension test (FET) is a sensitive but nonspecific indicator of carpal pathology [5]. With the wrist passively flexed, the examiner resists active finger extension. This loads the carpal joints. Pain in the dorsal aspect of the wrist or weak extension indicate an abnormal test. A normal FET is rarely seen with carpal instability (radiocarpal, midcarpal, or scaphoid rotatory instability) or Kienbock's disease [5], although an abnormal test does not provide information regarding the specific pathology.

Differential lidocaine injection

Differential lidocaine injections can be incorporated into the physical examination to help localize the source of pain [27,37].

Summary

The clinical examination of the wrist is still in a state of evolution. The significance of each maneuver, including the sensitivity and specificity of detecting distinct pathology, needs to be further clarified. Furthermore, the addition of other tests will likely be forthcoming.

References

[1] Cooney WP, Bishop AT, Linscheid RL. Physical examination of the wrist. In: Cooney WP, Dobyns JH, Linscheid RL, editors. The wrist: diagnosis and operative treatment. St. Louis: Mosby; 1997.
[2] Finkelstein H. Stenosing tendovaginitis at the radial styloid process. J Bone Joint Surg Am 1930;12:509–40.
[3] Wood MB, Linscheid RL. Abductor pollicis longus bursitis. Clin Orthop 1973;93:293–6.
[4] Grundberg AB, Reagan DS. Pathologic anatomy of the forearm: intersection syndrome. J Hand Surg [Am] 1985;10(2):299–302.
[5] Watson HK, Weinzweig J. Physical examination of the wrist. Hand Clin 1997;13(1):17–34.

[6] Watson HK, Ottoni L, Pitts EC, et al. Rotary subluxation of the scaphoid: a spectrum of instability. J Hand Surg [Br] 1993;18:62–4.
[7] Linscheid RL, Dobyns JH. Athletic injuries of the wrist. Clin Orthop Relat Res 1985;198:141–51.
[8] Linscheid RL, Dobyns JH. Physical examination of the wrist. In: Post M, editor. Physical examination of the musculoskeletal system. Chicago: Year Book Medical Publishers; 1987. p. 80–94.
[9] Friedman SL, Palmer AK. The ulnar impaction syndrome. Hand Clin 1991;7:295–310.
[10] Topper SM, Wood MB, Ruby LK. Ulnar styloid impaction syndrome. J Hand Surg [Am] 1997;22:699–704.
[11] Berger RA. Arthroscopic anatomy of the wrist and distal radioulnar joint. Hand Clin 1999;15(3):393–413.
[12] Linscheid RL. Examination of the wrist. In: Nakamura R, Linscheid RL, Miura T, editors. Wrist disorders. Current concepts and challenges. Tokyo: Springer-Verlag; 1992. p. 13–25.
[13] Raskin KB, Beldner S. Clinical examination of the distal ulna and surrounding structures. Hand Clin 1998;14(2):177–90.
[14] Watson HK. Triscaphe reconstruction. Presented at the American Research in Orthopedics. New Orleans (LA), March 1978.
[15] Watson HK, Ashmead D, Makhlouf V. Examination of the scaphoid. J Hand Surg [Am] 1988;13:657–60.
[16] Park MJ. Radiographic observation of the scaphoid shift. J Bone Joint Surg 2003;85:358–62.
[17] Wolfe SW, Crisco JJ. Mechanical evaluation of the scaphoid shift test. J Hand Surg [Am] 1994;19:762–8.
[18] Wolfe SW, Gupta A, Crisco JJ. Kinematics of the scaphoid shift test. J Hand Surg [Am] 1997;22:801–6.
[19] Easterling KJ, Wolfe SW. Scaphoid shift in the uninjured wrist. J Hand Surg [Am] 1994;19:604–6.
[20] Hwang JJ, Goldfarb CA, Gelberman RH, et al. The effect of dorsal carpal ganglion excision on the scaphoid shift test. J Hand Surg [Br] 1999;24(1):106–8.
[21] Lane L. The scaphoid shift test. J Hand Surg [Am] 1993;18:366–8.
[22] Lane L. The scaphoid shift test [letter to the editor]. J Hand Surg [Am] 1994;19:341.
[23] Shin AY, Battaglia MJ. Lunotriquetral instability: diagnosis and treatment. J Am Acad Orthop Surg 2000;8:170–9.
[24] Reagan DS, Linscheid RL, Dobyns JH. Lunotriquetral sprains. J Hand Surg [Am] 1984;9:502–14.
[25] Masquelet AC. L'examen clinique du poignet. Ann Chir Main Memb Super 1989;8:159–75 [French].
[26] Kleinman WB. Clinical examination of the ulnar side of the wrist. American Society for Surgery of the Hand Correspondence Club Newsletter. November 1985.
[27] Nelson DL. Additional thoughts on the physical examination of the wrist. Hand Clin 1997;13(1):35–7.
[28] Tubiana R, Thomine JM, Mackin E. Examination of the hand and wrist. Philadelphia: Mosby; 1995. p. 185–7.
[29] Lichtman DM, Schneider JR, Swafford AR, et al. Ulnar midcarpal instability—clinical and laboratory analysis. J Hand Surg [Am] 1981;6:515–23.
[30] Feinstein WK, Lichtman DM, Noble PC, et al. Quantitative assessment of the midcarpal shift test. J Hand Surg [Am] 1999;24:977–83.
[31] Lichtman DM, Brucker JD, Culp RW, et al. Palmar midcarpal instability: results of surgical reconstruction. J Hand Surg [Am] 1993;18:307–15.
[32] Lichtman DM, Gaenslen ES, Pollock GR. Midcarpal and proximal carpal instabilities. In: Lichtman DM, Alexander AH, editors. The wrist and its disorders. 2nd edition. Phildelphia: WB Saunders; 1997. p. 316–28.
[33] Stanley J, Saffar P. Wrist arthroscopy. Philadelphia: WB Saunders; 1994.
[34] Johnson RP, Carrera GF. Chronic capitolunate instability. J Bone Joint Surg [Am] 1986;68:1164–76.
[35] White SJ, Louis DS, Braunstein EM, et al. Capitatelunate instability: recognition by manipulation under fluoroscopy. AJR Am J Roentgenol 1984;143:361–4.
[36] Apergis EP. The unstable capitolunate and radiolunate joints as a source of wrist pain in young women. J Hand Surg [Br] 1996;21(4):501–6.
[37] Nelson DL, Manske PR. Lunotriquetral arthrodesis. In: Blair WF, editor. Techniques in hand surgery. Baltimore (MD): Williams and Wilkins; 1996. p. 855–64.

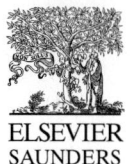

Distal Radius Fractures—Classification of Treatment and Indications for Surgery

Asif M. Ilyas, MD, Jesse B. Jupiter, MD*

Harvard Medical School, Orthopaedic Hand Service, Massachusetts General Hospital, Yawkey 2100, 55 Fruit Street, Boston, MA 02114, USA

Distal radius fractures remain an injury that fosters considerable interest and debate. It is an injury seen with high frequency, representing approximately one sixth of all fractures seen in emergency departments. Most are extracurricular and result from a fall. They typically present in a bimodal distribution with two distinct groups: children and the elderly. In the older population, it is more common in women and is attributed to postmenopausal osteoporosis.

Interest in distal radius fractures stems not only from its high incidence but also from the developing understanding of outcome variables and the influence of technology in evaluation and treatment. For years distal radius fractures were injuries assumed to warrant no more than a cast following Colles' [1] writings that they "will at some remote period again enjoy perfect freedom in all of its motions and be completely exempt from pain." Today, the literature is burgeoning with data, often contradictory, on the indications for operative and nonoperative management.

The goal of treatment for distal radius fractures is to obtain sufficient pain-free motion, allowing return to activities while minimizing the risk for future degenerative changes or disability. Multiple variables must be considered when evaluating a distal radius fracture and determining whether to operate. Closed reduction and casting has historically been the mainstay of treatment. However, the adequacy of closed treatment versus the need for operative intervention depends on several variables. These variables can be broadly divided into patient factors, fracture displacement, fracture stability, and associated injuries.

Classification

Any evaluation of fractures invokes the discussion of classifications. Traditionally, classification systems are used to categorize injuries and direct treatment based on expected outcome. Classifications are inherently meant to encompass the issue of fracture displacement and stability. In addition, they should provide a reproducible diagnosis with a high degree of intra- and interobserver reliability, take into account soft-tissue injuries, and offer prognostic considerations. Distal radius fractures more than any other fracture are wrought with various classifications. However, because of the large number of variables to consider and the spectrum of fracture characteristics of the distal radius, no one classification is adequate. Instead, different classifications have historically revealed certain important characteristics of distal radius fractures.

To be effective, a classification system must accurately categorize the fracture type and injury severity to serve as a guideline for treatment and prognosis [2]. Although the many classification systems have attempted to provide a more accurate representation of various distal radius fracture patterns, some have proven more useful than others in guiding treatment and predicting outcome.

Today, although many classification systems are of only historical interest, their review is relevant to the understanding and evolution of those more commonly used and their contributions to modern treatment.

* Corresponding author.
  E-mail address: jjupiter1@partners.org (J.B. Jupiter).

Gartland and Werley

In their sentinel article in 1951, Gartland and Werley [3] brought attention to the fact that many distal radius fractures were being ineffectively treated, leading to a high percentage of poor results. They created a detailed evaluation system and classification system that included consideration of intra-articular fractures and their implications. They showed that a large percentage of distal radius fractures are intra-articular, 88% in their population, with approximately one third yielding unsatisfactory results and one fifth showing evidence of posttraumatic arthrosis through radiograph, also in their series.

Lidstrom

In his detailed study on distal radius fractures published in 1959, Lidstrom [4] outlined that early classifications were based on:

1. The fracture line
2. The direction of displacement of the distal fragment
3. The degree of displacement of the fracture
4. The extent of articular involvement
5. Any involvement of the distal radioulnar joint

Lidstrom added a sixth criteria, the direction of displacement. He also expanded on the nature and extent of articular involvement.

Older and colleagues

In 1965 Older and colleagues [5] published a classification system that incorporated radial shortening of the distal fragment. This feature was later shown to be central to assessing fracture stability and providing prognostic information. In addition, the classification expanded on dorsal angulation, comminution, and the direction of displacement in a graded manner.

Frykman

In 1967, Frykman [6] introduced the involvement of the ulna in distal radius fractures. The classification system identified the individual involvement of the radioulnar joints and the presence or absence of a fracture of the ulna or ulnar styloid process. Aside from its significance in bringing the ulna into the discussion of distal radius fractures, the classification otherwise does not allow for quantification of the extent or direction of the initial fracture displacement, extent of comminution, or shortening, thereby limiting its ability to direct treatment and predict prognosis.

Thomas

After Barton's [7] description of dorsal fracture–dislocations, most classification systems focused instead on Colles' type distal radius fractures. In 1957, Thomas [8] included the volar fracture dislocation in his classification system of volarly displaced distal radius Smith fractures.

Melone

Recent classification systems have focused on developing accurate identification of intra-articular fragments. In 1984, Melone [9] heralded the contemporary classifications by observing that there were four components of the radiocarpal joint and that intra-articular fractures appeared to fall into five basic patterns. The four components included the radial shaft, radial styloid, dorsal medial fragment, and the palmar medial fragment. In addition, he termed the medial two components that attach to both the carpal bones distally and the ulna medially the *medial complex*. The extent and direction of these fragments form the basis of the classification and are a prognostic indicator of the fracture's stability.

Jenkins

In 1989, Jenkins [10] added to Melone's classification by adding the direction and distribution of comminution.

McMurtry and Jupiter

In 1990, McMurtry and Jupiter [11] defined an intra-articular fracture as including any fracture that extends into the radiocarpal or radioulnar joint and is displaced more than 1 mm, building on the findings of Knirk and Jupiter [12] that intra-articular step-off of greater than 1 mm can lead to radiocarpal arthrosis. These fractures were further divided into two-part, three-part, four-part, and five-part fractures if the part or fragment was large enough to be manipulated and internally fixed.

Universal classification

In 1990, a universal classification was proposed by Cooney [13] in a symposium on distal radius fractures. The classification was modeled after the Grartland and Werley system and divided groups into extra- versus intra-articular fractures and stable versus unstable fractures.

Mayo Clinic

An additional classification focusing on intra-articular fractures was developed by the Mayo Clinic in 1992. The Mayo classification focused on the role of specific articular contact areas. The classification was formulated to include the specific articular surfaces of the distal radius and highlight fracture components involving these articulations [14].

Association for the Study of Internal Fixation

The Swiss Association for the Study of Internal Fixation (AO/ASIF) group developed the "Comprehensive Classification of Fractures of Long Bones" to serve as a basis for treatment and evaluating results. It is organized in order of increasing severity of the bone and articular lesions. Each bone and segment of bone is given a designation. The three basic types include extra-articular fractures (type A), simple intra-articular fractures (type B), and complex intra-articular fractures (type C) [2]. Despite the exhaustive nature and extensive capabilities offered by the AO/ASIF classification, it is cumbersome, especially when treatment options are considered. However, its value in research and documentation cannot be overstated.

Fernandez

In 1993, Fernandez [15] developed a more simplified approach for classification that moved away from focusing on the fracture fragments and instead recognized that fracture patterns reflect specific mechanisms of injury. This system is designed to be practical, determine stability, include associated injuries, and provide general treatment recommendations (Fig. 1). The major groups include:

- Type 1 = Bending: the metaphyseal cortex fails because of tensile stresses with the opposite cortex undergoing a certain degree of comminution.
- Type 2 = Shearing: resulting in volar or dorsal fracture dislocation.
- Type 3 = Compression: leading to subchondral bone collapse with intra-articular extension.
- Type 4 = Avulsion: involving fractures of the radial or ulnar styloids.
- Type 5 = Combined: in high-energy injuries, combinations of bending, compression, shearing, or avulsion are encompassed.

Indications for surgery

The treatment plan for patients with distal radius fractures can be broken down broadly into the following criteria:

1. Patient factors
2. Fracture pattern
3. Fracture stability
4. Associated injuries

Patient factors

Patient factors must be taken into account when considering treatment options. Variables include lifestyle, mental attitude, associated medical conditions, and compliance with treatment. In addition, chronologic age should be considered but in the perspective of expected loading. Anticipated functional loading of the distal radius after recovery should influence the choice of method of stabilization far more than the absolute chronologic age of the patient alone.

Fracture pattern

For extra-articular distal radius fractures, adequacy of closed reduction is assessed by reducing the fracture to the normal radiographic parameters and maintaining them until the fracture heals [16]. Biomechanical studies have helped define the acceptable radiologic parameters of reduction relative to their association to function. Loss of radial inclination or radial shortening causes significant increase in stress across the lunate facet and disruption of distal radioulnar mechanics and distortion of the triangular fibrocartilage complex [17–19]. Malunions with angulations greater than 20° dorsally or volarly cause changes in the position of the carpus and higher load concentrations. A compensatory dorsal intercalary segmental instability forms with dorsal angulation and can result in marked alterations in carpal mechanics [20]. In addition, dorsal malunions often result in rotational deformities that can result in pronation and supination deficits [21]. Finally, malposition of a fracture has been shown to accelerate degenerative changes over the long-term [18,19,22].

For intra-articular distal radius fractures, articular congruity must be assessed in addition to the normal radiographic parameters of the distal radius. Several studies have shown that articular step-off of even 1 mm or more can result in late radiocarpal arthrosis [12,15,23,24]. The significance of this finding is relative because the presence of posttraumatic radiocarpal arthrosis alone does

Fracture type (adults) based on the mechanism of injury	Children fracture equivalent	Stability/ instability: high risk of secondary displacement after initial adequate reduction	Displacement pattern	No. of fragments	Associated lesions: carpal ligament, fractures, median, ulnar nerve, tendons, ipsilateral upper extremity, compartment syndrome	Recommended treatment
Type I: bending fracture of the metaphysis	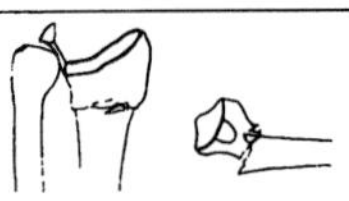 Distal forearm fracture: Salter II	Stable, unstable	Nondisplaced Dorsal (Colles-Pouteau) Volar (Smith) Proximal Combined	Always two main fragments + varying degree of metaphyseal comminution (instability)	Uncommon	Conservative (stable fractures) Percutaneous pinning (extra- or intrafocal) External fixation Exceptionally: bone graft
Type II: shearing fracture of the joint surface	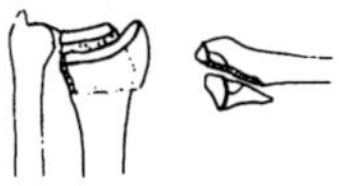 Salter IV	Unstable	Dorsal Radial Volar Proximal Combined	Two-part Three-part Comminuted	Less uncommon	Open reduction Screwplate fixation
Type III: compression fracture of the joint surface	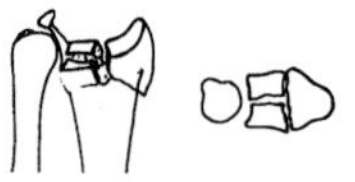 Salter III, IV, V	Stable, unstable	Nondisplaced Dorsal Radial Volar Proximal Combined	Two-part Three-part Four-part Comminuted	Common	Conservative closed, limited, arthroscopic assisted, or extensile open reduction Percutaneous pins combined external and internal fixation Bone Graft
Type IV: avulsion fractures, radiocarpal fracture, dislocation	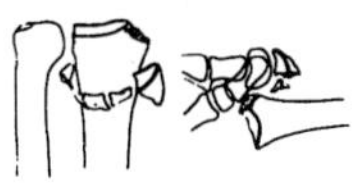 Rare	Unstable	Dorsal Radial Volar Proximal Combined	Two-part (radial styloid ulnar styloid) Three-part (volar, dorsal margin) Comminuted	Frequent	Closed or open reduction Pin or screw fixation Tension wiring
Type V: combined fractures (I, II, III, IV); high-velocity injury	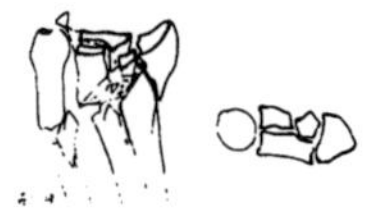 Rare	Unstable	Dorsal Radial Volar Proximal Combined	Comminuted and/or bone loss (frequently intraarticular, open, seldom extraarticular)	Always present	Combined method

Fig. 1. Practical, treatment-oriented classification of fractures of the distal radius and associated distal radioulnar joint lesions. (*From* Fernandez D, Jupiter J. Fractures of the distal radius, 2nd edition. New York: Springer; 2002. p. 48; with permission.)

not necessarily correlate with poor functional outcome [25]. In addition, discernment of 1 to 3 mm of step-off is has low interobserver reliability [26]. To assess articular step-off, reliable parameters must be developed and used to optimize identification.

Fracture displacement directs initial management of a distal radius fracture and requires accurate assessment of the position of the fracture after closed reduction and consideration of the biomechanical implications. With these variables in mind, guidelines for acceptable closed reduction have been formulated [27,28].

   Radial inclination: greater than or equal to 15° on posteroanterior view
   Radial length: less than or equal to 5 mm shortening on posteroanterior view
   Radial tilt: less than 15° dorsal or 20° volar tilt on lateral view
   Articular incongruity: less than to 2 mm of step-off

Fracture stability

If a fracture is reduced and the position is within the acceptable parameters of reduction as outlined, the next question is whether the fracture is stable. In other words, will the fracture pattern and soft tissue injuries allow the distal radius to maintain a reduced position in the acceptable alignment until union. Reliably determining factors that may lead to fracture instability at presentation would enable more timely surgical intervention and avoid unnecessary closed management and observation.

Radiographic signs that should alert the surgeon that the fracture is probably unstable and closed reduction will be insufficient include [15,29]:

   Dorsal comminution greater than 50% of the width laterally
   Palmar metaphyseal comminution
   Initial dorsal tilt greater than 20°
   Initial displacement (fragment translation) greater than 1 cm
   Initial radial shortening more than 5 mm
   Intra-articular disruption
   Associated ulna fracture
   Severe osteoporosis

Multiple studies examining distal radius fracture stability have validated these factors of instability. The definition of absolute instability has varied, with little consensus on specific criteria.

Cooney and colleagues [30] considered fractures that were widely displaced with extensive dorsal comminution, dorsal angulation greater than 20°, or extensive intra-articular involvement to have a significant chance of redisplacement after reduction. Weber [31] expanded this concept to include fractures with dorsal comminution that extended volar to the midaxial plane of the radius on the lateral radiograph. Jenkins [10] examined 121 distal radius fractures and found that the position of the fracture at presentation was the best predictor of position at union and that the lack of dorsal comminution was protective against dorsally angulated malunions. Abbaszadegan and colleagues [32] examined 267 fractures initially treated nonoperatively using stepwise regression analysis and found that initial radial shortening (greater than 4 mm) was the greatest prognostic indicator of instability. Lafontaine and colleagues [33] suggested five factors that indicated instability: (1) initial dorsal angulation greater than 20°, (2) dorsal comminution, (3) radiocarpal intra-articular involvement, (4) associated ulna fractures, and (5) age greater than 60 years. The study concluded that fractures presenting with three or more of these gravity factors correlated with loss of position despite cast immobilization.

Several subsequent studies have attempted to validate Lafontaine's criteria for instability. Hove and colleagues [34] analyzed 645 nonoperatively treated distal radius fractures, and using multiple regression analysis determined that the initial dorsal angulation, radial length, and patient age were all predictors of malunion. Leone and colleagues [35] also found that the degree of radial shortening and volar tilt were predictive of early instability, with dorsal comminution also approaching statistical significance. An interesting result showed that one-third of undisplaced fractures went on to fail, most of which occurred in those patients over the age of 65. Nesbitt et al. [36] also examined criteria of instability and found age (greater than 58 years old) to be the only statistically significant factor for instability.

More recently, examination of approximately 4000 distal radius fractures attempted to validate the known predictive factors and make a distinction between early and late fracture collapse. Mackenney and colleagues [37] found that the most important predictive factors were the age of the patient, dorsal comminution, and the position of the fracture at presentation. With increasing age, early and late instability increased proportionately.

Associated injuries

Several associated or secondary injuries may indicate operative intervention for distal radius fractures. Open fractures warrant operative management following well-established protocols of early irrigation and debridement followed by fixation of the fracture.

Various multi-injury patterns also warrant operative intervention, including bilateral distal radius fractures and ipsilateral concomitant fractures of the upper extremity. Examination of the ipsilateral elbow and shoulder should always be performed. Proximal fractures can have significant implications for rehabilitation considerations. In addition, distally, carpal fractures or dislocations should be sought and surgically treated, including scaphoid fractures [38,39].

Acute median nerve dysfunction is a common neurologic complication of distal radius fractures. Median nerve symptoms after distal radius fractures typically include pain and burning in the median distribution of the hand, often out of proportion and not responsive to elevation and narcotic analgesia. Compartment pressures have been measured acutely after distal radius fractures and found to be highest at approximately 2 to 4 hours after injury or immediately after reduction [40]. However, acute carpal tunnel syndrome is not associated with specific fracture patterns of the distal radius [41]. These symptoms may represent an acute or an acute on chronic carpal tunnel syndrome. Initial intervention should include reduction and splinting of the fracture. Symptoms that do not improve with reduction may represent direct injury or contusion to the nerve. Persistent or worsening symptoms warrant surgical fixation of the fracture and open carpal tunnel release.

Summary

Distal radius fractures are common injuries. Multiple classification systems exist that have helped identify different aspects of distal radius fracture that can affect its outcome. Identification of surgical indications includes consideration of patient factors, fracture reduction, fracture stability, and the presence of any associated injuries.

References

[1] Colles A. On the fracture of the carpal extremity of the radius. Edinburgh Med Surg 1814;10:182–6.
[2] Muller ME, Nazarian S, Koch P. AO classification of fractures. Berlin: Springer; 1987.
[3] Gartland JJ, Werley CW. Evaluation of healed Colles' fractures. J Bone Joint Surg Am 1951;33(4): 895–907.
[4] Lidstrom A. Fractures of the distal end of the radius. A clinical and statistical study of end results. Acta Orthop Scand Suppl 1959;41:1–118.
[5] Older TM, Stabler EU, Cassebaum WH. Colles' fracture: evaluation of selectin of therapy. J Trauma 1965;5:469–76.
[6] Frykman GK. Fracture of the distal radius including sequelae—shoulder hand finger syndrome. Disturbance in the distal radioulnar joint and impairment of nerve function. A clinical and experimental study. Acta Orthop Scand Suppl 1967;108:1–155.
[7] Barton JR. Views and treatment of an important injury of the wrist. Medical Examiner 1838;1:365–8.
[8] Thomas FB. Reduction of Smith's fracture. J Bone Joint Surg Br 1957;39:463–70.
[9] Melone CP. Articular fractures of the distal radius. Orthop Clin North Am 1984;15:217–36.
[10] Jenkins NH. The unstable Colles' fracture. J Hand Surg [Br] 1989;14:149–54.
[11] McMurtry RY, Jupiter JB. Fractures of the distal radius. In: Browner BD, Jupiter JB, Levine AM, et al, editors. Skeletal trauma. Philadelphia: Saunders; 1991. p. 1063–94.
[12] Knirk J, Jupiter J. Intraarticular fractures of the distal end of the radius in young adults. J Bone Joint Surg Am 1986;68(5):647–59.
[13] Cooney WP. Fracture of the distal radius: a modern treatment-based classification. Orthop Clin North Am 1993;24:211–6.
[14] Missakian ML, Cooney WP, Amadio PC, et al. Open reduction and internal fixation for distal radius fractures. J Hand Surg [Am] 1992;17:745–55.
[15] Fernandez DL. Fractures of the distal radius. Operative treatment. Instr Course Lect 1993;42:73–88.
[16] Friberg S, Lundstrom B. Radiographic measurements of the radio-carpal joint in normal adults. Acta Radiol Diagn (Stockh) 1976;2:249–56.
[17] Fourrier P, Bardy A, Roche G, et al. [Approach to a definition of malunion callus after Pouteau-Colles fractures]. Int Orthop 1981;4:299–305.
[18] Pogue DJ, Viegas SF, Patterson RM, et al. Effects of distal radius fracture malunion on wrist joint mechanics. J Hand Sur [Am] 1990;15:721–7.
[19] Adams BD. Effects of radial deformity on distal radioulnar joint mechanics. J Hand Surg [Am] 1993;18:492–8.
[20] Park MJ, Cooney WP, Hahn ME, et al. The effects of dorsally angulated distal radius fractures on carpal kinematics. J Hand Surg [Am] 2002;12(2): 223–32.
[21] Prommersberger KJ, Froehner SC, Schmitt RR, et al. Rotational deformity in malunited fractures of the distal radius. J Hand Surg [Am] 2004;29(1): 110–5.
[22] Short WH, Palmer AK, Werner FW, et al. A biomechanical study of distal radius fractures. J Hand Surg [Am] 1987;12:529–34.
[23] Geissler WB, Fernandez DL. Percutaneous and limited open reduction of the articular surface of the distal radius. J Orthop Trauma 1991;5(3): 255–64.
[24] Kopylov P, Johnell O, Redlund-Johnell I, et al. Fractures of the distal end of the radius in young adults: a 30-year follow-up. J Hand Surg [Br] 1993; 18(1):45–9.
[25] Catalano LW, Cole RJ, Gelberman RH, et al. Displaced intra-articular fractures of the distal aspect of the radius. Long-term results in young adults after open reduction and internal fixation. J Bone Joint Surg Am 1997;79(9):1290–302.
[26] Kreder HJ, Hanel DP, McKee M, et al. X-ray film measurements for healed distal radius fractures. J Hand Surg [Am] 1996;21:31–9.
[27] Graham TJ. Surgical correction of malunited fractures of the distal radius. J Am Acad Orthop Surg 1997;5:270–81.
[28] Nana AD, Joshi A, Lichtman DM. Plating of the distal radius. J Am Acad Orthop Surg 2005;13:159–71.
[29] Ruedi TP, Murphy WM, editors. AO principles of fracture management. New York: Thieme; 2000. p. 362.
[30] Cooney WP, Linscheid RL, Dobyns JH. External pin fixation for unstable Colles' fractures. J Bone Joint Surg Am 1979;61:840–5.
[31] Weber ER. A rational approach for the recognition and treatment of Colles' fracture. Hand Clin 1987;3: 13–21.
[32] Abbaszadegan H, Jonsson U, von Sivers K. Prediction of instability of Colles' fractures. Acta Orthop Scand 1989;60:646–50.
[33] Lafontaine M, Hardy D, Delince P. Stability assessment of distal radial fractures. Injury 1989;20: 208–10.
[34] Hove LM, Solheim E, Skjeie R, et al. Simultaneous scaphoid and distal radial fractures. J Hand Surg [Br] 1994;19(3):384–8.
[35] Leone J, Bhandari M, Adili A, et al. Predictors of early and late instability following conservative treatment of extra-articular distal radius fractures. Arch Orthop Trauma Surg 2004;124(1):38–41.
[36] Nesbitt KS, Failla JM, Les C. Assessment of instability factors in adult distal radius fractures. J Hand Surg [Am] 2004;29(6):1128–38.
[37] Mackenney PJ, McQueen MM, Elton R. Prediction of instability in distal radial fractures. J Bone Joint Surg Am 2006;88:1944–51.
[38] Trumble TE, Benirschke SK, Vedder NB. Ipsilateral fractures of the scaphoid and radius. J Hand Surg [Am] 1993;18(1):8–14.

[39] Hove LM, Solheim E, Skjeie R, et al. Prediction of secondary displacement in Colles' fracture. J Hand Surg [Br] 1994;19:731–6.

[40] Dresing K, Peterson T, Schmit-Neuerburg KP. Compartment pressure in the carpal tunnel in distal fractures of the radius. A prospective study. Arch Orthop Trauma Surg 1994;113(5):285–9.

[41] Bienek T, Kusz D, Cielinski L. Peripheral nerve compression neuropathy after fractures of the distal radius. J Hand Surg [Br] 2006;31(3):256–60.

Distal Radius Fractures: Nonoperative and Percutaneous Pinning Treatment Options

Wade Gofton, MD, MEd, FRCSC, Allan Liew, MD, FRCSC*

Department of Orthopaedic Surgery, University of Ottawa, The Ottawa Hospital—Civic Campus, 1053 Carling Avenue, Ottawa, Ontario K1Y 4E9, Canada

Nonoperative treatment of distal radial fractures by reduction and immobilization remains the most common form of treatment, as seen in many epidemiological studies in the literature. In this article, the indications, technique, predictors of failure, outcomes, and complications are reviewed. A variety of treatment options have been proposed for distal radial fractures that are predicted, or subsequently identified, to be too unstable for nonoperative management. Percutaneous pinning is an effective option for select fractures. The authors also review the indications, described techniques, complications and outcomes associated with this treatment option.

Nonoperative management

Historically, many authors have described a high rate of satisfaction and good results based on subjective outcomes, regardless of radiographic appearance, after nonoperative management of distal radius fractures [1,2]. When validated objective and subjective outcomes scores are used, it becomes clear that significant functional deficiencies are correlated with poor reductions at intermediate and long-term follow-up [3–7]. There are significant changes in radiocarpal stress concentration and distribution with malalignment of the distal radius [8,9]. Malalignment of the distal radius can also lead to distal radio-ulnar joint incongruity, limiting forearm rotation [8–13]. In an early retrospective review of 565 distal radius fractures, Cooney and colleagues [4] found that malunion was frequently associated with pain, limited range of motion, and decreased strength. The basic science data, in conjunction with longer-term radiographic and functional outcomes measures, clearly support the treatment of distal radius fractures with more than just benign neglect in most patients.

Nonoperative treatment by reduction and immobilization remains the most common treatment, based on the incidence of appropriate fracture types, as seen in many epidemiological studies in the literature. The indications, technique, predictors of failure, outcomes, and complications are reviewed below.

Indications for nonoperative treatment

Successful nonoperative management of distal radius fractures is dependent on appropriate injury pattern and patient selection. Most distal radial fracture classification schemes are based on the location of the fracture, number of articular fragments, involvement of the distal ulna, and direction of angulation. Analysis of the biomechanical and functional outcome literature suggests that predicting the success of nonoperative treatment may be better determined by a different set of radiographic parameters and patient factors.

Clinical outcome studies and the biomechanic literature [8,9] demonstrate that maintenance of palmar tilt [14–16] (normally 11°), ulnar variance (normally −2 mm) and radial height [15,17,18] (normally 12 mm) are probably the most important factors in attaining acceptable patient outcomes. An articular gap of less than 2 mm [19],

* Corresponding author.

E-mail address: aliew@ottawahospital.on.ca (A. Liew).

and a step of 1 mm or less is required to reduce the risk of residual pain and wrist dysfunction [20]. Failure to achieve these goals in a cogent, functional patient, following a reduction if required, suggests that nonoperative management may not be able to achieve the desired outcomes. The authors' suggested minimal requirements for an acceptable reduction are ulnar variance negative or neutral (or within 2 mm of the unaffected contralateral wrist), less than 10° of angulation from the normal volar tilt in either the volar or dorsal direction, radial inclination greater than 15°, and a congruent articular surface (Fig. 1A, B).

Accurately evaluating these radiographic parameters requires standardized postero-anterior and lateral views in the neutral position, and may include comparative views of the unaffected wrist. Computed tomography improves the reliability of injury characterization for intra-articular fractures, frequently altering the treatment plan [21,22]. The addition of three-dimensional CT reconstructions is of value in the assessment of complex intra-articular injuries, particularly for coronal plane fractures and central die punch fractures [23].

If the fracture is minimally displaced, reduction and immobilization may not be necessary [24,25]; however, some authors have demonstrated displacement in initially undisplaced fractures, suggesting that treatment without immobilization requires careful patient selection and monitoring [26]. The indications for nonoperative management advocated by the authors of this article include patients presenting with a fracture in acceptable position, or patients in whom the fracture can be maintained in an acceptable position following reduction.

The indications for nonoperative management may be broader in the elderly, low-demand patient for several reasons. The fracture often represents a low-energy fragility fracture with less articular involvement. Frequently, there are associated comorbid factors that increase the risks associated with operative management. In this population, there appears to be less correlation between radiographic and functional outcomes, with the evidence suggesting that most distal radius fractures in older patients may be treated conservatively with satisfactory functional outcomes likely [1,2,6].

Reduction techniques

Adequate pain control is necessary when a closed reduction is required. This can be accomplished with a hematoma block, intravenous regional anesthetic (Bier block), or interscalene block. Occasionally, neuroleptic or general anesthesia is required; however, regional techniques are preferred where possible. Although no one particular regional technique has been demonstrated to be clearly superior or clinically safer, there is evidence to suggest that hematoma blocks provide inferior pain control and may compromise reduction [27].

After achieving adequate analgesia, in-line traction facilitates relaxation of the forearm musculature. The use of finger-traps and the gentle application of weights may assist in achieving this with relative pain control, but has not been

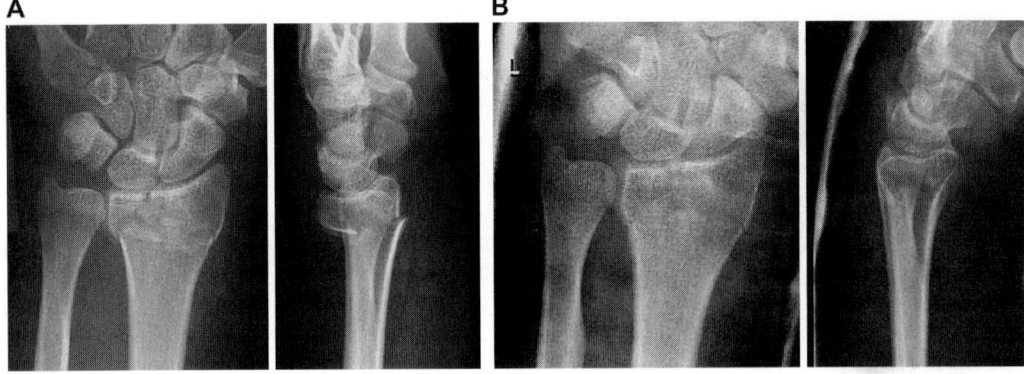

Fig. 1. (*A*) Intra-articular distal radius fracture in a 36-year-old female. Closed reduction is indicated based on patient function and radiographic measurements. (*B*) Postreduction radiographs demonstrate acceptable reduction based on radiographic criteria.

demonstrated to improve reduction rates or long-term outcomes [28]. Required manipulation will depend on the presenting fracture, but for the typical dorsally angulated fracture with minimal displacement of the volar cortex, the reduction can be obtained by direct pressure on the distal fragment from the dorsal surface to correct the angulation. When there is significant dorsal translation associated with the angulation, the technique starts with increasing the dorsal angulation to ease the volar translation or "unlocking" of the volar cortex if overlapped. This is followed by direct pressure on the distal fragment to correct the angulation. Longitudinal traction with palmar flexion of the wrist effects a reduction of the fracture [29]. The volar and dorsal rim of the radius can be palpated to give an estimate of the correction of volar tilt before cast application.

The ideal position of immobilization has been debated. The traditional Cotton-Loder position, with extreme flexion and ulnar deviation, has been associated with an increased incidence of reflex sympathetic dystrophy, and is therefore not recommended. Gupta [30] reported that in a prospective randomized trial of 204 patients who had acceptable initial reduction, casting with the wrist in dorsiflexion had the least subsequent loss of reduction, especially for dorsal angulation, and the best early functional outcome. Although the position of forearm rotation may play a role [31,32], van der Linden and Ericson [33] suggest that the position of immobilization is likely not as important as the initial displacement and reduction in determining outcome.

A short-arm cast or splint is sufficient for immobilization, demonstrating equivalent radiographic and functional outcomes in both the pediatric and adult populations when compared with above-elbow immobilization [34–36]. Non-circumferential immobilization is appropriate when swelling, potential compartment syndrome, or patient reliability is a concern. Functional bracing is more expensive, and for most fracture patterns has failed to demonstrate a significant difference in reduction or functional outcome [37,38]; however, with a minimally displaced fracture in a young patient, it may provide greater satisfaction with improved functional outcomes [39].

Follow-up and aftercare

Despite an adequate initial reduction and immobilization, redisplacement is common, caused by deforming forces across the wrist as well as individual patient factors. Significant indirect deforming forces across the fracture include the long flexor and extensor tendons. Deforming forces directly influencing fracture fragments include the brachioradialis, which has a consistent pattern of insertion on the radial side of the styloid and may contribute to the secondary displacement of this fragment [11].

Adequately reduced distal radius fractures require follow-up radiographs to assess for redisplacement and healing. Although fractures requiring reduction are at greatest risk of redisplacement, even undisplaced fractures, particularly in the elderly osteopaenic patient, are at risk for displacement [26]. Loss of reduction most commonly occurs during the second week of cast treatment [6,40,41] or later [25], especially in the elderly [25]. This suggests that the timing and number of follow-up visits needs to be individualized to both the patient and fracture.

For minimally displaced and stable fractures, the period of immobilization may be shortened, provided that radiographs show satisfactory healing. Vang and colleagues [42] observed no difference in dorsal angulation, radial length, range of motion, grip strength, or pain between 3 or 5 weeks of immobilization at 1-year follow-up. For those fractures that are less stable, immobilization to at least 6 weeks is indicated [6,25,40].

When a loss of reduction is observed, a repeat reduction may be attempted; however, Schmalholz [43] demonstrated that a recurrence of deformity is common. He observed that dorsal angulation could be corrected in only 41% of patients, and that radial length could only be corrected in 11% of patients, and he concluded that in patients requiring a repeat reduction, cast immobilization may be insufficient definitive treatment [43].

Another important aspect of aftercare is the recognition that this fracture pattern often represents a pathologic injury. Low-energy distal radius fractures have been strongly associated with osteoporosis; thus patients presenting with this injury should be appropriately investigated and treated if required [44,45].

Predicting successful nonoperative treatment

Difficulty obtaining adequate correction of intra-articular displacement and maintaining axial stability throughout the course of treatment are the two major limitations of nonoperative management. Successful nonoperative treatment requires careful patient selection, an initial satisfactory reduction, and maintenance of reduction throughout the follow-up period to final fracture healing. It is evident that certain fractures lack the inherent stability for this to occur.

It was initially felt that the ability to achieve an acceptable reduction was important in predicting functional outcome [16]; however, in many instances the fracture settles back toward the original injury film alignment, despite an adequate initial radiographic reduction [25]. Leung and colleagues [15] demonstrated that the functional outcome in redisplaced fractures was worse than those without redisplacement, suggesting that being able to determine the factors of fracture stability may be important in determining those patients who may be successfully managed nonoperatively.

Cooney and colleagues considered displaced fractures with dorsal comminution (especially if beyond the mid-axial plane [46]), dorsal angulation greater than 20°, or extensive intra-articular involvement, to have a significant risk of redisplacement following reduction [47]. Abbaszadegan and colleagues [48] considered radial shortening greater than 4 mm a hallmark of potential instability. Lafontaine has suggested five factors that contribute to instability: (1) initial dorsal angulation greater than 20°, (2) dorsal comminution, (3) radiocarpal intra-articular involvement, (4) associated ulnar fractures, and (5) age greater than 60 years (Fig. 2A, B). He concluded that patients who had three or more factors correlated with loss of position despite cast immobilization [49], suggesting that these patients either need to be monitored closely, or considered for another form of fracture stabilization.

Several authors have suggested that the severity of initial radial shortening may be the most reliable indicator of instability [40,41,43,48]. Mackenny and colleagues [50] observed that patient age, comminution, and the ulnar variance at presentation to be important predictive factors. Their findings suggest that dorsal angulation is only a predictor of instability with minimally displaced fractures, as it is superseded by radial shortening in displaced fractures. Nesbitt and colleagues [51] found that only patient age was a statistically significant factor in predicting secondary displacement, with patients older than 58 found to be at a 50% risk of secondary displacement. Leone and colleagues [26] have suggested that early and late instability may be predicted by different factors, with risk of early displacement predicted by radial shortening and dorsal tilt, and risk of late displacement also including patient age. Researchers continue to work toward the development of a validated method of prospectively quantifying the risk of displacement and failure of conservative management [50].

At present, we can conclude that radial shortening, followed by dorsal comminution, is most predictive of instability. Increasing age significantly increases the risk of both early and late loss of reduction, even with minimal initial displacement. In situations where the prereduction radiographs predict for a low probability of successful nonoperative treatment, the patient should be counseled as such;, however, this still

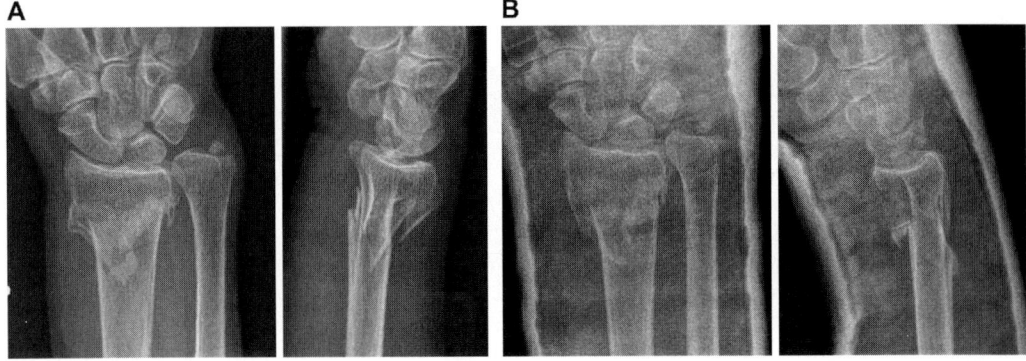

Fig. 2. (*A*) Isolated distal radius fracture in an 82-year-old independently functioning woman. Radiographic measurements predict low probability of successful closed reduction as definitive treatment. (*B*) Radiographs after attempted closed reduction. Although volar tilt is restored, axial stability cannot be maintained as predicted on prereduction films with resultant unacceptable reduction.

does not preclude an attempt at closed reduction and close follow-up.

Adjunctive modalities such as ultrasound and electrical stimulation have been postulated to quicken healing and subsequently prevent redisplacement. Kristiansen and colleagues [52] reported a randomized controlled trial on the use of low-intensity ultrasound for distal radius fractures treated with a cast. There was less loss of reduction in the test group, and earlier fracture stability achieved, with no loss of reduction after 12 versus 25 days in the controls. Total time to union was also shorter, at 9 versus 14 weeks [52].

Complications

Complications associated with this injury may be diverse and unexpectedly frequent [4,41,53]. The complications may be associated with the injury itself [54], its management, or failure to restore the anatomy, which may lead to midcarpal instability or post-traumatic arthritis [19,55]. Cooney and colleagues [4] presented one of the most complete reviews of complications associated with distal radius fractures. They attributed the majority of complications to inadequate restoration of radial length or a secondary loss of reduction.

The most common complication was compression neuropathies, which may present on an acute or delayed basis and may be severe enough to warrant operative release. Bienek and colleagues [56] reported a 20% incidence of delayed carpal tunnel symptoms in 60 patients treated with closed reduction and casting, but did not find a correlation between symptoms and fracture type or final radiographic findings.

The next most commonly observed complication was malunion, for which we have previously discussed the potential risk factors. Other complications include residual wrist and hand stiffness, which demands early interventions to preserve hand function and restore wrist function as soon as possible after the immobilization period. Attrition ruptures of the extensor pollicis longus (EPL) tendon have been observed, and Helal and colleagues [57] reported a higher risk of rupture in undisplaced versus displaced fractures, and postulated that an intact extensor retinaculum may be a contributing cause.

Complex regional pain syndrome (CRPS) of both Types I and II have also been observed. Fortunately relatively infrequent, it remains a significant clinical concern and an important contributor to long-term unsatisfactory results in distal radial fractures [7]. Although there is some evidence to suggest that treatment with vitamin C during the course of immobilization may reduce the risk of CRPS [58], the evidence is weak at best [59]. At present, prevention may be best achieved by early range of motion of the affected and adjacent joints where possible.

Outcomes

Despite the large body of literature on the subject, results of the nonoperative management of distal radius fractures remain conflicted. A recent Cochrane review has found insufficient evidence to recommend any particular method of reduction, or duration and type of immobilization for distal radial fractures [60,61]. As our appreciation for the importance of functional outcomes improves, studies are increasingly demonstrating that our outcomes are not completely satisfactory [4,16,31,62]. What is clear is that in most instances, restoration of the normal anatomy is important for the restoration of function, and thus patient satisfaction [5,6].

Radiographic factors predictive of instability may also be linked to function, with several studies reporting that the preservation of radial length was most important for the preservation of function [3,7,63], followed by palmar angulation [3,64]. Loss of radial length can lead to ulnar impaction or dysfunction of the distal radial ulnar joint, with limited range of motion in pronation and supination, depending on the volar or dorsal subluxation of the ulnar head within the sigmoid notch [12]. Warwick and colleagues [7] demonstrated that the functional limitations of lost radial length persisted even after 10 years. Residual dorsal angulation can precipitate ulnar impaction [9,65], midcarpal instability [55], and altered stress concentrations, which may lead to early arthritis [8,9].

Good radiographic parameters do not always result in good functional results. In a large retrospective review, Altissimi and colleagues [62] demonstrated that whereas 87% of fractures had good-to-excellent radiographic outcomes, subjective results demonstrated that those that had poor radiographic outcomes still reported 80% good and excellent subjective outcomes. Poor outcomes were more common in malunions (14.5% versus 6%), and included at least one of the following: (1) distal radio-ulnar joint pain, (2) radial deviation of the wrist, (3) dorsal angulation, (4) prominent ulnar styloid, (5) nerve compression, (6) osteoarthritis, or (7) reduced grip strength [62]. More recent work has suggested that outcomes may be more dependant on patient factors, with elderly patients of lower functional demand more tolerant of persistent radiographic abnormalities [1].

Summary

The literature continues to support nonoperative management of many distal radial fractures. The goals of a return to normal function and patient satisfaction are most likely to be achieved through the restoration of anatomy facilitating normal radiocarpal and distal radio-ulnar joint function. This is best achieved through appropriate patient selection and monitoring during the course of treatment. Patient factors (physiologically >65, osteoporosis) or initial radiographic factors predictive of instability (loss of radial length and dorsal angulation) should be considered for alternate forms of management where applicable, because residual deformity leads to reduced outcomes, particularly in the young, active patient.

Percutaneous pinning of distal radius fractures

A variety of treatment options have been proposed for distal radial fractures that are predicted, or subsequently identified, to be too unstable for nonoperative management. Percutaneous pinning is an effective option for select fractures. Below the authors review the indications, described techniques, complications, and outcomes associated with this treatment option.

Indications

Percutaneous pinning may be indicated for younger patients who have reduced or reducible fractures with predicted or proven instability. It has been demonstrated to provide good outcomes in younger patients who have reducible intra- or extra-articular fracture patterns [66–69]. In elderly osteoporotic patients [70], and in severely comminuted intra-articular fractures [67] this technique has less favorable results, and is therefore considered inappropriate. Fractures without significant shortening, comminution of the volar cortex, and that have failed closed reduction or redisplaced with regards to dorsal angulation, are ideal for percutaneous pinning techniques, which has been recommended as a simple method of improving fracture stability with minimal morbidity [71,72].

Technique

Percutaneous pinning is performed with adequate anesthesia, fluoroscopy, and a sterile operating environment. Numerous techniques have been described; these can be broadly categorized into extra-focal or intra-focal (passing through the fracture site) techniques. Irrespective of the preferred method of fixation, the selected technique should achieve fracture stability, minimize injury to nerves, vessels, and tendons, and avoid injury to the articular surface [73].

With initial percutaneous pinning techniques, an adequate reduction was achieved through closed reduction techniques followed by the insertion of Kirschner wires (K-wires) across the fracture to stabilize the distal segment [74]. Naidu [75] subsequently demonstrated that a crossed wire technique using two parallel styloid pins and a third pin from the dorsal-ulnar corner provided the greatest biomechanic stability of these extra-focal techniques.

In 1976, Kapandji [76] described a method of K-wire osteosynthesis in which two wires were inserted intrafocally from the dorsal side, levered distally to obtain an adequate reduction, then advanced through the volar cortex proximally to buttress the distal segment. Fritz and colleagues [77] subsequently modified this technique with the addition of a styloid pin. Ruschel and Albertoni's [78] modification of Kapandji's technique added a lateral intrafocal pin for restoration of radial inclination and shift. Walton and colleagues [79] describe a different modification of Kapandji's original technique using intrafocal, intramedullary K-wires.

The authors' preferred technique is similar to the modified Kapandji technique described by Ruschel and Albertoni [78]. After a closed reduction, two intrafocal dorsal K-wires are placed and manipulated to effect a reduction. An intrafocal pin is inserted from the radial side if there is significant radial shift or loss of inclination. After confirmation of satisfactory reduction by fluoroscopy, the fragments are further neutralized by a trans-radial styloid pin. A neutralization pin inserted from the dorsal-ulnar aspect across the fracture may also be used (Fig. 3A, B). All K-wires are placed through small stab incisions with blunt dissection down to bone, to minimize tendon entrapment and nerve injury.

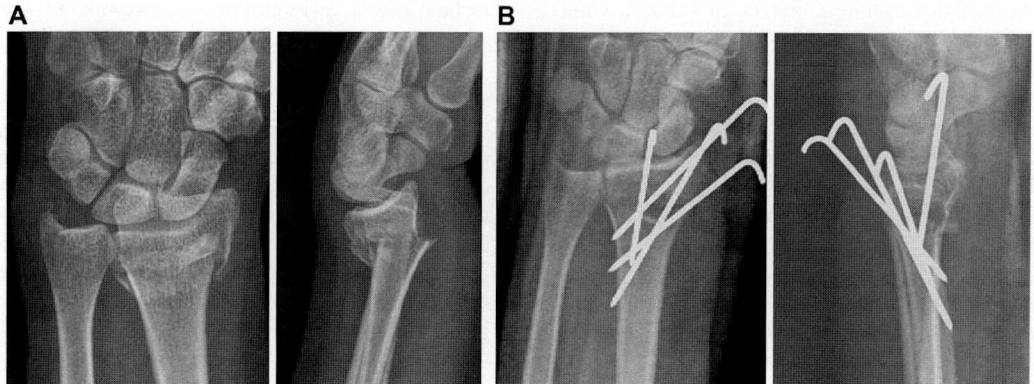

Fig. 3. (*A*) Initial radiographs of an isolated distal radius fracture in a 42-year-old female. Radiographic measurements predict for low probability of success with nonoperative management. (*B*) After an unsuccessful closed reduction and casting, patient undergoes percutaneous pinning using the modified Kapandji technique. Resultant radiographs demonstrate successful restoration of ulnar variance, radial inclination, and volar tilt.

Postoperative supplemental support with a volar slab is beneficial for patient comfort, while allowing for early functional exercises of the hand and wrist. The need for, and method of, pin site care remains controversial [80], but patients need to be monitored regularly for potential infection and to ensure maintenance of reduction. The timing of pin removal is also controversial, but the authors prefer to remove them between 4 to 6 weeks, with evidence of early radiographic union.

Complications

Complications include those previously described for nonoperative treatment, as well as those directly attributed to the use of percutaneous pins, such as tendon tethering, injury or rupture, pin migration, nerve injury, and pin-site infection.

Superficial radial nerve irritation and injury is relatively common. Singh and colleagues [81] reported a 20% rate of injury to the superficial radial nerve in a retrospective review of 40 patients treated with K-wires through the radial styloid. Hochwald and colleagues [82] demonstrated that the rate of injury could be reduced using a limited open technique to place the K-wires.

Percutaneous pin tract infections are also common, which can lead to serious sequelae if left untreated. Hargreaves and colleagues [83] reported that infection rates were lower if the ends of the K-wires were buried beneath the skin surface, compared with those protruding through the skin, especially if the pins were maintained for greater than 8 weeks.

Outcomes

Despite the large body of literature on the treatment of distal radius fractures, there are few evidence-based guidelines to direct the surgeon to choose one treatment technique over another [60]. Although many studies on the use of percutaneous K-wires for the stabilization of distal radius fractures have been published [66–68,84,85], they often include a heterogeneous group of fracture patterns and treatment regimes. Of those studies published, percutaneous fixation in appropriate fracture conditions can lead to very good outcomes.

Although some studies have demonstrated no significant difference in outcomes between percutaneous pinning and casting alone [69,84], results may be difficult to interpret because of the inclusion of an elderly population group. Clancey and colleagues [67] found better radiographic outcomes in younger patients, and recommended this technique be used for simple fracture patterns without comminution. This conclusion has been supported by recent studies, with Rodriguez-Merchan [71] demonstrating improved radiographic and functional outcomes in a group of patients between 45 and 65 years of age with a crossed-wire percutaneous technique, whereas Azzopardi and colleagues [70] did not observe a significant radiographic or functional improvement in a review of patients over the age of 60. They concluded that although this technique maybe of value in younger patients, K-wires did not gain sufficient purchase in osteopaenic bone to improve outcomes [70].

Reviewing an extra-focal K-wire technique (two parallel styloid pins), Rosati and colleagues [73] demonstrated good radiographic and functional outcomes without tendon or nerve injury. Best results were observed in younger patients and simple metaphyseal fractures; poor prognostic indicators included age over 50, a die punch fragment, associated ulnar fracture, and inability to achieve an adequate reduction [73].

Reviews of intra-focal K-wire techniques demonstrate it to be effective in maintaining reduction and function, but less effective in the elderly population. A large, heterogeneous European review [86] demonstrated good outcomes with the Kapandji technique. In a smaller review, Greatting and Bishop [72] found excellent or good results in 60% of their over-65 patients and in 79% of their under-65 patients. Ebraheim and colleagues [87] similarly demonstrated excellent or good results in 80% of their over-65 patients and 86% of their under-65 patients, using an intra-focal technique with trans-styloid pin augmentation. In a younger population, Ruschel and Albertoni [78] observed a mild loss of reduction with 95% excellent and good functional results at the 1-year mark with a modified Kapandji technique. Using intrafocal intramedullary K-wires, Walton and colleagues [79] demonstrated 95% excellent or good outcomes using radiographic and functional outcome scoring systems. With their encouraging results in a patient group with an average age of 60, they concluded that the intramedullary buttress may have reduced the reliance of K-wire purchase on osteoporotic bone for fracture stability.

A number of studies have attempted to compare extra-focal and intra-focal techniques. Lenoble and colleagues [85] demonstrated that with Kapandji pinning and early mobilization there was a better initial radiographic reduction with subsequent partial loss of reduction and radial shortening when compared with trans-styloid pins. The Kapandji group had increased pain and reflex sympathetic dystrophy rates with better early range of motion, although this became statistically insignificant after 6 weeks [85]. Strohm and colleagues [88], however, observed a small but significant radiographic and functional advantage, with fewer complications and reduced fluoroscopic time with a modified Kapandji technique and early motion when compared with a trans-styloid pinning technique.

Percutaneous pinning has also been demonstrated to be as effective as external fixation for unstable distal radius fractures. Ludvigsen and colleagues [89] prospectively compared percutaneous pinning and casting with external fixation, demonstrating no significant differences in outcomes or complications in a mixed-age population. Harley [90] subsequently performed a similar prospective comparison restricted to patients under the age of 65 who had unstable distal radial fractures (AO type C2 and C3). They observed no difference in radiographic or clinical outcomes between treatment groups, except that three patients treated with external fixation developed RSD.

Percutaneous techniques have also been compared with open techniques. In a randomized controlled trial, Kreder and colleagues [91] demonstrated that reducible intra-articular fracture patterns managed with indirection reduction and percutaneous fixation techniques resulted in a more rapid return of function and better functional outcomes than those treated with open reduction and fixation techniques. Although this study used mixed forms of percutaneous fixation, it clearly demonstrated the importance of soft-tissue preservation in optimizing outcomes for distal radial fractures, provided that intra-articular step and gap deformities were minimized.

Summary

Percutaneous pinning demonstrates good reproducible outcomes with minimal risk in appropriately selected fracture patterns. It is well-suited for younger patients who have unstable but reducible extra or intra-articular distal radial fractures. This technique can provide adequate fracture stability, and soft-tissue and vascular preservation, in addition to minimal patient morbidity, which may facilitate a more rapid return to function compared with more invasive methods of treatment.

References

[1] Anzarut A, Johnson JA, Rowe BH, et al. Radiologic and patient-reported functional outcomes in an elderly cohort with conservatively treated distal radius fractures. J Hand Surg [Am] 2004;29(6):1121–7.

[2] Young BT, Rayan GM. Outcome following nonoperative treatment of displaced distal radius fractures

in low-demand patients older than 60 years. J Hand Surg [Am] 2000;25(1):19–28.
[3] Batra S, Gupta A. The effect of fracture-related factors on the functional outcome at 1 year in distal radius fractures. Injury 2002;33(6):499–502.
[4] Cooney WP III, Dobyns JH, Linscheid RL. Complications of Colles' fractures. J Bone Joint Surg Am 1980;62(4):613–9.
[5] McQueen M, Caspers J. Colles fracture: does the anatomical result affect the final function? J Bone Joint Surg Br 1988;70(4):649–51.
[6] Chang HC, Tay SC, Chan BK, et al. Conservative treatment of redisplaced Colles' fractures in elderly patients older than 60 years old—anatomical and functional outcome. Hand Surg 2001;6(2):137–44.
[7] Warwick D, Field J, Prothero D, et al. Function ten years after Colles' fracture. Clin Orthop Relat Res 1993;295:270–4.
[8] Pogue DJ, Viegas SF, Patterson RM, et al. Effects of distal radius fracture malunion on wrist joint mechanics. J Hand Surg [Am] 1990;15(5):721–7.
[9] Short WH, Palmer AK, Werner FW, et al. A biomechanical study of distal radial fractures. J Hand Surg [Am] 1987;12(4):529–34.
[10] McCallister WV, Smith JM, Knight J, et al. A cadaver model to evaluate the accuracy and reproducibility of plain radiograph step and gap measurements for intra-articular fracture of the distal radius. J Hand Surg [Am] 2004;29(5):841–7.
[11] Koh S, Andersen CR, Buford WL Jr, et al. Anatomy of the distal brachioradialis and its potential relationship to distal radius fracture. J Hand Surg [Am] 2006;31(1):2–8.
[12] Ishikawa J, Iwasaki N, Minami A. Influence of distal radioulnar joint subluxation on restricted forearm rotation after distal radius fracture. J Hand Surg [Am] 2005;30(6):1178–84.
[13] Kihara H, Palmer AK, Werner FW, et al. The effect of dorsally angulated distal radius fractures on distal radioulnar joint congruency and forearm rotation. J Hand Surg [Am] 1996;21(1):40–7.
[14] Gliatis JD, Plessas SJ, Davis TR. Outcome of distal radial fractures in young adults. J Hand Surg [Br] 2000;25(6):535–43.
[15] Leung F, Ozkan M, Chow SP. Conservative treatment of intra-articular fractures of the distal radius–factors affecting functional outcome. Hand Surg 2000;5(2):145–53.
[16] Gartland JJ Jr, Werley CW. Evaluation of healed Colles' fractures. J Bone Joint Surg Am 1951;33(4):895–907.
[17] Trumble TE, Schmitt SR, Vedder NB. Factors affecting functional outcome of displaced intra-articular distal radius fractures. J Hand Surg [Am] 1994;19(2):325–40.
[18] Kopylov P, Johnell O, Redlund-Johnell I, et al. Fractures of the distal end of the radius in young adults: a 30-year follow-up. J Hand Surg [Br] 1993;18(1):45–9.

[19] Knirk JL, Jupiter JB. Intra-articular fractures of the distal end of the radius in young adults. J Bone Joint Surg Am 1986;68(5):647–59.
[20] Karnezis IA, Panagiotopoulos E, Tyllianakis M, et al. Correlation between radiological parameters and patient-rated wrist dysfunction following fractures of the distal radius. Injury 2005;36(12):1435–9.
[21] Johnston GH, Friedman L, Kriegler JC. Computerized tomographic evaluation of acute distal radial fractures. J Hand Surg [Am] 1992;17(4):738–44.
[22] Katz MA, Beredjiklian PK, Bozentka DJ, et al. Computed tomography scanning of intra-articular distal radius fractures: does it influence treatment? J Hand Surg [Am] 2001;26(3):415–21.
[23] Harness NG, Ring D, Zurakowski D, et al. The influence of three-dimensional computed tomography reconstructions on the characterization and treatment of distal radial fractures. J Bone Joint Surg Am 2006;88(6):1315–23.
[24] Abbaszadegan H, Conradi P, Jonsson U. Fixation not needed for undisplaced Colles' fracture. Acta Orthop Scand 1989;60(1):60–2.
[25] Dias JJ, Wray CC, Jones JM. The radiological deformity of Colles' fractures. Injury 1987;18(5):304–8.
[26] Leone J, Bhandari M, Adili A, et al. Predictors of early and late instability following conservative treatment of extra-articular distal radius fractures. Arch Orthop Trauma Surg 2004;124(1):38–41.
[27] Handoll HH, Madhok R, Dodds C. Anaesthesia for treating distal radial fracture in adults. Cochrane Database Syst Rev 2002;3:CD003320.
[28] Earnshaw SA, Aladin A, Surendran S, et al. Closed reduction of Colles' fractures: comparison of manual manipulation and finger-trap traction: a prospective, randomized study. J Bone Joint Surg Am 2002;84(3):354–8.
[29] Bartosh RA, Saldana MJ. Intraarticular fractures of the distal radius: a cadaveric study to determine if ligamentotaxis restores radiopalmar tilt. J Hand Surg [Am] 1990;15(1):18–21.
[30] Gupta A. The treatment of Colles' fracture. Immobilisation with the wrist dorsiflexed. J Bone Joint Surg Br 1991;73(2):312–5.
[31] Sarmiento A, Pratt GW, Berry NC, et al. Colles' fractures. Functional bracing in supination. J Bone Joint Surg Am 1975;57(3):311–7.
[32] Wahlstrom O. Treatment of Colles' fracture. A prospective comparison of three different positions of immobilization. Acta Orthop Scand 1982;53(2):225–8.
[33] van der Linden W, Ericson R. Colles' fracture. How should its displacement be measured and how should it be immobilized? J Bone Joint Surg Am 1981;63(8):1285–8.
[34] Webb GR, Galpin RD, Armstrong DG. Comparison of short and long arm plaster casts for displaced fractures in the distal third of the forearm in children. J Bone Joint Surg Am 2006;88(1):9–17.

[35] Bohm ER, Bubbar V, Yong HK, et al. Above and below-the-elbow plaster casts for distal forearm fractures in children. A randomized controlled trial. J Bone Joint Surg Am 2006;88(1):1–8.

[36] Bong MR, Egol KA, Leibman M, et al. A comparison of immediate postreduction splinting constructs for controlling initial displacement of fractures of the distal radius: a prospective randomized study of long-arm versus short-arm splinting. J Hand Surg [Am] 2006;31(5):766–70.

[37] Stewart HD, Innes AR, Burke FD. Functional cast-bracing for Colles' fractures. A comparison between cast-bracing and conventional plaster casts. J Bone Joint Surg Br 1984;66(5):749–53.

[38] Tumia N, Wardlaw D, Hallett J, et al. Aberdeen Colles' fracture brace as a treatment for Colles' fracture. A multicentre, prospective, randomised, controlled trial. J Bone Joint Surg Br 2003;85(1):78–82.

[39] O'Connor D, Mullett H, Doyle M, et al. Minimally displaced Colles' fractures: a prospective randomized trial of treatment with a wrist splint or a plaster cast. J Hand Surg [Br] 2003;28(1):50–3.

[40] Hove LM, Solheim E, Skjeie R, et al. Prediction of secondary displacement in Colles' fracture. J Hand Surg [Br] 1994;19(6):731–6.

[41] Altissimi M, Mancini GB, Azzara A, et al. Early and late displacement of fractures of the distal radius. The prediction of instability. Int Orthop 1994;18(2):61–5.

[42] Vang HF, Staunstrup H, Mikkelsen S. A comparison of 3 and 5 weeks immobilization for older type 1 and 2 Colles' fractures. J Hand Surg [Br] 1998;23(3):400–1.

[43] Schmalholz A. Closed rereduction of axial compression in Colles' fracture is hardly possible. Acta Orthop Scand 1989;60(1):57–9.

[44] Hung LK, Wu HT, Leung PC, et al. Low BMD is a risk factor for low-energy Colles' fractures in women before and after menopause. Clin Orthop Relat Res 2005;435:219–25.

[45] Wigderowitz CA, Cunningham T, Rowley DI, et al. Peripheral bone mineral density in patients with distal radial fractures. J Bone Joint Surg Br 2003;85(3):423–5.

[46] Weber ER. A rational approach for the recognition and treatment of Colles' fracture. Hand Clin 1987;3(1):13–21.

[47] Cooney WP. Management of Colles' fractures. J Hand Surg [Br] 1989;14(2):137–9.

[48] Abbaszadegan H, Jonsson U, von SK. Prediction of instability of Colles' fractures. Acta Orthop Scand 1989;60(6):646–50.

[49] Lafontaine M, Hardy D, Delince P. Stability assessment of distal radius fractures. Injury 1989;20(4):208–10.

[50] Mackenney PJ, McQueen MM, Elton R. Prediction of instability in distal radial fractures. J Bone Joint Surg Am 2006;88(9):1944–51.

[51] Nesbitt KS, Failla JM, Les C. Assessment of instability factors in adult distal radius fractures. J Hand Surg [Am] 2004;29(6):1128–38.

[52] Kristiansen TK, Ryaby JP, McCabe J, et al. Accelerated healing of distal radial fractures with the use of specific, low-intensity ultrasound. A multicenter, prospective, randomized, double-blind, placebo-controlled study. J Bone Joint Surg Am 1997;79(7):961–73.

[53] Atkins RM, Duckworth T, Kanis JA. Algodystrophy following Colles' fracture. J Hand Surg [Br] 1989;14(2):161–4.

[54] Belsole RJ, Hess AV. Concomitant skeletal and soft tissue injuries. Orthop Clin North Am 1993;24(2):327–31.

[55] Taleisnik J, Watson HK. Midcarpal instability caused by malunited fractures of the distal radius. J Hand Surg [Am] 1984;9(3):350–7.

[56] Bienek T, Kusz D, Cielinski L. Peripheral nerve compression neuropathy after fractures of the distal radius. J Hand Surg [Br] 2006;31(3):256–60.

[57] Helal B, Chen SC, Iwegbu G. Rupture of the extensor pollicis longus tendon in undisplaced Colles' type of fracture. Hand 1982;14(1):41–7.

[58] Zollinger PE, Tuinebreijer WE, Kreis RW, et al. Effect of vitamin C on frequency of reflex sympathetic dystrophy in wrist fractures: a randomised trial. Lancet 1999;354(9195):2025–8.

[59] Amadio PC. Vitamin C reduced the incidence of reflex sympathetic dystrophy after wrist fracture. J Bone Joint Surg Am 2000;82(6):873.

[60] Handoll HH, Madhok R. Closed reduction methods for treating distal radial fractures in adults. Cochrane Database Syst Rev 2003;1:CD003763.

[61] Handoll HH, Madhok R. Conservative interventions for treating distal radial fractures in adults. Cochrane Database Syst Rev 2003;2:CD000314.

[62] Altissimi M, Antenucci R, Fiacca C, et al. Long-term results of conservative treatment of fractures of the distal radius. Clin Orthop Relat Res 1986;206:202–10.

[63] Villar RN, Marsh D, Rushton N, et al. Three years after Colles' fracture. A prospective review. J Bone Joint Surg Br 1987;69(4):635–8.

[64] Tsukazaki T, Iwasaki K. Ulnar wrist pain after Colles' fracture. 109 fractures followed for 4 years. Acta Orthop Scand 1993;64(4):462–4.

[65] Friedman SL, Palmer AK. The ulnar impaction syndrome. Hand Clin 1991;7(2):295–310.

[66] Ring D, Jupiter JB. Percutaneous and limited open fixation of fractures of the distal radius. Clin Orthop Relat Res 2000;375:105–15.

[67] Clancey GJ. Percutaneous Kirschner-wire fixation of Colles' fractures. A prospective study of thirty cases. J Bone Joint Surg Am 1984;66(7):1008–14.

[68] Mah ET, Atkinson RN. Percutaneous Kirschner wire stabilisation following closed reduction of Colles' fractures. J Hand Surg [Br] 1992;17(1):55–62.

[69] Shankar NS, Craxford AD. Comminuted Colles' fractures: a prospective trial of management. J R Coll Surg Edinb 1992;37(3):199–202.

[70] Azzopardi T, Ehrendorfer S, Coulton T, et al. Unstable extra-articular fractures of the distal radius: a prospective, randomised study of immobilisation in a cast versus supplementary percutaneous pinning. J Bone Joint Surg Br 2005;87(6): 837–40.

[71] Rodriguez-Merchan EC. Plaster cast versus percutaneous pin fixation for comminuted fractures of the distal radius in patients between 46 and 65 years of age. J Orthop Trauma 1997;11(3):212–7.

[72] Greatting MD, Bishop AT. Intrafocal (Kapandji) pinning of unstable fractures of the distal radius. Orthop Clin North Am 1993;24(2):301–7.

[73] Rosati M, Bertagnini S, Digrandi G, et al. Percutaneous pinning for fractures of the distal radius. Acta Orthop Belg 2006;72(2):138–46.

[74] Willenegger H, Uggenbuhl A. [Operative treatment of certain cases of distal radius fracture]. Helv Chir Acta 1959;26(2):81–94 [German].

[75] Naidu SH, Capo JT, Moulton M, et al. Percutaneous pinning of distal radius fractures: a biomechanical study. J Hand Surg [Am] 1997;22(2):252–7.

[76] Kapandji A. L'osteosyntese par double embrochage intra-focal: Traitment fonctionnel des fractures non articulaires de l'"extremite inferieure du radius. Ann Chir 1976;30:903–8.

[77] Fritz T, Wersching D, Klavora R, et al. Combined Kirschner wire fixation in the treatment of Colles' fracture. A prospective, controlled trial. Arch Orthop Trauma Surg 1999;119(3–4):171–8.

[78] Ruschel PH, Albertoni WM. Treatment of unstable extra-articular distal radius fractures by modified intrafocal Kapandji method. Tech Hand Up Extrem Surg 2005;9(1):7–16.

[79] Walton NP, Brammar TJ, Hutchinson J, et al. Treatment of unstable distal radial fractures by intrafocal, intramedullary K-wires. Injury 2001; 32(5):383–9.

[80] Temple J, Santy J. Pin site care for preventing infections associated with external bone fixators and pins. Cochrane Database Syst Rev 2004;1: CD004551.

[81] Singh S, Trikha P, Twyman R. Superficial radial nerve damage due to Kirschner wiring of the radius. Injury 2005;36(2):330–2.

[82] Hochwald NL, Levine R, Tornetta P III. The risks of Kirschner wire placement in the distal radius: a comparison of techniques. J Hand Surg [Am] 1997;22(4): 580–4.

[83] Hargreaves DG, Drew SJ, Eckersley R. Kirschner wire pin tract infection rates: a randomized controlled trial between percutaneous and buried wires. J Hand Surg [Br] 2004;29(4):374–6.

[84] Stoffelen DV, Broos PL. Closed reduction versus Kapandji-pinning for extra-articular distal radial fractures. J Hand Surg [Br] 1999;24(1):89–91.

[85] Lenoble E, Dumontier C, Goutallier D, et al. Fracture of the distal radius. A prospective comparison between trans-styloid and Kapandji fixations. J Bone Joint Surg Br 1995;77(4):562–7.

[86] Nonnenmacher J, Kempf I. [Role of intrafocal pinning in the treatment of wrist fractures]. Int Orthop 1988;12(2):155–62 [French].

[87] Ebraheim NA, Ali SS, Gove NK. Fixation of unstable distal radius fractures with intrafocal pins and trans-styloid augmentation: a retrospective review and radiographic analysis. Am J Orthop 2006; 35(8):362–8.

[88] Strohm PC, Muller CA, Boll T, et al. Two procedures for Kirschner wire osteosynthesis of distal radial fractures. A randomized trial. J Bone Joint Surg Am 2004;86(12):2621–8.

[89] Ludvigsen TC, Johansen S, Svenningsen S, et al. External fixation versus percutaneous pinning for unstable Colles' fracture. Equal outcome in a randomized study of 60 patients. Acta Orthop Scand 1997;68(3):255–8.

[90] Harley BJ, Scharfenberger A, Beaupre LA, et al. Augmented external fixation versus percutaneous pinning and casting for unstable fractures of the distal radius–a prospective randomized trial. J Hand Surg [Am] 2004;29(5):815–24.

[91] Kreder HJ, Hanel DP, Agel J, et al. Indirect reduction and percutaneous fixation versus open reduction and internal fixation for displaced intra-articular fractures of the distal radius: a randomised, controlled trial. J Bone Joint Surg Br 2005;87(6):829–36.

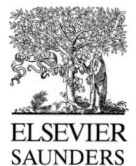

External Fixation of Distal Radius Fractures

Jubin B. Payandeh, MD, FRCS(C),
Michael D. McKee, MD, FRCS(C)*

*Division of Orthopaedics, Department of Surgery, 55 Queen Street East,
Suite 800, Toronto, Ontario, Canada M5C 1R6*

Fractures of the distal radius are the most common fractures that occur in patients between ages 15 and 75 years [1]. The mechanism of injury usually involves a fall onto the outstretched hand in an elderly patient whose bone quality is diminished by osteoporosis. In younger patients, high-energy injury mechanisms lead to wide displacement and marked comminution in bone of normal quality [2]. In either case, associated injuries (both systemic and of the upper extremity) must be identified and treated appropriately. Specifically, fractures of the distal radius may be associated with open wounds, tendon rupture, neurologic insult, or vascular injury. Treatment of these injuries must coincide with fracture care.

Many methods for treating displaced distal radius fractures are available. All forms of treatment involve obtaining fracture reduction, which may then be maintained with casting, functional bracing, external fixation, percutaneous pinning, internal fixation, or a combination of these methods. This article discusses the indications and technique of fracture treatment with external fixation and, when required, adjuvant percutaneous pins. The authors believe that most fractures failing closed reduction and casting can be treated successfully with this method including those with a displaced articular component.

Patient evaluation

The initial evaluation of a patient who has a distal radius fracture begins with reviewing their pertinent medical history and screening for associated injury. Physical examination must include an evaluation of the soft tissue injury, including the identification of open wounds and an assessment of neurovascular function. When a patient has been assessed, provisional splinting and high-quality radiographs should be obtained. The initial radiographs direct the surgeon toward the treatment method most likely to yield a successful outcome.

Several classification schemes have been proposed for distal radius fractures, although their practical usefulness, reproducibility, and applicability are controversial [3]. Important points to consider are:

- Fracture displacement
- Intra-articular or partial articular involvement
- Associated ulna fracture or disruption of the distal radioulnar joint
- An overall assessment of bone quality and comminution

In evaluating radiographs, the following parameters should be noted, which determine if the reduction is acceptable:

- Radial length
- Radial inclination
- Lateral tilt
- Intra-articular step or gap

Table 1 outlines normal parameters and what is generally considered acceptable reduction criteria for young, active individuals. The acceptability of reduction varies with the physiologic health and functional demands of the patient [4].

The goals of treatment for a patient who has a distal radius fracture include obtaining and maintaining an acceptable reduction to bony

---

* Corresponding author.
 E-mail address: mckeem@smh.toronto.on.ca (M.D. McKee).

Table 1
Acceptable reduction paramaters

Radiographic parameter	Normal	Acceptable
Radial length	±2 mm comparing level of lunate facet to ulnar head	No more than 2 mm of shortening relative to ulnar head
Radial inclination	20° as measured from lunate facet to radial styloid	No less than 10°
Lateral tilt	11° of volar tilt	Neutral
Intra-articular step or gap	None	Less than 2 mm of either

Data from Knirk JL, Jupiter J. Intra-articular fracture of the distal end of the radius in young adults. J Bone Joint Surg Am 1986;68:647–59.

union as previously defined. Surgeons must also consider the soft tissue component of the injury. Open wounds that are typically on the volar side must be addressed with operative irrigation and debridement at injury and then followed up closely to ensure healing. The wrist and fingers are subject to stiffness after fracture treatment and must be mobilized when adequate bony stability is obtained. Occasionally in the acute setting an associated nerve injury occurs, most commonly median, that requires exploration and decompression.

Treatment algorithm

Treatment is initiated after the initial assessment. Displaced fractures of the distal radius, regardless of configuration, deserve an attempt at closed reduction and casting. Even fractures that require immediate operative treatment, such as those with open injuries, should be reduced closed in the emergency department. Decreasing the deformity will relieve pressure on the surrounding soft tissues and neurovascular structures and provide some pain relief. More information is gained from viewing postreduction radiographs, which help in planning the definitive treatment and fixation. The authors typically use a hematoma block with local anesthetic that can be supplemented with intravenous narcotics or conscious sedation in a monitored setting. An appropriate reduction maneuver is performed and a moulded plaster slab is applied.

Postreduction radiographs are assessed to determine if an acceptable reduction has been achieved using the criteria specified in Table 1. If the reduction is not acceptable, a second reduction can be attempted. Adjuvants can be used to facilitate reduction, such as finger traps and a skilled assistant. If the second attempt fails, the patient should undergo operative treatment. Which fractures will fail closed treatment can often be predicted based on the initial fracture pattern. Severe comminution of the dorsal cortex usually leads to failure to obtain or maintain an acceptable reduction [5,6]. In these cases, a provisional reduction and splinting should be obtained while the patient is prepared for the operating room.

For patients requiring operative treatment of displaced distal radius fractures, including intra-articular fractures, the authors advocate external fixation with percutaneous pins as first-line treatment. This recommendation is based on randomized, controlled trials that show a more rapid return of function and better functional outcome with this treatment compared with open reduction and conventional plate fixation for displaced fractures that fail closed reduction [7,8]. The caveat is that the goals of an acceptable reduction, including intra-articular step or gap, must be met during the procedure. The surgeon may have to resort to open reduction and internal fixation to achieve these goals in approximately 5% to 10% of cases. This recommendation does not apply to dorsal or volar shear fractures, which should be treated primarily with open reduction and plate fixation [9].

Operative technique

The operative technique the authors use is closed reduction with the application of an external fixator that may be supplemented with percutaneous pins or bone grafting. The patient is positioned supine on the operating table and anesthetized. A hand table is used on the operative side and the authors apply, but not necessarily inflate, a tourniquet on the upper arm. The hand, wrist, and forearm are prepared and draped in a sterile fashion (Fig. 1).

The authors use a small external fixator and 2-mm K-wires. Intraoperative image intensification is mandatory for this procedure. They prefer to use a small C-arm, which the surgeon can manipulate to obtain anteroposterior and lateral views once the patient has been draped. A small fragment set is available if closed reduction fails and an open procedure is required.

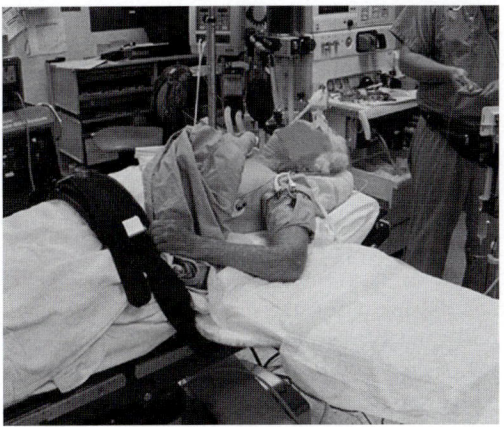

Fig. 1. The patient is positioned supine with a hand table and tourniquet on the operative side.

Initially, a closed reduction maneuver should be performed to correct significant deformity. An assistant provides countertraction at the elbow and the surgeon manipulates the hand and wrist first with inline traction. Most fractures can be reduced with slight volar and ulnar deviation of the hand and wrist. Manipulating the fracture fragments directly with digital pressure is often helpful. A rolled towel can be placed under the wrist to act as a fulcrum with which the deformity can be corrected. If the fracture fragments are incarcerated, the deformity may need to be exaggerated initially to unlock the fragments [10]. The major fracture displacement must be reduced before the external fixator is applied because, once applied, the wrist is difficult to manipulate. Using the image intensifier during the reduction is invaluable.

When the provisional reduction has been achieved, the external fixator can be applied. Two pins are inserted into the radial shaft proximal to the zone of injury and another two pins are inserted into the second metacarpal. The plane of the pins should be varied to construct a quadrangular frame. For the radial pins, a small incision is made and the soft tissues are bluntly dissected down to bone. Right-angle retractors are used so the pins can be inserted under direct vision to protect surrounding structures. For the second metacarpal, the pins are radially based to avoid the extensor mechanism. Once the pins are in place, they should be checked for purchase and their length and position verified using the image intensifier.

The frame assembly begins with two short bars between the radial and metacarpal pins, respectively. The connections can then be tightened. The authors use carbon-fiber bars, which are radiolucent, to facilitate adequate radiographs. Then a long bar connecting the radial and metacarpal pins is applied on one side with the connectors loosened. The reduction maneuver is then reapplied and an assistant tightens the connectors on the single bar. The reduction is verified using the image intensifier and, once achieved, a second bar is added to the frame construct and tightened (Fig. 2A, B).

When applying an external fixator, extreme positions of the wrist should be avoided. The goal is to restore radiographic parameters, most importantly radial length, to an acceptable position (see Table 1). The reduction, especially residual intra-articular deformity, often must be fine-tuned using percutaneous pins or bone grafting.

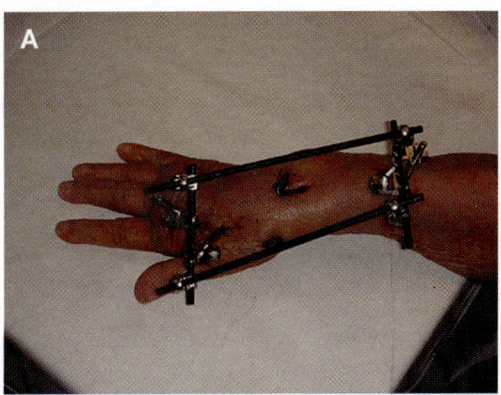
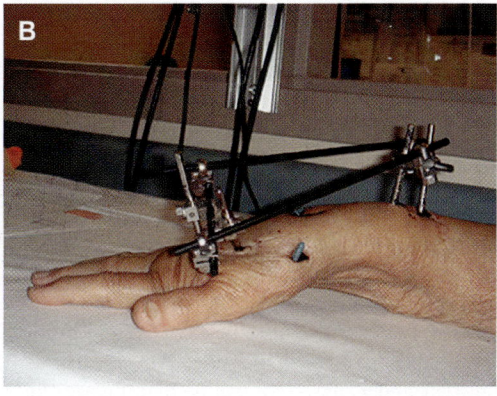

Fig. 2. (*A, B*) This patient has had a fixator applied and percutaneous pins inserted for an open, displaced, and intra-articular distal radius fracture.

Percutaneous K-wires are a useful adjuvant to external fixation for treating these fractures. The pins are inserted when the reduction has been achieved and the fixator applied. Commonly, pins are inserted in the radial styloid and dorsally. The fracture fragments can be manipulated either directly with the pin or indirectly by using them as a buttress. Although pins can be passed from the volar side, this is not recommended because of the proximity of important neurovascular structures.

The authors insert the pins using the image intensifier to guide placement. If the fractured fragments are of sufficient size and the bone quality is good, the pins are passed through the distal fragment. Once the distal fragment is engaged with the pin, the authors use live image intensification to manipulate the captured fragment into the desired position. Once this position is gained, the pin is advanced proximally into the shaft, catching the opposite cortex. Typically, two or three pins are used.

If the bone quality is poor or the distal fragments are small because of comminution, the K-wires can be used as a buttress. This procedure involves passing the wire through the fracture site and then using it as a lever to improve the fracture position with image control. The wire is then advanced proximally to either the opposite cortex or, if not possible, the medullary canal [11].

When the ulna is fractured distally, causing the carpus or distal radius to drift in the ulnar direction, an ulnar-sided pin can be used. This pin is inserted using image control through the ulnar styloid or fracture to act as a buttress. Ulnar styloid fractures are not routinely fixed. If obvious clinical or radiographic instability of the distal radioulnar joint occurs after radial fracture fixation, the ulnar styloid may require fixation.

After the wires are passed and the fracture acceptably reduced, the wires are bent at the skin level to prevent migration and ease their removal. The skin should be relaxed with a small incision around the pin entry site if any tension is present.

When a depressed articular fragment cannot be improved or manipulated with traction or a percutaneous pin, direct elevation and bone grafting is another option [12]. Where exactly the fragment is located should be determined from the anteroposterior and lateral views. A small incision is made below the fragment to be elevated and blunt dissection is performed to bone. An elevator is then used under image control to manipulate the articular fragment to an acceptable position. The defect created during this elevation is then filled with either bone graft or graft substitute. Bone graft can be obtained from the iliac crest through a separate small incision. Alternatively, several bone graft substitutes are available, including calcium phosphate bone cements [13].

Before the conclusion of this procedure, the surgeon must determine if the goals of treatment have been achieved, which should be an acceptable reduction according to the criteria listed in Table 1. Rarely, in 5% to 10% of cases, achieving this goal is not possible using the methods described previously and the surgeon must consider converting to open reduction with internal fixation.

Case example

Fig. 3 shows radiographs of an elderly woman who fell while at church and was brought to the emergency department with an isolated injury to her wrist. She had a 2-cm open wound on the volar/ulnar side of her wrist. The initial radiographs show significant radial shortening, loss of radial angulation, dorsal displacement, comminution, and intra-articular extension. The open wound demanded emergent operative treatment with debridement and reduction. An external fixator was applied after provisional reduction. In this case, the wrist tended to translate in an ulnar direction after the fixator was applied. The authors restored the ulnar buttress with an intramedullary K-wire.

Postoperative care

The authors dress the pin sites with Vaseline-coated gauze followed by dry gauze, and then wrap the forearm and wrist in a soft bandage. They do not order a specific pin care regimen, other than keeping the sites clean and dry, and have found that minimal perturbation of the pin sites is ideal. Plain radiographs are obtained in the recovery room. Patients who have an isolated injury are discharged from the hospital the same day, whereas others stay longer depending on their associated injuries. Patients return to the clinic within 2 weeks and again 6 weeks postoperatively. At each visit, plain radiographs are taken. The frame and pins are usually removed in the clinic at 6 weeks if the radiograph shows fracture union and a supervised physiotherapy program is initiated to regain wrist motion and strength. Patients are encouraged to maintain motion of their shoulder, elbow, and fingers while the frame is in place. The authors

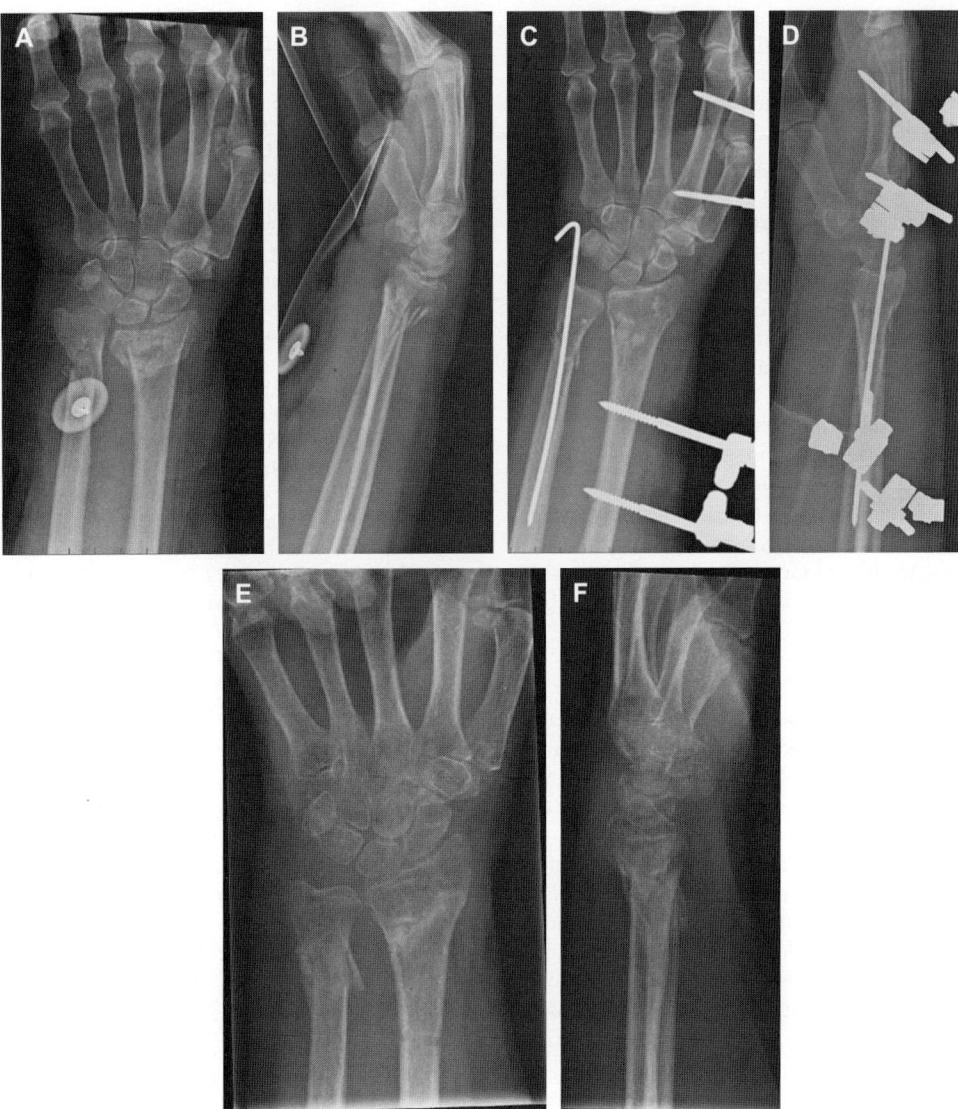

Fig. 3. (*A*, *B*) Anteroposterior and lateral radiographs after open wrist injury. (*C*, *D*) Anteroposterior and lateral radiographs after operative treatment with external fixator application and percutaneous ulnar K-wire. (*E*, *F*) Anteroposterior and lateral radiographs 6 weeks after the removal of hardware.

then follow-up their patients at 3 and 6 months, or longer if specific problems associated with the injury are present.

Results

Treating displaced distal radius fractures, including those with an articular component, with external fixation and percutaneous pins typically yields good results [7,8]. A recent randomized controlled trial showed that percutaneous fixation had superior results compared with open reduction and internal fixation; patients experienced improvement in function and pain scores at all points of follow-up. Those treated with indirect reduction scored a mean of 6 points better on the musculoskeletal function assessment. Grip strength is also superior in those treated with external methods, by a mean of 10.1 lb. Outcomes were equivalent in terms of restoring radiographic parameters. Range of motion measurements were also the same with the injured wrist, losing on average 20° of flexion compared with the uninjured side [7]. This trial evaluated internal fixation using conventional, nonlocking plates. Whether the use of locking plates improves outcomes for these injuries has not been determined.

Pin tract infections can occur with percutaneous fixation methods in 20% of patients. Most can be treated with an oral antibiotic prescription and local pin care. Occasionally, pin replacement, irrigation, and debridement are required for deep infections. Patients treated with either internal or external means may rarely develop a complex regional pain syndrome after treatment of a distal radius fracture [14].

The fractures are usually healed by 6 to 8 weeks. Fracture malunion, even when treated by expert surgeons, occurs in approximately 10% of cases. Although extra-articular deformity can be corrected with osteotomy, persistent articular step or gap deformity of more than 2 mm increases the risk for developing wrist arthritis by 10 times [15].

Discussion

External fixation supplemented with percutaneous pins is an excellent option for treating displaced fractures of the distal radius, with reliably good results, a low reoperation rate, and a low complication rate. These fractures are common and this treatment method is familiar to orthopaedic surgeons. The key to success is to restore anatomic parameters of the distal radius while minimizing insult to the soft tissue envelope. All fractures, except shear fractures, failing closed treatment can be treated with external means. If these fail to produce an acceptable reduction, open reduction may rarely be required.

Although locked plates are becoming increasingly popular for treating these fractures, whether they improve functional results compared with conventional implants or external fixation methods has not been determined in a direct comparative study.

References

[1] Emmett JE, Breck LW. A review and analysis of 11,000 fractures seen in a private practice of orthopaedic surgery. J Bone Joint Surg Am 1958;40:1169–75.

[2] Larsen CF, Lauritsen J. Epidemiology of acute wrist trauma. Int J Epidemiol 1993;22:911–6.

[3] Kreder HJ, Hanel DP, McKee M, et al. Consistency of AO fracture classification for the distal radius. J Bone Joint Surg Br 1996;78:726–31.

[4] Beumer A, McQueen MM. Fractures of the distal radius in low-demand elderly patients: closed reduction of no value in 53 of 60 wrists. Acta Orthop Scand 2003;74:98–100.

[5] McQueen MM, Hajducka C, Court-Brown CM. Redisplaced unstable fractures of the distal radius: a prospective randomised comparison of four methods of treatment. J Bone Joint Surg Br 1996; 78:404–9.

[6] McQueen MM, McLaren A, Chalmers J. The value of remanipulating Colles' fractures. J Bone Joint Surg Br 1986;68:232–3.

[7] Kreder HJ, Hanel DP, Agel J, et al. Indirect reduction and percutaneous fixation versus open reduction and internal fixation for displaced intra-articular fractures of the distal radius. J Bone Joint Surg Br 2005;87(6):829–36.

[8] Kreder HJ, Agel J, Mckee MD, et al. A randomized, controlled trial of distal radius fractures with metaphyseal displacement but without joint incongruity: closed reduction and casting versus closed reduction, spanning external fixation, and optional percutaneous K-wires. J Orthop Trauma 2006; 20(2):115–21.

[9] Jupiter JB, Fernandez DL, Toh CL, et al. Operative treatment of volar intra-articular fractures of the distal end of the radius. J Bone Joint Surg Am 1996;78(12):1817–28.

[10] Handoll HH, Madhok R. Closed reduction methods for treating distal radial fractures in adults. Cochrane Database Syst Rev 2003;1:CD003763.

[11] Kapandji A. [Intra-focal pinning of fractures of the distal end of the radius 10 years later]. Ann Chir Main 1987;6(1):57–63 [French].

[12] Axelrod T, Paley D, Green J, et al. Limited open reduction of the lunate facet in comminuted intra-articular fractures of the distal radius. J Hand Surg [Am] 1988;13(3):372–7.

[13] Sanchez-Sotelo J, Munuera L, Madero R. Treatment of fractures of the distal radius with a remoldable bone cement: a prospective, randomized study using Norian SRS. J Bone Joint Surg Br 2000;82(6): 856–63.

[14] Chaise F, Friol JP, Gainse E. [The post-fracture painful wrist]. Ann Chir 1994;48(1):88–90 [French].

[15] Knirk JL, Jupiter J. Intra-articular fracture of the distal end of the radius in young adults. J Bone Joint Surg Am 1986;68:647–59.

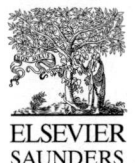

Plating for Distal Radius Fractures

Paul A. Martineau, MD, FRCSC[a], Gregory K. Berry, MD, FRCSC[b], Edward J. Harvey, MD, MSc, FRCSC[b],*

[a]*University of Washington, Seattle, WA 98195, USA*
[b]*McGill University Division of Orthopedic Surgery, Montreal, Quebec, Canada*

No area of fracture management has had such a recent explosion of new treatment modalities as distal radius plating. This explosion has largely been implant- and industry-driven, with little evidence-based research guiding the way. A perceived difficulty with commonly used modalities by the orthopedic community has been enough to drive an entire new set of options for distal radius fixation. A drift from dorsal to volar plating has occurred that has been unexamined by randomized research. Segment specific fixation has been a new mindset that has resulted in a novel plate line and has caused other manufacturers to redesign their product lines. Other novel approaches for proposed problems include locking plates, nail-plate combinations, and others. This article outlines some of these options with a literature opinion and a clarification from the authors. A treatment plan for common fractures of the distal radius is also outlined.

Discussion

Several studies clearly show that restoration of normal anatomy after this fracture provides more optimal function [1–8]. In addition, functional outcome scores have shown that patients who have no anatomic reduction function poorly [2,9]. Malunion of the distal radius has been associated with pain, stiffness, weak grip strength, and carpal instability in a significant percentage of patients [4]. Long-term consequences include degenerative arthritis in up to 50% of patients with even minimal displacement in the young adult population [10]. As surgical treatment (plating in particular) ensures more consistent correction of displacement and maintenance of reduction there has been a trend to operative treatment of these fractures in both the elderly and the young population.

Currently, several established surgical options are available for displaced distal radius fractures [11–22]. The choice of surgical technique for reduction and fixation will depend on fracture displacement, joint surface involvement, patient age, bone quality, handedness, occupation, and avocation. Surgeon experience and preference will also dictate the treatment method. Unfortunately, little high quality literature exists on which to base these treatment decisions [13].

Plating techniques

Volar plates versus dorsal plates

Because of a high rate of complications with dorsal plate placement and with the advent of new fixed-angle screw-plate designs, volar fixation has become the standard approach for distal radius fractures with joint congruity [23–29]. The placement of dorsal plates has been associated with complications in the past. Stiffness and tendon rupture have been reported [9,16,20,30,31]. The effect of the incision and approach with attendant scar is difficult to separate from the actual dorsal location of a plate. Certainly, a volar plate placement through a flexor carpi radialis approach affords a soft tissue layer

* Corresponding author. McGill University Health Center, Department of Orthopaedic Surgery, Montreal General Hospital, Room B5.159.5, 1650 Cedar Ave., Montreal, Quebec, Canada, H3G 1A4.

E-mail address: edward.harvey@muhc.mcgill.ca (E.J. Harvey).

between the skin and the plate that may have greater depth than a dorsal approach. In the authors' institution, the use of multiple plates for open reduction internal fixation (ORIF) of distal radius fractures is common because of the higher energy fractures seen at a level-one trauma center. But dorsal and volar plates are often used in revision cases, patients treated later than 3 weeks, or referral patients from other institutions where some osteoporotic comminuted fractures may need this treatment modality. The authors tend to use the volar plate (or a radial styloid plate) initially, without distal screws, and then apply one or more dorsal plates as needed (Fig. 1). The distal volar screws are then used as needed, with the new locking plates often useful in these special cases (Fig. 1D). In the authors' experience, the newer near-anatomic volar plates

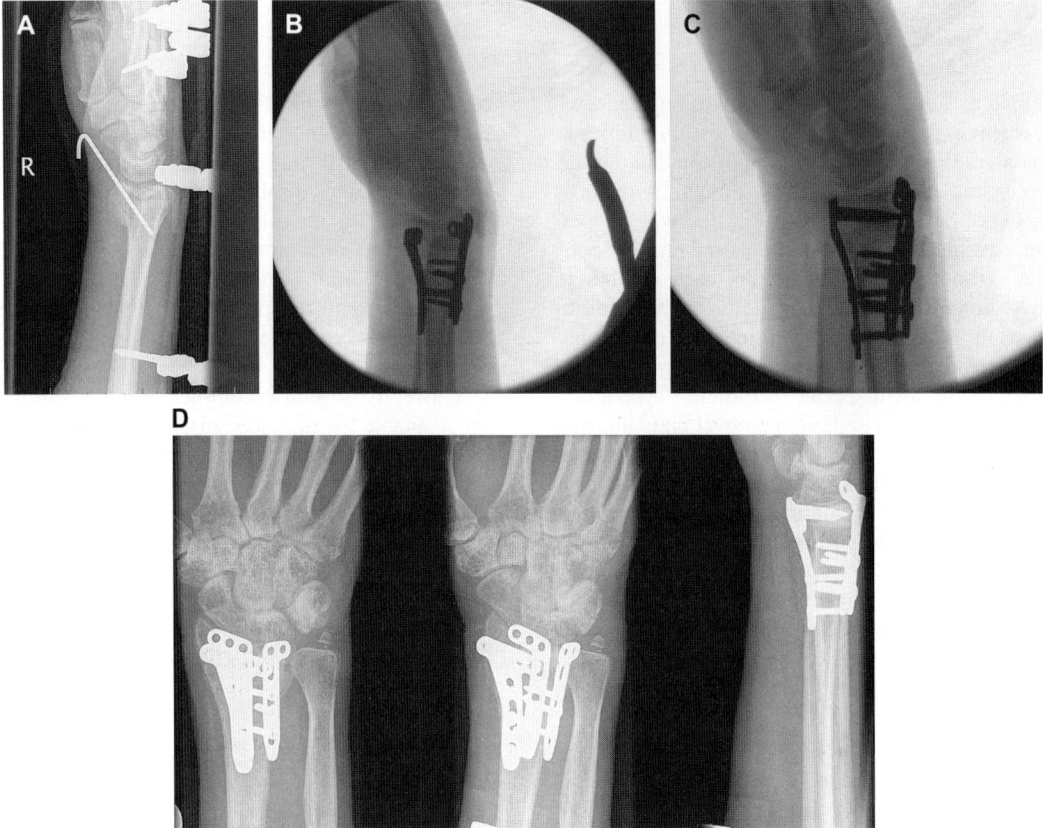

Fig. 1. (*A*) High-energy injury initially treated 5 weeks before referral with a spanning external fixator and K-wire pinning. The wrist has subluxed volarly and joint incongruity is present because of both volar translation (gap) and dorsal marginal impaction (angulation). Multiple dorsal joint lines are obvious on this lateral image. Because of the late presentation, this reduction would be difficult to accomplish from only a dorsal or volar approach. (*B*) Surgeons elected to fix this fracture from both a dorsal and volar approach. The volar approach is performed first with application of the plate in a buttress fashion. The wrist is then approached dorsally. Although the fracture is exposed to allow manipulation of fragments, the dorsal wrist capsular attachments should not be completely stripped from the dorsal rim of the radiocarpal joint primarily. After freeing all fracture lines, the application of one or more dorsal plates in buttress fashion will often extrude the dorsal comminution distally. The intact dorsal capsule aids in lining up the joint line as the bone fragments are sandwiched between the plates. In this case, an allograft bone graft was inserted to aid in pushing the joint distally. (*C*) After the joint is aligned, the volar plate is used to lock the fragments in position with the distal row locking screws. Because of the distal dorsal plate placement to enable reduction, the distal row of screws could not be safely placed. (*D*) The joint can be seen to be well reduced 3 years after fixation. The graft has consolidated and the patient has returned to work.

have proven to be more efficacious in aiding dorsal reduction without the need to worry about volar translation.

Volar plates generally fall into four functional categories: buttress plates (with or without distal screws), tine or blade plates, fixed-angled locking plates, and polyaxial locking plates [11,24,32–34]. Volar buttress plates are the traditional plate designs used to treat distal radius volar shear fractures and can be used with or without screw fixation in the distal fragment. Because the screws are not locked in the plate construct, they do not resist angular motion effectively. In normal bone, or even osteoporotic bone without comminution, a locked device provides no advantage and a normal buttress plate can be used. Blade plates have one or several tines that are part of the plate extending in a perpendicular direction to the main body of the plate. They offer the advantage of high strength and stiffness but the disadvantage of having to be placed in a position predetermined by the shape and position of the tines on the plate. The operating surgeon in some cases can shape these plates to better fit the articular contours. Fixed-angle locking plates are implants with screws or pegs that lock into the plate at a fixed trajectory. The peg or screw head usually has a thread to engage the corresponding screw hole in the plate. Pegs are smooth and are intended for subchondral support only, whereas screws allow direct purchase of bone fragments. Fixed-angled locking plate designs have improved strength characteristics compared with traditional nonlocking plates to resist angular motion. Finally, if the locking pegs or screws are placed as distal as possible to provide subchondral support of the distal fragment, the construct will be more effective at maintaining length [11].

Polyaxial locking plates allow an independent trajectory to be selected for each distal screw or peg. They display all the same advantages of fixed-angled locking plates but have the advantage of matching the distal fixation to the variable geometry and surface contour of the distal radius. In addition, polyaxial-locking plates can adapt the distal fixation to independently address each intra-articular fragment. Finally, the ability to adjust the screw or peg trajectories means that the plate does not have to be located in a specific position. They do tend to be thicker and more prominent than the standard locking plate design and differ radically from manufacturer to manufacturer. Early biomechanical reports show a large variability in the actual rigidity of the plate–screw construct and the surgeon should become familiar with these reports before deciding on an optimal plate. Both fixed-angled and polyaxial-locking plate designs are available with more than a single row of distal fixation to potentially provide additional distal fragment fixation strength and improve subchondral support. However, no evidence exists supporting the need for this plate design feature. In fact, very little evidence-based research promotes the use of locking plate in general for the distal radius.

Although the advent of volar locking plates for treating distal radius fractures may seem like a panacea, their use is not without complications. Reports of the complications of volar plates are beginning to appear in the literature [35,36]. Volar plating is not immune to the extensor tendon complications that affect dorsal plates [35]. At least one newer study with low profile dorsal plates [15] shows that patients can expect to have 80% of their range of motion and strength after dorsal plating for distal radius fractures. Moreover, 93% of the patients will have good-to-excellent functional outcomes. The authors believe that the specific plate used might cause complications from dorsal plating, rather than the technique itself, therefore supporting a dorsal approach for dorsally angulated distal radius fractures.

Fragment-specific fixation

Fragment-specific fixation is designed to independently stabilize each major fracture element using an implant specifically designed for each fragment. Similar to volar-locking plates, subchondral support and rigidity can be enhanced, in this case using a combination of small implants designed for each main distal radius fracture component, with implants taking into consideration the complex three-dimensional geometry of the distal radius [16,21,34,37,38]. Fragment-specific fixation also takes advantage of increased rigidity provided by implants placed in orthogonal planes. Dodds and colleagues [37] compared fragment specific fixation to external fixation augmented with K-wire fixation and found equivalent stability in their three-part fracture model [37]. However, the fragment-specific fixation displayed significantly more stability in their four-part fracture model.

Few clinical reports exist supporting the use of fragment-specific fixation. Konrath and Bahler [16] reported on the results with a fragment specific system on 27 patients with a minimum 2-year follow-up [16]. Results were encouraging, with high reported patient satisfaction and low implant-related complications (three cases required hardware removal during the study period, no reported cases of tendon ruptures). Similarly, Schnall and colleagues [21] reported on 37 patients treated with a fragment-specific distal radius fracture system with equally positive clinical and radiographic results. Fragment-specific fixation using AO 2-mm plates (Synthes, Paoli, Pennsylvania) was associated with extensor tendonitis and extensor tendon rupture in patients requiring cutting of the 2-mm plates [39]. Benson and colleagues [38] assessed the clinical, radiographic, and functional outcome with fragment-specific fixation in a retrospective review of 81 patients with 85 intra-articular distal radius fractures who were treated with fragment-specific fixation. Radiographic alignment was maintained between immediate postoperative and final follow-up films, and no cases of symptomatic arthritis were seen at the final follow-up evaluation. Based on these results, Benson and colleagues consider fragment-specific fixation a reasonable alternative with good-to-excellent results with respect to range of motion, grip strength, radiographic alignment, and satisfaction scores.

At least one manufacturer advocates radial styloid reduction before lunate reduction and fixation for fragment-specific fixation. Most case reports associated with this technique show excellent reduction in short- and medium-term follow-up periods. The need for anatomic reduction of the lunate may be lost on some surgeons with this technique. The intact lunate fossa articulation is infinitely more useful as a secondary reconstruction platform than the radioscaphoid articulation. In a biomechanical study, Taylor and colleagues [34] found no significant difference in load to failure between the systems with respect to ulnar, radial, or overall fragment displacement. Fragment-specific fixation had improved stiffness characteristics only with respect to the smaller ulnar-sided fragment.

Locking versus nonlocking plates

The locking nature of the screw–plate construct produces fixation even in bone defects and osteopenic bone and permits early range of motion exercises. In contrast to external fixation and percutaneous pinning, no tethering of muscle, tendon, or capsule occurs with plate fixation and therefore motion of the wrist and fingers is uninhibited. These advantages would suggest that plate fixation with a volar fixed-angle device should permit earlier and more aggressive rehabilitation and more rapid regain of function when compared with stabilization with external fixation or percutaneous pinning, although this has not been studied systematically. Rapid and effective recovery of function is important in both the young, active population and the elderly population, who often live alone and require both hands to function independently.

Another advantage of a locked plate is the ability to perform indirect reduction (Fig. 2) [40]. The distal fragment of an A-type fracture, or after fixation of the intra-articular portion of a C-type fracture, may be brought into appropriate palmar tilt through placing the plate off the bone during fixation to the distal piece. Bringing the plate to the bone for proximal fixation performs the indirect reduction.

Whether locking plates provide an advantage, even in comminuted osteoporotic fractures, although intuitively obvious, has yet to be proven. The authors looked at radiographs from 211 distal radius fractures treated with one of three surgical options: nonspanning external fixator (NSEF), plates (ORIF), or pinning (closed reduction and percutaneous pinning [CRPP]). A large group (107) was treated with either locked or unlocked plates. Of the 211 fractures, 104 (49.3%) were type A fractures, 12 (5.7%) were type B factures, and 95 (45.0%) were type C fractures. ORIF was able to significantly improve nearly all of the radiographic parameters, including joint surface congruity. All three treatment methods maintained the reduction obtained at surgery until healing. ORIF of comminuted, intra-articular, distal radius fractures produces good radiographic results, whereas NSEF and CRPP of less complex fractures also provide good results. The ORIF group had a discernable difference in obtaining reduction for palmar tilt, radial inclination, radial length, and posteroanterior and lateral articular gaps, and posteroanterior and lateral articular steps. Although this is a retrospective study, a measured difference certainly seems present even in a study where the more severe cases were placed with bias into the locked-plate group. This certainly needs to be explored in a prospective manner.

Although indications for using locked plates are still to be defined, several are seen in the authors' practice for the use of these plate—comminution,

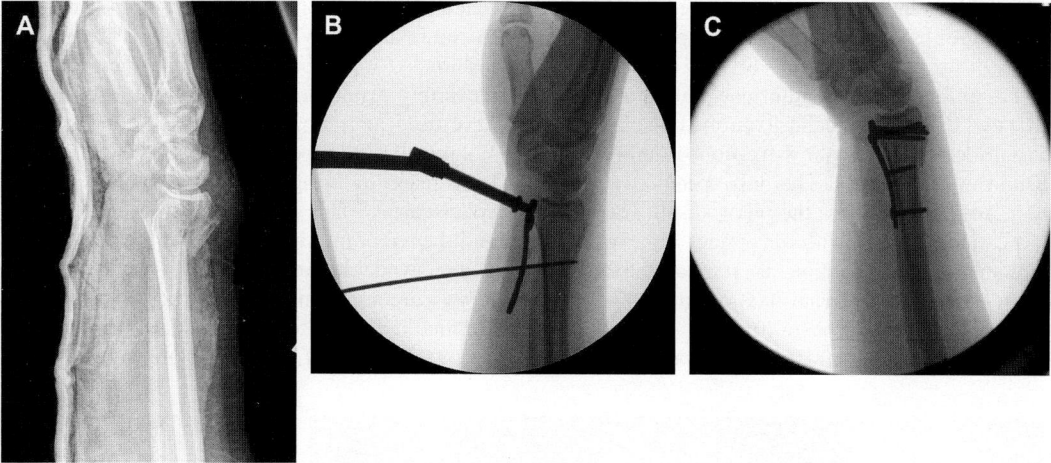

Fig. 2. (*A*) Lateral radiograph of a metaphyseal–diaphyseal comminuted fracture of the distal radius. 25° of dorsal tilt is present in this postreduction radiograph. (*B*) Surgeons elected to perform a volar plating after ORIF for this patient. Through an flexor carpi radialis approach, the distal fragment has a volar plate applied to it with the proximal portion of the plate off of the bone. After reduction in the operating room, 10° of dorsal tilt is still present in this patient's radius. Screw placement is checked on intraoperative fluoroscopy to ensure that the distal locking screws are not more than 3 to 4 mm proximal to the joint line for optimal biomechanical stability. (*C*) The distal screws are applied and the plate is then pushed down to the bone and held in place initially with a nonlocked screw. The distal fragment is then tilted more volarly. 10° of volar tilt can now be seen at the radiocarpal joint. If the initial distal subchondral row of screws is applied with the proximal plate ulnar on the radius, another reduction will also take place.

osteoporosis, early mobilization, and revision surgery are good indications. Old fractures needing reduction are also best treated with these plates because of the inherent soft tissue tightness that tends to make the old deformity recur with the use of conventional plates.

Special plates

The use of internal distraction plating or bridge plating for distal radius fractures was first introduced by Burke and Singer [41]. Treating high-energy comminuted distal radius fractures continues to be challenging. In particular, fracture patterns extending into the diaphyses of the radius and ulna represent unique treatment challenges. In addition, polytrauma patients requiring load-bearing through the wrist to assist with mobilization can also benefit from the bridge-plating technique. Finally, this internal fixator can potentially decrease the nursing requirements for these patients when compared with external fixation. The technique was further expanded by Ruch and colleagues [42,43], who described the use of a 3.5-mm plate (Synthes, Paoli, Pennsylvania) to span from the intact radial diaphysis to the third metacarpal. The bride-plating technique provides strong fixation and allows for distraction across impacted articular segments. The technique can be combined with a limited definitive articular fixation approach for fracture patterns with intra-articular extension.

The technique of bridge plating of the distal radius was recently further refined. Hanel and colleagues [44] described a variant of the technique using 2.4-mm AO plates passed extra-articularly through the second dorsal compartment and secured onto the dorsal–radial aspect of the radial diaphysis and the second metacarpal. They reported on their experience with bridge plating using either a 2.4-mm titanium mandibular reconstruction plate or, later in the series, a 2.4-mm stainless steel plate specifically designed to be a distal radius bridge plate (DRB plate, Synthes, Paoli, Pennsylvania).

The desire to provide stable fracture fixation combined with minimal soft tissue dissection to potentially decrease soft tissue/implant-related complications has led to the development of novel intramedullary implants for treating distal radius fracture. Divergent screws, fixed-angled locking screws, and minimally invasive insertion techniques may allow for earlier patient rehabilitation. Although promising early results have been reported by a limited number of surgeons in small patient groups, longer-term follow-up is required for these novel implants [45,46].

The authors have found bridge plating to be of little use. Fragment-specific fixation and volar and dorsal locking plates allow fixation of almost all distal radius fractures. The only specific fracture with any difficulty is the very distal fracture dislocation pattern with no intact rim, which allows dorsal dislocation if standard fixation devices are used. External fixation augmentation will not hold this type of fracture beyond the operating room. Unfortunately, patients who sustain this type of fracture are often unreliable to return to follow-up appointments in a timely fashion. Using a bridge plate for these patients inevitably results in a wrist fusion. The authors have used another technique with good success. Volar plates may be used, if necessary, as a buttress plate to bring anatomic reduction to the volar cortex. This may require several K-wires and the use of multiple plates, but the new locking plates available are adequate. Only proximal screws are used initially and then filled in with the final reduction to lock the distal fragment (see Fig. 2). Before this occurs, a plate is used on the

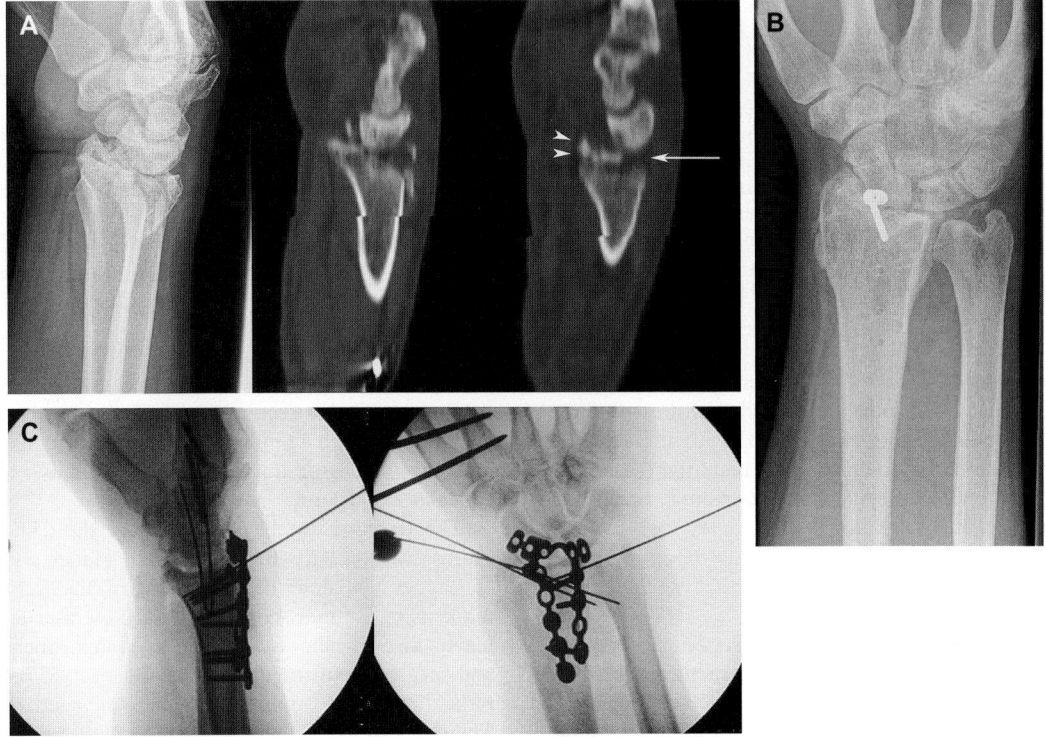

Fig. 3. (*A*) 40-year-old male who fell 70 ft from a crane into a quarry and sustained multiple injuries, including this wrist fracture. The lateral radiograph shows a comminuted distal intra-articular fracture with splaying of the metaphysis. Multiple CT scan cuts all show multiple intra-articular fragments (*small arrowheads*) and dorsal subluxation of the carpus. The dorsal rim of the radius is nonexistent because of the high-energy injury. (*B*) Dorsal approach confirms the CT reports. Even with an external fixator in place with multiple K-wires, the carpus continued to dislocate dorsally. A pi-plate (Synthes, Paoli, Pennsylvania) has been placed over the distal radius and the proximal row of the carpus, immediately stopping the carpus from subluxating. Range of motion with the plate in place is from neutral to 40° of palmar flexion. Because of the type of patient that usually sustains this type of injury, the authors are happier with its use than the spanning internal plate to the metacarpals [44] The authors have found that this type of patient tends to miss follow-up appointments, which would result in a functional fusion with a spanning plate. (*B*) The patient was lost to follow-up after his 3 month appointment and reappeared after 2 years complaining of loss of dorsiflexion. He had his pate removed. A small fragment of nonunion was found on the dorsal rim of the wrist and fixed in place with a screw. The patient was seen 1 year later and had returned to his job in construction with 40° of palmar flexion and 30° of dorsiflexion. Long-term osteoarthritis cannot be prevented with this type of injury, but the authors have found that this type of fixation favors range of motion in these patients and can enable them to return to work for several years.

dorsal side. A pi-plate from the Synthes distal radius set is used in an unconventional manner through a standard 3 to 4 interval; it is placed over the first carpal row without contouring (Fig. 3). Care is taken to prevent further stripping of the soft tissue at the radiocarpal joint to use the joint capsule and ligaments as an indirect aid to reduction. No screws are placed distally to the radiocarpal articulation, but the first carpal row and the intact soft tissue on the dorsum of the wrist permit reduction. Obviously a block to dorsiflexion is present, but palmar flexion is permitted and encouraged after the locking screws are placed on the volar plate in the distal fragment.

Plate type (titanium versus stainless)

Most implants currently used to treat distal radius fractures are made either of stainless steel or titanium alloys. The most commonly used stainless steels are 316L and 22-13-5 as designated by the American Standard for Testing and Materials. Stainless steel is essentially an alloy containing iron, carbon, nickel, and molybdenum [47].

Earlier implants made out of commercially pure titanium have been replaced with titanium alloys to improve their mechanical strength. The most commonly used titanium alloys used today are Ti-6Al-7Nb and Ti-6Al-4V. These alloys display excellent corrosion resistance, biocompatibility, decreased implant stiffness, and diminished stress shielding compared with stainless steel [47].

Concerns have been expressed about the increased occurrence of tendon irritation and adhesions with the use of titanium implants in the hand and wrist. However, research with dorsal plating of the distal radius in animal models has yielded conflicting results. Sinicropi and colleagues [48] found that dorsal plating using titanium plates in their canine radius model produced greater inflammatory peritendinous response than matched stainless steel implants. However, Cohen and

Table 1
Authors' choice for plates in common fracture types

Fracture type	Chosen treatment
Extra-articular	
	A volar fixed angled locking plate.
Intra-articular	
Partial (B-type) volar	A volar buttress plate is an effective method of fixation of isolated volar lip shearing injuries.
Partial (B-type) dorsal	If percutaneous reduction and pinning is attained- a volar fixed angled or polyaxial locking plate. Volar treatment of dorsal lip fractures requires purchase into the distal fragment and distally inclined locking screws to provide subchondral support of the dorsal articular surface. If the dorsal fragment is small and or comminuted the addition of a dorsal buttress plate may be required.
Radial styloid	A volar fixed-angle locking plate or fragment specific fixation.
Lunate fossa	A volar fixed-angled locking plate or polyaxial locking plate to provide adequate subchondral support to each of the common intra-articular fracture patterns. Comminution necessitates dorsal reduction then a fragment specific plate is used as well.
Lunate fossa split and displaced	A volar locking plate or polyaxial locking plate to provide adequate subchondral support to each of the common intra-articular fracture patterns. However, when attempting to treat complex intra-articular fracture patterns, different plate designs and alternate fixation options should be readily available and familiar to the surgeon undertaking such cases.
Comminuted (C2-3)	An extended volar locking plate plus or minus a dorsal plates in a fragment specific manner. If severe comminution the volar and dorsal plates may be substituted with a distal radius bridge plate depending on the extent of comminution and energy of the trauma.
Comminuted (C2) osteoporotic	An extended volar locking plate or distal radius bridge plate depending on the extent of comminution and energy of the trauma.
Comminuted with non-reconstructable dorsal rim	Volar plate with dorsal pi-plate extending over the first carpal row.

colleagues [30] in a canine model of dorsal plating, and Nazzal and colleagues [49] in a rabbit model, did not find any difference with the use of stainless steel or titanium. In fact, titanium plates around the distal radius seem to have been condemned on the basis of one small case series. The authors performed a review including a small subset of matched patients (40) for morphologically identical distal radius plates composed of either stainless or titanium alloy placed by a single surgeon. Although this is a retrospective study, no correlation was found between complications and the material of the implant or the approach.

Summary

The authors have made several decisions over the years regarding choice of implants (Table 1) that are currently in use in their center. Obviously, specific equipment and reduction choices must be made within the capabilities of the operating surgeon, but the wide array of options and approaches means that almost all distal radius fractures can be fixed and held in place with ORIF. Whether this procedure is required or can reliably be accomplished with good functional outcome is open to debate until clinically relevant questions are answered by appropriately powered well-designed studies. Whether plate placement and the newer locking devices have given ORIF a better outcome for the patients has yet to be determined.

References

[1] Knirk JL, Jupiter JB. Intra-articular fractures of the distal end of the radius in young adults. J Bone Joint Surg Am 1986;68(5):647–59.

[2] Pogue DJ, Viegas SF, Patterson RM, et al. Effects of distal radius fracture malunion on wrist joint mechanics. J Hand Surg [Am] 1990;15(5):721–7.

[3] Prommersberger KJ, Lanz U. [Biomechanical aspects of malunited distal radius fracture. A review of the literature]. Handchir Mikrochir Plast Chir 1999;31(4):221–6 [German].

[4] McQueen M, Caspers J. Colles fracture: does the anatomical result affect the final function? J Bone Joint Surg Br 1988;70(4):649–51.

[5] Kapoor H, Agarwal A, Dhaon BK. Displaced intra-articular fractures of distal radius: a comparative evaluation of results following closed reduction, external fixation and open reduction with internal fixation. Injury 2000;31(2):75–9.

[6] Kazuki K, Kusunoki M, Yamada J, et al. Cineradiographic study of wrist motion after fracture of the distal radius. J Hand Surg [Am] 1993;18(1):41–6.

[7] Board T, Kocialkowski A, Andrew G. Does Kapandji wiring help in older patients? A retrospective comparative review of displaced intra-articular distal radial fractures in patients over 55 years. Injury 1999;30(10):663–9.

[8] Stoffelen DV, Broos PL. Closed reduction versus Kapandji-pinning for extra-articular distal radial fractures. J Hand Surg [Br] 1999;24(1):89–91.

[9] Gliatis JD, Plessas SJ, Davis TR. Outcome of distal radial fractures in young adults. J Hand Surg [Br] 2000;25(6):535–43.

[10] Taleisnik J, Watson HK. Midcarpal instability caused by malunited fractures of the distal radius. J Hand Surg [Am] 1984;9(3):350–7.

[11] Drobetz H, Bryant AL, Pokorny T, et al. Volar fixed-angle plating of distal radius extension fractures: influence of plate position on secondary loss of reduction—a biomechanic study in a cadaveric model. J Hand Surg [Am] 2006;31(4):615–22.

[12] Gradl G, Jupiter JB, Gierer P, et al. Fractures of the distal radius treated with a nonbridging external fixation technique using multiplanar k-wires. J Hand Surg [Am] 2005;30(5):960–8.

[13] Handoll HH, Madhok R. Surgical interventions for treating distal radial fractures in adults. Cochrane Database Syst Rev 2003;3:CD003209.

[14] Hastings H 2nd, Leibovic SJ. Indications and techniques of open reduction. Internal fixation of distal radius fractures. Orthop Clin North Am 1993;24(2):309–26.

[15] Kamath AF, Zurakowski D, Day CS. Low-profile dorsal plating for dorsally angulated distal radius fractures: an outcomes study. J Hand Surg [Am] 2006;31(7):1061–7.

[16] Konrath GA, Bahler S. Open reduction and internal fixation of unstable distal radius fractures: results using the trimed fixation system. J Orthop Trauma 2002;16(8):578–85.

[17] McQueen MM. Non-spanning external fixation of the distal radius. Hand Clin 2005;21(3):375–80.

[18] McQueen MM, Simpson D, Court-Brown CM. Use of the Hoffman 2 compact external fixator in the treatment of redisplaced unstable distal radial fractures. J Orthop Trauma 1999;13(7):501–5.

[19] Orbay JL, Touhami A. Current concepts in volar fixed-angle fixation of unstable distal radius fractures. Clin Orthop Relat Res 2006;445:58–67.

[20] Rikli DA, Regazzoni P. The double plating technique for distal radius fractures. Tech Hand Up Extrem Surg 2000;4(2):107–14.

[21] Schnall SB, Kim BJ, Abramo A, et al. Fixation of distal radius fractures using a fragment-specific system. Clin Orthop Relat Res 2006;445:51–7.

[22] Tornetta P 3rd, Klein DM, Stein AB, et al. Distal radius fracture. J Orthop Trauma 2002;16(8):608–11.

[23] Jupiter JB, Fernandez DL, Whipple TL, et al. Intra-articular fractures of the distal radius: contemporary perspectives. Instr Course Lect 1998;47:191–202.

[24] Kamano M, Honda Y, Kazuki K, et al. Palmar plating for dorsally displaced fractures of the distal radius. Clin Orthop Relat Res 2002;397:403–8.

[25] Rikli DA, Regazzoni P. Fractures of the distal end of the radius treated by internal fixation and early function. A preliminary report of 20 cases. J Bone Joint Surg Br 1996;78(4):588–92.

[26] Jupiter JB. Plate fixation of fractures of the distal aspect of the radius: relative indications. J Orthop Trauma 1999;13(8):559–69.

[27] Campbell DA. Open reduction and internal fixation of intra articular and unstable fractures of the distal radius using the AO distal radius plate. J Hand Surg [Br] 2000;25(6):528–34.

[28] Heim D. [Plate osteosynthesis of distal radius fractures–incidence, indications and results]. Swiss Surg 2000;6(6):304–14 [German].

[29] Hove LM, Nilsen PT, Furnes O, et al. Open reduction and internal fixation of displaced intra-articular fractures of the distal radius. 31 patients followed for 3-7 years. Acta Orthop Scand 1997;68(1):59–63.

[30] Cohen MS, Turner TM, Urban RM. Effects of implant material and plate design on tendon function and morphology. Clin Orthop Relat Res 2006;445: 81–90.

[31] Lenoble E, Dumontier C, Goutallier D, et al. Fracture of the distal radius. A prospective comparison between trans-styloid and Kapandji fixations. J Bone Joint Surg Br 1995;77(4):562–7.

[32] Jupiter JB, Fernandez DL, Toh CL, et al. Operative treatment of volar intra-articular fractures of the distal end of the radius. J Bone Joint Surg Am 1996; 78(12):1817–28.

[33] Keating JF, Court-Brown CM, McQueen MM. Internal fixation of volar-displaced distal radial fractures. J Bone Joint Surg Br 1994;76(3):401–5.

[34] Taylor KF, Parks BG, Segalman KA. Biomechanical stability of a fixed-angle volar plate versus fragment-specific fixation system: cyclic testing in a C2-type distal radius cadaver fracture model. J Hand Surg [Am] 2006;31(3):373–81.

[35] Benson EC, DeCarvalho A, Mikola EA, et al. Two potential causes of EPL rupture after distal radius volar plate fixation. Clin Orthop Relat Res 2006; 451:218–22.

[36] Rozental T, Blazar P. Functional outcome and complications after volar plating for dorsally displaced, unstable fractures of the distal radius. J Hand Surg [Am] 2006;31(3):359–65.

[37] Dodds SD, Cornelissen S, Jossan S, et al. A biomechanical comparison of fragment-specific fixation and augmented external fixation for intra-articular distal radius fractures. J Hand Surg [Am] 2002; 27(6):953–64.

[38] Benson LS, Minihane KP, Stern LD, et al. The outcome of intra-articular distal radius fractures treated with fragment-specific fixation. J Hand Surg [Am] 2006;31(8):1333–9.

[39] Jakob M, Rikli DA, Regazzoni P. Fractures of the distal radius treated by internal fixation and early function. A prospective study of 73 consecutive patients. J Bone Joint Surg Br 2000;82(3):340–4.

[40] Prommersberger KJ, van Schoonhoven J, Lanz UB. A radiovolar approach to dorsal malunions of the distal radius. Tech Hand Up Extrem Surg 2000; 4(4):236–43.

[41] Burke EF, Singer RM. Treatment of comminuted distal radius with the use of an internal distraction plate. Tech Hand Up Extrem Surg 1998;2(4): 248–52.

[42] Ginn TA, Ruch DS, Yang CC, et al. Use of a distraction plate for distal radial fractures with metaphyseal and diaphyseal comminution. Surgical technique. J Bone Joint Surg Am 2006;88(Suppl 1 Pt 1):29–36.

[43] Ruch DS, Ginn TA, Yang CC, et al. Use of a distraction plate for distal radial fractures with metaphyseal and diaphyseal comminution. J Bone Joint Surg Am 2005;87(5):945–54.

[44] Hanel DP, Lu TS, Weil WM. Bridge plating of distal radius fractures: the Harborview method. Clin Orthop Relat Res 2006;445:91–9.

[45] Brooks KR, Capo JT, Warburton M, et al. Internal fixation of distal radius fractures with novel intramedullary implants. Clin Orthop Relat Res 2006;445: 42–50.

[46] Orbay JL, Touhami A, Orbay C. Fixed angle fixation of distal radius fractures through a minimally invasive approach. Tech Hand Up Extrem Surg 2005;9(3):142–8.

[47] Mudgal CS, Jupiter JB. Plate and screw design in fractures of the hand and wrist. Clin Orthop Relat Res 2006;445:68–80.

[48] Sinicropi SM, Su BW, Raia FJ, et al. The effects of implant composition on extensor tenosynovitis in a canine distal radius fracture model. J Hand Surg [Am] 2005;30(2):300–7.

[49] Nazzal A, Lozano-Calderon S, Jupiter JB, et al. A histologic analysis of the effects of stainless steel and titanium implants adjacent to tendons: an experimental rabbit study. J Hand Surg [Am] 2006;31(7): 1123–30.

Management of Post-Traumatic Malunion of Fractures of the Distal Radius

Bradley E. Slagel, MD, Suriya Luenam, MD, David R. Pichora, MD, FRCSC*

Division of Orthopaedic Surgery, Kingston General Hospital, Room 9-311, 76 Stuart Street, Queen's University, Kingston, Ontario, K7L 2V7, Canada

Fractures of the distal radius are a common occurrence, composing 10% to 12% of all fractures [1,2]. In spite of being seen as routine, a large retrospective study found that only 2.9% of 2132 individuals who had Colles' fractures were free from permanent loss of function [2]. Malunion and post-traumatic arthritis are the most commonly seen sequelae. After reviewing several studies, Amadio and Botte [3] quoted a pooled average malunion rate of 23.5% for conservatively treated distal radius fractures. In those managed operatively the risk decreased to 10.1% [3].

Distal radius malunion has been extensively reviewed in the literature, with several articles elucidating the natural history, evaluation, and treatment options [3–12]. In this article the authors strive to provide an overview of the literature surrounding distal radius malunions, while highlighting areas that have not been reviewed as extensively; including intra-articular malunion, computer-assisted techniques, bone graft alternatives, and volar fixed-angle plate osteosynthesis.

Extra-articular malunion

Anatomy

The anatomy of the distal radius and its associated radiographic measurements are well-known (Fig. 1). The distal radius typically has a radial tilt of 11° to 12° volar, a radial inclination of 22° to 23°, and a radial length of 11 to 12 mm [13–17]. Often the ulnar variance is used in place of measuring radial length [18]. The normal ulnar variance varies among individuals, and is best determined by comparison with the contralateral limb.

Graham [19] has defined acceptable parameters of the distal radius as: ulnar variance of less than 5 mm compared with the contralateral wrist, radial inclination on the posteroanterior (PA) radiograph greater than 15°, and radial tilt measured on the lateral radiograph between 15° dorsal and 20° volar.

Kinematics

Eighty percent of the joint reactive force across the wrist is borne by the radiocarpal joint [20]. Radial shortening has been associated with alteration of force transfer across the wrist, pain, and decreased rotation. Loss of radial length is seen by some as the most important cause of symptoms in distal radius malunion [1,6,21]. Palmer and Werner [22] have shown an increase of 18% to 42% in the force borne by the distal ulna, with a relative shortening of 2.5 mm of the radius. As the radius shortens relative to the ulna, the triangular fibrocartilage complex (TFCC) becomes tighter and the distal radioulnar joint (DRUJ) is disrupted, leading to pain and loss of forearm rotation [23–25]. Shortening of 6 to 8 mm causes the ulna to impinge on the triquetrum or the extreme ulnar aspect of the lunate [6,26–28]. Bronstein and colleagues [29] found that 10 mm of shortening resulted in a mean 47% loss of pronation and 29% loss of supination. The DRUJ was effectively locked by ulnocarpal abutment at 15 mm of shortening. In a study of 61 Colles'

* Corresponding author.
  E-mail address: pichorad@kgh.kari.net (D.R. Pichora).

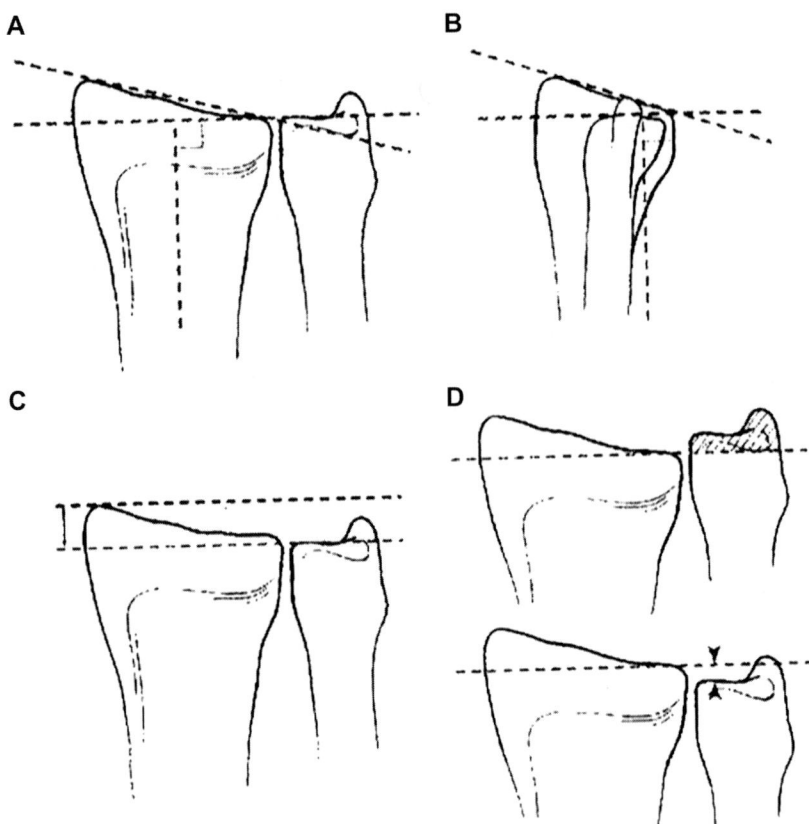

Fig. 1. Standard measurements of the distal radius. (*A*) Radial inclination. (*B*) Volar tilt. (*C*) Radial length. (*D*) Ulnar variance. (*From* Sharpe F, Stevanovic M. Extra-articular distal radial fracture malunion. Hand Clinics 2005;21:472; with permission.)

fractures, Jenkins and Mintowt-Czyz [30] found that a mean shortening of 4.7 mm led to increased wrist pain. Four to 5 mm of shortening appears to be a threshold to the onset of wrist symptoms. There is general agreement that radial shortening of greater than 5 mm leads to unsatisfactory outcomes [1,7–10,23,25,28–33].

Dorsal angulation is by far the most common deformity seen in distal radius malunion [3]. Despite its frequency, there is a vast disagreement in the acceptable parameters of dorsal angulation, ranging from 0° to 30° [1,7,8,16,23,28,32,34,35]. As dorsal angulation increases, the load distribution shifts from volar-radial to dorsal-ulnar [10,20,22,36–38]. In a cadaveric study, Short and colleagues [20] demonstrated that the load through the ulna increased from 21% at 10° of volar tilt to 67% at 45° of dorsal tilt. At 30° of dorsal angulation, 50% of the load was borne by the ulna. In a similar study, Miyake and colleagues [38] concluded that osteotomy to decrease abnormal wrist loading should be conducted when dorsal angulation exceeds 20°. Increased dorsal tilt also affects the DRUJ and the midcarpal joint. Abnormalities of statistical significance in rotation and instability of the DRUJ have been demonstrated at 20° to 30° of dorsal angulation [39,40]. Bronstein and colleagues [29] did not find a significant change in forearm rotation as dorsal tilt increased to 30°. They suggested that the decreased rotation observed clinically may relate to subacute capsular scarring. As dorsal tilt increases, there is a tendency for the midcarpal joint to compensate by flexing, leading to painful synovitis at the midcarpal level and a dorsal intercalary segment instability (DISI) type deformity [7,16,41,42]. This deformity is classed into a lax, reducible form that corrects with osteotomy, and a nonreducible form that remains unchanged with osteotomy [3]. Increased volar tilt

(Smith's fracture) leads to decreased wrist extension and dorsal subluxation of the ulnar head, which restricts supination [7,27].

Change in the radial inclination of the wrist affects grip strength, range of motion in radial/ulnar deviation, and distribution of load on the wrist. A deformity of the radial inclination alters the position of the carpal tunnel, and thus the flexor tendons, leading to a mechanical disadvantage and weaker grip strength [7,30,43,44]. Disabling decreases in ulnar deviation of the wrist are seen at radial inclinations less than or equal to 0° [3,7]. Pogue and colleagues [26] have shown that as radial inclination decreases, there is increased load borne by the lunate facet and decreased load borne by the scaphoid facet. In their long-term follow-up of distal radius fractures, Altissimi and colleagues [31] found that 100% of their fair and poor results had less than 5° of radial inclination.

Goals and indications

The goal of extra-articular osteotomy is to re-establish the normal kinematics of the midcarpal, radiocarpal, and distal radioulnar joints. This is accomplished by restoring palmar tilt in the sagittal plane and radial inclination in the coronal plane, correcting any rotational malalignment in the horizontal plane, and restoring radial length and DRUJ congruity [6]. It is not sufficient to proceed with osteotomy simply because the radiographic parameters previously mentioned have not been met. Many individuals who have distal radius malunion remain functional and symptom-free [4,8,10]. The decision to proceed with osteotomy should be based on the presence of a symptomatic malunion, or a deformity so severe that pain and dysfunction are inevitable. The indications for extra-articular reconstruction of distal radius malunions include [5,20,23,26,36,45,46]

- Poor radiographic features, including: dorsal tilt >20°, displaced fractures with carpal malalignment (>15° of dorsal angulation of lunate on lateral radiograph), incongruity of the DRUJ, >5 mm of ulnar variance
- Pain—radiocarpal, midcarpal or distal radioulnar
- Decreased range of motion
- Cosmetic deformity
- Young, active individuals who have poor radiographic features, deemed to be at high risk to develop pain, loss of motion and function, and post-traumatic arthritis

Reconstruction is relatively contraindicated in those who have poor general health, advanced post-traumatic arthritis, advanced osteoporosis, and dystrophy [6]; other salvage options may be considered.

Surgical techniques

Dorsally displaced malunion

Opening wedge osteotomy with iliac crest or radius bone graft is the most widely recommended technique for treating distal radius malunion [47,48]. Conventionally, this is accomplished through a dorsal-radial–based opening wedge osteotomy that hinges on the volar-ulnar side of the metaphysis, a procedure that has been repeatedly described in the literature [6–8,10,11]. Recently, with the availability of fixed-angle plates, there is interest in performing these dorsal-opening osteotomies via a volar approach with volar fixation. Computer-assisted distal radius osteotomies are new additions to the options for correcting dorsal distal radius malunions. These are conceptually based on the opening wedge osteotomy and are discussed in detail later.

An alternative option is to perform a closing wedge osteotomy of the radius, which eliminates the need for separate-site bone graft, thus decreasing patient morbidity [49,50]. This is especially advantageous in older patients and in those who have osteopenia and who are at risk of failure of fixation. It is not recommended, however, for high-level athletes or heavy manual workers, because the associated radial shortening may cause decreased grip strength [51]. Traditionally, the radial closing wedge osteotomy was performed with either simultaneous or subsequent resection of the ulnar head, to accommodate closure of the corrective osteotomy and alleviate ulnocarpal impingement symptoms. Unfortunately, this can result in ulnar stump subluxation and instability [52]. An ulnar shortening osteotomy, which preserves the DRUJ and TFCC, may be a better solution [53]. Wada and colleagues [51] reported good functional and radiographic outcomes of five patients treated for symptomatic distal radius malunion with simultaneous radial closing wedge and ulnar shortening osteotomies. The ulnar shortening osteotomy should be performed before completing the reduction and internal fixation of the radius fragments, because the intact ulna will act as a strut, preventing correction of the distal radius [51,54].

Regardless of the chosen surgical method, the prerequisites for a successful outcome include the correct indications, optimal surgical timing, and a meticulous surgical technique. The optimal time to proceed with correction of extra-articular distal radius malunion has evolved over the past 20 years. Initially it was felt that a delay in intervention was most prudent, because many people retain excellent function and are pain-free in spite of radiologic deformity [5,7,8,26,31]. It was also recognized, however, that a delay in treatment leads to soft-tissue contracture [55,56] and dysfunction of the distal radial ulnar joint [8,57,58], ultimately making surgery more difficult and potentially compromising the final result. Jupiter and Ring [5] addressed this dilemma in their retrospective study comparing 10 early (6–14 weeks) and 10 late reconstructions (30–48 weeks). The overall functional and radiographic outcomes were similar, although early intervention significantly reduced the delay in returning to work. The greatest advantage to early reconstruction was ease of correction, because the soft tissues remained compliant. Early osteotomy was recommended for those who have high functional demands, regardless of age. In the correction of long-standing malunion the authors have found, along with others [59], that releasing the brachioradialis and if also needed, the pronator quadratus tendons, may be instrumental to achieving appropriate corrections.

Volarly displaced malunion

Given the rarity of Smith's fractures as compared with Colles' fractures, it is not surprising that the literature is sparse in studies detailing the correction of volarly angulated malunions. The most common technique for correcting volarly displaced distal radius malunions is with a volar opening wedge osteotomy. The technique is similar to a dorsal opening wedge osteotomy, and is well-described in the retrospective review conducted by Shea and colleagues [60]. They found significant improvement in grip strength, forearm supination and pronation, and wrist extension following the corrective osteotomy.

An alternative technique has been described by Thiavaios and McKee [61], who advocate the use of a sliding osteotomy for volar malunions. They use a volar approach and make an oblique osteotomy designed to recreate the original fracture. The distal fragment is then slid into the appropriate position and fixed with Kirschner wires (K-wires). A ridge of bone remains anteriorly on the proximal fragment, which is removed and used as bone graft if necessary. A contoured volar buttress plate T-plate is applied as definitive fixation. Their results showed significant increases in grip strength, range of motion, and functional outcome [61]. They emphasize that volar malunions are fundamentally different from dorsal malunions, in that there is a lesser degree of impaction and metaphyseal bone loss in Smith's fractures, which allows for a sliding correction that often does not require bone graft.

Disorders of the distal radioulnar joint associated with distal radial malunion

Incongruity, impaction, and instability of the distal radioulnar joint are common causes of pain and limited forearm rotation in distal radius malunion [10]. These may present in isolation or in combination. Careful clinical assessment of the joint is necessary to localize the source of ulnar-sided pain. Several procedures have been described to treat DRUJ dysfunction, including the Darrach procedure [62–66], the hemiresection and interposition arthroplasty [10,67], matched distal resection of the ulna [68–70], Sauvé-Kapandji procedure [63,71,72], and ulnar head replacement [10,65,73,74]. Each of these procedures has encountered mixed results, which has led to controversy regarding the optimal treatment.

When symptomatic intra-articular incongruity of the DRUJ is seen on plain radiographs or CT scans, a resection arthroplasty, a Sauvé-Kapandji procedure, or a prosthetic replacement is indicated, depending on the severity of the degenerative changes and the patient's age, hand dominance, and occupation [10]. Total resection of the ulnar head (the Darrach procedure) still has a place in the treatment of derangement or osteoarthritis of the DRUJ in elderly patients. In this age group, the disadvantages of this operation (reduction of grip strength, ulnar impingement, and painful radioulnar instability) are remarkably well-tolerated [62,75]. Several studies suggest that overaggressive resection of the ulna (>30 mm) may potentiate symptomatic radioulnar impingement, a complication less likely in patients who have an ulnar stump that resides within the sigmoid notch cavity [66,76–79]. Ulnar stump morphology may also be an important determinant of whether impingement is symptomatic. If the ulnar osteotomy has sharp edges, the forces producing impingement are concentrated in a focal area, and may be more likely to produce symptoms. Contact stress may be diminished by rounding or tapering the ulnar stump [68,69]. The sheath of the extensor carpi ulnaris tendon should be closed carefully to prevent dorsal subluxation. Radioulnar impingement after distal ulna resection may manifest radiographically as a shallow groove or scalloping of the ulnar side of the radius and sclerosis of the ulnar stump [76,77,79]. To confirm radioulnar impingement, Lees and Scheker [80] have suggested obtaining a radiograph of the forearm taken with the patient holding a 2.2-kg weight with the shoulder adducted, the elbow flexed to 90°, and the forearm in neutral rotation.

Radioulnar instability is often recognized as a dorsal deformity of the wrist and forearm, and has also been identified as a source of pain [81]. Although frequently described as dorsal subluxation of the ulna, the deformity is better understood as volar subluxation of the radius relative to the ulna when the forearm is pronated [82,83].

A variety of procedures have been developed to address the adverse sequelae of painful radioulnar instability. Arthroplasty of the DRUJ is increasingly used to treat the failed Darrach operation, and appears to produce acceptable clinical results while maintaining functional pronosupination [10]. Further follow-up will be required to determine the durability of prosthetic replacement of the DRUJ. The Sauvé-Kapandji procedure [63,71,72] (fusion of the distal radioulnar joint with creation of a proximal ulnar pseudarthrosis) has several theoretical advantages over the Darrach procedure. It preserves a more physiologic pattern of force transmission from the hand to the forearm by maintaining the ulnocarpal buttress, preserving the TFCC and the origin of the ulnocarpal ligaments, and allowing the extensor carpi ulnaris to remain in its compartment. Although there are conflicting results, most authors recommend that this technique be used in younger patients who have high functional demands on the wrist and forearm [65,84–87]. The Sauvé-Kapandji procedure should be regarded as a reliable method for restoring forearm rotation, but as inconsistent at relieving pain [88].

Much has been written about problems of the ulnar stump associated with the Sauvé-Kapandji procedure [71,89,90]. Pain and clicking of the ulnar stump is common, but is often described as a minor inconvenience [71,86,89]. Instability of the ulnar stump post–Sauvé-Kapandji may be caused by secondary incompetence of the static (interosseous membrane) and dynamic (extensor carpi ulnaris [ECU], flexor carpi ulnaris [FCU], and pronator quadratus) supports of the ulnar stump. Intraperiosteal resection has been advocated in an attempt to increase stability [90]. It would seem logical that Kapandji's recommendation of leaving a short distal ulnar fragment, fashioning the ulnar gap as far distally as possible, and creating a pseudarthrosis of approximately 10 mm, would reduce instability and retain grip strength [71]. The incidence of bridging heterotopic calcification of the pseudarthrosis may be reduced by careful periosteal resection, the elimination of "sawdust," and soft-tissue interposition [10,27]. Some studies indicate that there is no increased risk of ossification in the pseudarthrosis when an intraperiosteal excision is accomplished [88].

A partial resection of the ulnar head or Bowers hemiresection interpositional technique should be reserved for patients who make low demands on the wrist [10]. The Bowers hemiresection does not alter the ulnar variance, and therefore an additional ulnar shortening procedure, either at the styloid level or at the ulnar shaft, should be done with this procedure to prevent impingement of the ulnar styloid on the carpus [9,10].

The recently developed ulnar head prosthesis has been used to prevent radioulnar instability and maintain ulnar support for the carpus after ulnar head resection. A normally oriented sigmoid notch and adequate soft-tissue coverage are required to maintain the congruity of the prosthesis. Thus a radial osteotomy is required in the presence of metaphyseal deformity [10,91]. The ulnar prosthesis can also be used in combination with an annular ligament reconstruction for the treatment of patients who have painful radioulnar impingement following Darrach or Sauvé-Kapandji procedures [10].

Extra-articular incongruity of the distal radioulnar joint is managed by restoration of radial anatomy and reorientation of the sigmoid notch to the ulnar head with a radial osteotomy. If osteotomy has restored full passive pronation and supination, a stable DRUJ, and a normal anatomic relationship between the sigmoid notch and the ulnar head, then no additional surgery is necessary [10]. Arthroscopic evaluation and repair of the TFCC are indicated, however, if the DRUJ remains unstable [52].

In cases with only axial shortening, ulnocarpal impaction is managed by restoring the radioulnar length discrepancy to a physiological ulnar variance, as dictated by the study of the radiographs of the patient's unaffected wrist. A shortening osteotomy of the ulna is preferred if there is an ulnar variance of greater than 2 mm, whereas the more minimally invasive arthroscopic partial ulnar head resection (wafer) is an alternative if the ulnar variance is less [52,65,92]. If the wafer procedure is used, one must be certain that the full circumference of the ulnar head is resected; however, in cases with additional wear of the luno-triquetral ligament, an ulnar shortening osteotomy to stabilize the entire ulnocarpal complex is recommended [52]. Prerequisites for a shortening osteotomy of the ulna are a well-oriented sigmoid notch in both the frontal and the sagittal plane, and an absence of intra-articular step-offs or degenerative changes [9,10].

Intra-articular malunion

Intra-articular involvement (radiocarpal or radioulnar) is present in approximately 60% of distal radius fractures [57]. Cadaveric studies have shown that contact stress is significantly increased with 1 mm of lunate facet depression [93] and 3 mm of intra-articular step from a coronal fracture (simulated dorsal Barton's) [94]. There is a large body of clinical literature indicating that intra-articular incongruity greater than 1 or 2 mm leads to radiographic signs of arthritis and a poor result [95–101]. In a randomized controlled trial of distal radius fracture treatment, Kreder and colleagues [95] observed that the likelihood of arthritis was 10.4 times greater in those who had an articular step greater than 2 mm, as compared with those who had a step of less than 2 mm. Knirk and Jupiter [99] found a 91% incidence of radiographic arthritis in those who had an intra-articular step greater than 1 mm, and a 100% incidence in those who had a step greater than 2 mm. Trumble and colleagues [100] noted that the single most important factor precluding a good functional outcome is joint incongruity. Others, however, have found that patient function was not hindered, despite joint incongruity and radiographic arthritis [102,103]. In addition to arthritis, malunited Barton's fractures often result in volar or dorsal carpal subluxation [8]. Collapse of the lunate facet is associated with palmar rotation of the lunate, frequently resulting in a volar intercalary segment instability (VISI) type of carpal instability [7].

Goals and indications

The goals of intra-articular osteotomy are restoration of articular congruity and preservation of articular cartilage to maintain a functional, pain-free wrist. The indications for correction of intra-articular malunion are [4,61,104–106]: (1) articular incongruity of 2 mm or greater on PA view of distal radius, and (2) articular incongruity in the coronal plane with subluxation of the radiocarpal joint.

Some advocate operating if 1 mm of incongruity is present [93,100]. Intra-articular osteotomy is contraindicated in those who have established, advanced arthrosis; or slight malunions in relatively nonarticular areas (between the scaphoid and lunate facets); in low-demand and infirm patients; in those greater than 70 years of age who have few symptoms and adequate function; and in those who have complicating factors (poor bone stock, mutilating soft-tissue injury) [45,104].

Imaging

The majority of authors reporting on distal radius malunion are in agreement on the indications for osteotomy and the importance of decreasing the intra-articular step to less than 1 to 2 mm. This becomes irrelevant, however, if one is unable to measure the intra-articular step. Kreder and colleagues [107] and Cole and colleagues [108] both found poor intraclass correlation coefficients (ICC) for intra- and interobserver agreement on articular step deformity as seen on plain films. In fact, 24% of plain radiographs classified at less than 2 mm of intra-articular step were found to have greater than 2 mm of displacement on CT scan [108]. Agreement on CT images was found to be "substantial" to "almost perfect" [108]. CT scanning is thus recommended to assess intra-articular deformity.

Surgical technique

There have been relatively few articles in the English literature describing intra-articular osteotomy [5,45,61,104,105]. The reluctance to address intra-articular malunion may be related to concerns regarding limited exposure, inadequate fixation, difficulty recreating the fracture, and possible osteonecrosis caused by compromised blood supply to the osteotomized fragment [105]. The retrospective case series conducted by Ring and colleagues [105] contains 23 patients, and is the largest of the intra-articular distal radius malunion studies. The remainder of the studies contain 5 or fewer patients [5,45,61]. Conceptually all authors used the same operative technique. The fracture is approached from the side of greatest displacement. The original fracture line is recreated either with an osteotome or an oscillating saw. Marx and Axelrod [45] recommend using a dull instrument to differentiate between the hyaline cartilage (firm) and fibrocartilage (soft) on the joint surface. They then suggest removing the fibrocartilage to better appreciate the joint step and to reapproximate the fracture line with K-wires before making the osteotomy. If a dorsal approach is used, the reduction may be observed both fluoroscopically and by direct vision through a dorsal capsulotomy [45,104,105]. If a volar approach is used, the volar radiocarpal ligaments are left intact, and the articular surface is visualized through the osteotomy [104,105]. The authors have found a combination of both volar and dorsal approaches to be helpful on occasion. After having reduced the osteotomized fragment, it is then secured using K-wires, screws, or plate fixation. Given the small numbers of patients in these studies, Ring and colleagues [105] likely have the most reliable results. They had an average follow-up of 38 months postinjury (minimum 24 months). All osteotomies healed without evidence of osteonecrosis. There was significant improvement in range of motion, grip strength (85% of contralateral side), articular congruity, and ulnar variance. There were 19 excellent/good results according to the systems of Fernandez [27] and Gartland and Werley [13]; however, according to the Mayo modification of the Green and O'Brien system [109], there were only 10 excellent/good results. The Green and O'Brien modification is very strict and consistently produces poorer results than the other scoring systems. The authors interpret this difference as indicating that intra-articular osteotomy restores useful function, but rarely restores normal function of the wrist [105].

Intra-articular malunions must have relatively simple geometric patterns to permit reconstruction via intra-articular osteotomy [4]. In cases of multiple intra-articular fragments or die-punch injuries, restoration of the joint surface is quite difficult. Radiolunate [110] and radioscapholunate [4] arthrodeses are salvage options in these patients that allow them to retain some of their wrist motion.

Although perfection cannot be expected, intra-articular osteotomy produces symptomatic and functional improvement in most patients. It remains to be seen whether or not long-term arthrosis will be decreased by correction of the intra-articular malunion. It is important to carefully select the patients who will benefit most from the procedure. Those who have high likelihood of rapid articular surface degeneration and those who have symptomatic malunions but only mild articular cartilage degeneration are appropriate candidates [107]. Individuals who have severe cartilage degeneration, low functional demand, and the elderly are unlikely to benefit from osteotomy, and would be better served by nonoperative treatment and a salvage procedure in the future if necessary.

Intra-articular osteotomy is best performed as soon as the deformity is recognized, in order to preserve the articular surface and facilitate fracture re-creation and fragment reduction [4,7,8,45,104,105]. Because fracture callus is relatively easy to remove within 4 to 6 weeks of injury, the procedure is facilitated by operating within 6 weeks [7,45].

Evolving trends

Computer-assisted techniques

The importance of accurate preoperative planning has been stressed by many [28,101,111–113]. Plain radiographs provide an accurate appreciation of deformity in the coronal and sagittal planes, but are inadequate for complex three-dimensional deformities [100,114]. Several authors have recommended preoperative CT scan to better understand the deformity [108,115]. Three separate authors have attempted to combine CT scanning with computer technology to improve pre-operative planning [101,116,117].

Jupiter and colleagues [101] were the first group to incorporate computer technology with distal radius malunion correction. They reported a case series of five patients wherein computer-aided design/computer-aided manufacturing (CAD/CAM) technology was used to make synthetic bone models replicating the patient's deformity. These models were used to conduct trial osteotomies to gain "hands-on" experience as well as provide the dimensions required for bone graft, and the size and shape of internal fixation. Jupiter and colleagues felt that this technique had potential for providing a more predictable outcome, thus limiting residual disability and its inherent expense.

The authors' group has had a strong interest in computer modeling and computer-assisted techniques for distal radius osteotomies. Athwal and colleagues [116] reported our case series of six computer-assisted distal radius osteotomies. This technique involves conducting CT scans of both the malunited and the contralateral forearms. The scans are then imported into a computer, a virtual osteotomy is created in the malunited bone, and the osteotomized bone is aligned to the contralateral, normal radius. A digitized fixation plate is then positioned in a satisfactory position and the plan saved (Fig. 2). The computer system is brought into the operating theater. The surgeon registers the in vivo malunited distal radius to the virtual model on the computer. Using a calibrated drill, the two proximal and two distal pilot holes for the fixation plate are predrilled with image guidance, as dictated by the preoperative plan. The radius is osteotomized at the predetermined location using image guidance. The plate is then fixed to the distal fragment and the distal fragment/plate complex is distracted until the proximal holes align with the pilot holes drilled in the radius, indicating that the planned correction has been attained. The plate is fixed to the proximal radius and the osteotomy defect is filled with iliac crest cancellous bone graft.

The preoperative goal of this computer-assisted distal radius osteotomy (based on the contralateral radius) was 23° of radial inclination, 10° of volar tilt, and +1.5 mm of ulnar variance. The average postoperative alignment averaged 21° of radial inclination, 9° of volar tilt, and +1.9 mm of ulnar variance. In a follow-up study, the authors [118] have found that there is a proximal radius deformity in distal radius malunions that tends toward radioulnar convergence (Fig. 3). Using standard surgical methods, this convergence is instinctively corrected; however, when using the computer planning method, one must ensure that the radial bow is corrected to match the contralateral side as well. The importance of thorough preoperative planning and precise surgical technique has been well-documented [61,93,94,102,108]. The most significant advantages of this technique of computer-assisted distal radius osteotomy are that it serves as both a means of preoperative planning and as a system of intraoperative guidance.

Rieger and colleagues [117] recently published their case series of 11 patients who underwent distal radius osteotomy assisted by virtual reality preoperative planning. Their technique also involves undergoing a CT scan of both forearms. The images are transferred to a computer, and ultimately to a virtual reality work station that allows the surgeon to practice the osteotomy in a virtual reality setting. The contralateral radius is mirrored onto the osteotomized radius to determine the appropriate correction. The virtual wedge-shaped gap in the osteotomy defect is

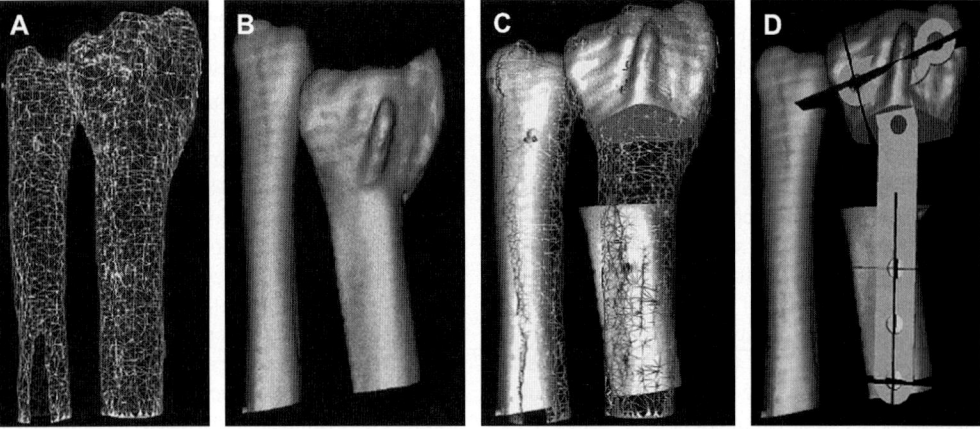

Fig. 2. Computer-assisted distal radius osteotomy planning. (*A*) Computer-assisted 3-dimensional surgical planner uses the contralateral wrist as a template. (*B*) The malunited wrist undergoes a (*C*) virtual osteotomy and is aligned to the template. (*D*) The surgical planner then digitizes a plate onto the realigned radius and saves the coordinates and orientations of the screw holes for intraoperative referencing. (*From* Athwal GS, Ellis RE, Small CF, et al. Computer-assisted distal radiusosteotomy. J Hand Surg 2003;28A:952–3; with permission from The American Society for Surgery of the Hand.)

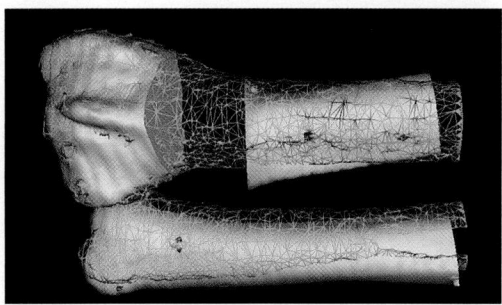

Fig. 3. Radioulnar convergence in distal radius malunion. After having performed the virtual osteotomy, the proximal fragment (*solid*) remains ulnarly deviated compared with the superimposed opposite limb (*mesh*). (*From* Vasarhelyi EM, Athwal GS, Ellis RE, et al. Multiple bone fragment correction in computer-assisted osteotomy to restore the radial bow of a malunion of the distal radius. Presented at Adrian E. Flatt Residents and Fellows Conference, American Society for Surgery of the Hand. New York, September 8, 2004; with permission.)

then calculated, and a synthetic template of stereolithography material is manufactured. During surgery, the osteotomy is performed at the level determined during the virtual procedure. The manufactured spacer is then placed in the defect to produce the appropriate correction. A volar plate is fixated to the bone and the spacer is replaced with bone graft. This procedure ultimately serves as a means of preoperative planning as well as an intraoperative guide to reduction.

Computer-assisted distal radius osteotomy and virtual reality-assisted distal radius osteotomy appear to have potential for improving upon the unassisted methods of correction, because they assist both in the planning phase and in intraoperative guidance. The study of the authors' group and the Rieger and colleagues study cannot be compared directly because their outcomes are reported differently; however, in both cases, all of their patients were satisfied, showed improved range of motion, and were corrected to normal radiographic parameters [116,117]. A larger series of patients will be required to determine whether or not these techniques demonstrate significant improvements on the unassisted techniques.

Volar fixed-angle plate osteosynthesis

The introduction of volar fixed-angle plating in 2000 has provided an effective means of treating dorsal and volar distal radius fractures [119]. The volar approach is less disruptive to the nearby tendons than the dorsal approach, because there is more space available for the plate on the volar surface of the distal radius [120]. The use of a fixed-angle plate permits the surgeon to place the plate on the unstable (volar) side of the fracture [119,121,122]. Traditionally structural corticocancellous iliac crest structural bone graft has been required to stabilize distal radius osteotomies [3,7,9,10,28,100,116]. Volar fixed-angle plating permits the surgeon to use cancellous bone graft rather than cortical graft, because thicker, stronger plates may be placed in the volar space [59,120]. Although mentioned in three review articles [4,12,123], it was not until recently that a clinical study of volar fixed-angle plating for distal radius osteotomy was published [59].

Malone and colleagues [59] conducted a case series of four distal radius malunions corrected by volar fixed-angle plates (SCS/V plate, Avanta Orthopaedics, San Diego, California). A volar approach was used, and the distal plate holes were predrilled. The osteotomy was then made, and the distal portion of the plate was applied to the bone. The plate and distal fragment were then moved as a unit, and normal anatomy was restored using plate reduction technique. The proximal sliding hole was secured to allow for slight modifications. Once the surgeon was satisfied with the position, the remaining proximal holes were filled with screws, and cancellous bone graft was placed into the osteotomy defect. Their patients were splinted for 2 weeks and then weaned out of the splint as tolerated. At an average follow-up of 13.5 months Malone and colleagues found improved disabilities of the arm, shoulder, and hand (DASH) scores (from 30 to 7, retrospectively completed), and improved visual analog pain scores from 4.5 to 1 (also retrospective). Final radiographic parameters were 2° of dorsal tilt, 24° of radial inclination, and 1 mm of ulnar variance. These values were unchanged from postoperative radiographs. Bone graft incorporation was seen at an average of 12 weeks.

This study demonstrates that volar fixed-angle plating maintains correction with the use of cancellous bone graft. The plate, however, does not seem to have the strength required to be used to obtain the reduction. Malone and colleagues describe that the contour of the plate changed during the procedure, presumably during the reduction maneuver and fixation [59]. Regardless, the volar fixed-angle plating technique shows promise as a method of fixation that may reduce the need for cortical bone graft. Use of a stronger plate or a different reduction technique would likely improve the volar tilt.

The authors, having observed two cases of flexor tendon rupture, have found that although volar plating may decrease the risk of problems associated with hardware prominence, it certainly does not eliminate them completely. Further study is required in this area.

Bone graft alternatives

The use of autogenous iliac crest cancellous or corticocancellous bone graft is fairly standard in distal radius osteotomies [28,124]. Several problems have been identified and documented regarding this approach, including donor site morbidity, delayed union at the bone-graft interfaces, and size mismatch between the graft and the osteotomy defect [125,126]. One means of avoiding structural corticocancellous graft is to use a locking plate with cancellous bone graft, as described above. This requires reliance on the locking plate to transmit the axial force from the distal to the proximal radius, because the cancellous graft does not provide structural support [59]. The authors have gradually moved from corticocancellous to cancellous graft use combined with a locking plate, and have thus far found positive results.

During the past few years several different types of substitutive grafts have been used in opening wedge osteotomies as substitutes for bone graft [127,128]. The main advantages of bone graft substitutes are shorter surgical times and decreased iliac crest morbidity [129]. Carbonated hydroxyapatite and calcium phosphate have been reported as bone substitutes for corrective distal radius osteotomy [129,130]. These should be used in conjunction with K-wires or plates, because their structural support is inadequate on their own [131–133]. The proper containment of this biosynthetic material should be enhanced by the presence of the volarly positioned pronator quadratus muscle and dorsally by an extensor retinaculum flap [129]. Luchetti and colleagues [129] found a minimal loss of volar tilt with use of carbonated hydroxyapatite and K-wires, but this did not prove to be a problem clinically.

Another option is to avoid grafting altogether. Wieland and colleagues [127] reported successful correction of malunions in 47 patients, achieved by an opening wedge osteotomy with stable buttress plate fixation without bone grafting. All osteotomies healed without evidence of nonunion within 3 months. Reduction was maintained postoperatively, in spite of patients being mobilized after 10 days. This technique seems very attractive; however, its reproducibility has not yet been evaluated.

To the best of the authors' knowledge, there have not been any studies published on osteoinductive materials (eg, bone morphogenic protein) in distal radius osteotomies. We have relied thus far on autograft, and have little experience with graft substitutes. The limited number of clinical studies currently limits adequate comparison of these alternatives to conventional autogenous bone graft. Further study is required to validate these techniques.

Summary

The treatment of distal radius malunions is continually evolving. The advent of new computer technologies, plating systems, and bone graft substitutes will likely have a significant impact upon the way distal radius malunions are corrected in the near future. Prevention of malunion through optimal fracture management remains the best option.

References

[1] Lidstrom A. Fractures of the distal end of the radius. Acta Orthop Scand 1959;41S:58–118.
[2] Bacorn RW, Kurtzke JF. Colles' fracture: a study of two thousand cases from the New York state workmen's compensation board. J Bone Joint Surg Am 1953;35:643–58.
[3] Amadio PC, Botte MJ. Treatment of malunion of the distal radius. Hand Clin 1987;3(4):541–61.
[4] Ring D. Treatment of the neglected distal radius fracture. Clin Orthop 2005;431:85–92.
[5] Jupiter JB, Ring D. A Comparison of early and late reconstruction of malunited fractures of the distal end of the radius. J Bone Joint Surg Am 1996;78:739–48.
[6] Jupiter JB, Masem M. Reconstruction of post-traumatic deformity of the distal radius and ulna. Hand Clin 1988;4(3):377–90.
[7] Fernandez DL. Malunion of the distal radius: current approach to management. Instr Course Lect 1993;42:99–113.
[8] Fernandez DL. Reconstructive procedures for malunion and traumatic arthritis. Orthop Clin North Am 1993;24(2):341–63.
[9] Hutchinson F III. Malunions of the distal radius: treatment options. J South Orthop Assoc 1995;4(1):53–68.
[10] Jupiter JB, Fernandez DL. Complications following distal radial fractures. Instr Course Lect 2002;51:203–19.

[11] Sharpe F, Stevanovic M. Extra-articular distal radial fracture malunion. Hand Clin 2005;21:469–87.
[12] Fernandez DL, Wolfe W. Chapter 16—Distal radius fractures. In: Green DP, Hotchkiss RN, Pederson WC, et al, editors. Green's operative hand surgery, vol. 1. 5th edition. Philadelphia: Elsevier Churchill Livingstone; 2005. p. 645–710.
[13] Gartland JJ Jr, Werley CW. Evaluation of healed Colles' fractures. J Bone Joint Surg Am 1951;33: 895–907.
[14] Dowling JJ, Sawyer B. Comminuted Colles' fractures: evaluation of method of treatment. J Bone Joint Surg Am 1961;43:657–68.
[15] Friberg S, Lundstrom B. Radiographic measurements of the radiocarpal joint in normal adults. Acta Radiol Diagn (Stockh) 1976;17(2):249–56.
[16] Taleisnik J, Watson HK. Midcarpal instability caused by malunited fractures of the distal radius. J Hand Surg [Am] 1984;9:350–7.
[17] Scheck M. Long-term follow-up of treatment comminuted fractures of the distal end of the radius by transfixion with Kirschner wires and cast. J Bone Joint Surg Am 1962;44:337–51.
[18] Palmer AK, Glisson RR, Werner FW. Ulnar variance determination. J Hand Surg [Am] 1982;7: 376–9.
[19] Graham T. Surgical correction of malunited fractures of the distal radius. J Am Acad Orthop Surg 1997;5(5):270–81.
[20] Short WH, Palmer AK, Werner FW, et al. A biomechanical study of distal radial fractures. J Hand Surg [Am] 1987;12:529–34.
[21] Milch H. Treatment of disabilities following fracture of the lower end of the radius. Clin Orthop 1963;29:157–63.
[22] Palmer AK, Werner FW. Biomechanics of the distal radioulnar joint. Clin Orthop 1984;18:26–35.
[23] af Ekenstam F, Hagert CG, Engkvist O, et al. Corrective osteotomy of malunited fractures of the distal end of the radius. Scand J Plast Reconstr Surg 1985;19:175–87.
[24] Melone CP Jr. Articular fractures of the distal radius. Orthop Clin North Am 1984;15:217–36.
[25] Adams BD. Effects of radial deformity on distal radioulnar joint mechanics. J Hand Surg [Am] 1993;18:492–8.
[26] Pogue DJ, Viegas SF, Patterson RM, et al. Effects of distal radius fracture malunion on wrist joint kinematics. J Hand Surg [Am] 1990;15:721–7.
[27] Fernandez DL. Radial osteotomy and Bowers arthroplasty for malunited fractures of the distal end of the radius. J Bone Joint Surg Am 1988;70: 1538–51.
[28] Fernandez DL. Correction of post-traumatic wrist deformity in adults by osteotomy, bone-grafting, and internal fixation. J Bone Joint Surg Am 1982; 64:1164–78.
[29] Bronstein AJ, Trumble TE, Tencer AF. The effects of distal radius fracture malalignment on forearm rotation: a cadaveric study. J Hand Surg [Am] 1997;22:258–62.
[30] Jenkins NH, Mintowt-Czyz WJ. Mal-union and dysfunction in Colles' fracture. J Hand Surg [Br] 1988;13:291–3.
[31] Altissimi M, Antenucci R, Fiacca C, et al. Long-term results of conservative treatment of fractures of the distal radius. Clin Orthop 1986;206:202–10.
[32] DePalma AF. Comminuted fractures of the distal end of the radius treated by ulnar pinning. J Bone Joint Surg Am 1952;34:651–62.
[33] Linscheid RL, Dobyns JH. Radiolunate arthrodesis. J Hand Surg [Am] 1985;10:821–9.
[34] Hobart MH, Kraft GL. Malunited Colles' fracture. Am J Surg 1941;53:55–60.
[35] Bora FW Jr, Osterman AL, Zielinski CJ. Osteotomy of the distal radius with a biplanar iliac bone graft for malunion. Bull Hosp Jt Dis Orthop Inst 1984;44:122–31.
[36] Kazuki K, Kusunoki M, Yamada J, et al. Cineradiographic study of wrist motion after fracture of the distal radius. J Hand Surg [Am] 1993;18:41–6.
[37] Kazuki K, Kusunoki M, Shimazu A. Pressure distribution in the radiocarpal joint measured with a densitometer designed for pressure sensitive film. J Hand Surg [Am] 1991;16:401–8.
[38] Miyake T, Hashizume H, Inoue H, et al. Malunited Colles' fracture. Analysis of stress distribution. J Hand Surg [Br] 1994;19(6):737–42.
[39] Hirahara H, Neale PG, Lin YT, et al. Kinematic and torque-related effects of dorsally angulated distal radius fractures and the distal radial ulnar joint. J Hand Surg [Am] 2003;28:614–21.
[40] Kihara H, Palmer AK, Werner FW, et al. The effect of dorsally angulated distal radius fractures on distal radioulnar joint congruency and forearm rotation. J Hand Surg [Am] 1996;21:40–7.
[41] Linscheid RL. Kinematic considerations of the carpal joint. Clin Orthop 1986;202:27–39.
[42] Taleisnik J. Post-traumatic carpal instability. Clin Orthop 1980;149:73–82.
[43] Fernandez DL, Capo JT, Gonzalez E. Corrective osteotomy for symptomatic increased ulnar tilt of the distal end of the radius. J Hand Surg [Am] 2001;26:722–32.
[44] Tang JB, Ruy J, Omokawa S, et al. Biomechanical evaluation of wrist motor tendons after fractures of the distal radius. J Hand Surg [Am] 1999;24: 121–32.
[45] Marx RG, Axelrod TS. Intraarticular osteotomy of distal radius malunions. Clin Orthop 1996;327: 152–7.
[46] Linscheid RL, Dobyns JH, Beabout JW, et al. Traumatic instability of the wrist. Diagnosis, classification, and pathomechanics. J Bone Joint Surg Am 1972;54:1612–32.
[47] Sennwald G, Fischer M. Correction du cal vicieux du radius distal par ostéotomie de glissement-avancement. Ann Chir Main 1993;12:214–9.

[48] Watson H, Castle T. Trapezoidal osteotomy of the distal radius for unacceptable articular angulation after Colles' fractures. J Hand Surg [Am] 1988;13: 837–43.
[49] Posner MA, Ambrose L. Malunited Colles' fractures: correction with a biplanar closing wedge osteotomy. J Hand Surg [Am] 1991;16:1017–26.
[50] Viso R, Wegener EE, Freeland AE. Use of a closing wedge osteotomy to correct malunion of dorsally displaced extra-articular distal radius fractures. Orthopedics 2000;23:721–4.
[51] Wada T, Tsuji H, Iba K, et al. Simultaneous radial closing wedge and ulnar shortening osteotomy for distal radius malunion. J Hand Surg [Am] 2004; 29:264–72.
[52] Lindau T. Treatment of injuries to the ulnar side of the wrist occurring with distal radial fractures. Hand Clin 2005;21:417–25.
[53] Oskam J, Bongers KM, Karthaus AJM, et al. Corrective osteotomy for malunion of the distal radius—the effect of concomitant ulnar shortening osteotomy. Arch Orthop Trauma Surg 1996;115: 219–22.
[54] Wada T, Tsuji H, Iba K, et al. Simultaneous radial closing wedge and ulnar shortening osteotomy for distal radius malunion. Techn Hand Upper Extrem Surg 2005;9(4):184–94.
[55] Bunnell S. Surgery of the hand. 2nd edition. Philadelphia: J.B. Lippincott; 1948. p. 681–2.
[56] Fernandez DL, Albrecht HU, Saxer U. Die Korrekturosteotomie am distalen Radius bei posttraumatischer Fehlstellung. Arch Orthop Unfallchir 1977;90:199–211.
[57] Frykman G. Fracture of the distal radius including sequelae-shoulder-hand-finger syndrome, disturbance in the distal radioulnar joint and impairment of nerve function. Acta Orthop Scand Suppl 1967; 108:1–153.
[58] Cooney WP, Dobyns JH, Linscheid RL. Complications of Colles' fractures. J Bone Joint Surg Am 1980;43:657–68.
[59] Malone KJ, Magnell T, Freeman DC, et al. Surgical correction of dorsally angulated distal radius malunions with fixed angle volar plating: a case series. J Hand Surg [Am] 2006;31:366–72.
[60] Shea K, Fernandez DL, Jupiter JB, et al. Corrective osteotomy for malunited, volarly displaced fractures of the distal end of the radius. J Bone Joint Surg Am 1997;79:1816–26.
[61] Thivaios GC, McKee MD. Sliding osteotomy for deformity correction following malunion of volarly displaced distal radial fractures. J Orthop Trauma 2003;17(5):326–33.
[62] Darrach W. Partial excision of lower shaft of ulna for deformity following Colles' fracture. Ann Surg 1913;57:764–5.
[63] Bieber EJ, Linscheid RL, Dobyns JH, et al. Failed distal ulnar resections. J Hand Surg [Am] 1988;13: 193–200.
[64] Nolan WB, Eaton RG. A Darrach procedure for distal ulnar pathology derangements. Clin Orthop 1992;275:85–9.
[65] Gaebler C, McQueen MM. Ulnar procedures for post-traumatic disorders of the distal radioulnar joint. Injury 2003;34:47–59.
[66] Tulipan DJ, Eaton RO, Eberhart RE. The Darrach procedure defended: technique redefined and long term follow-up. J Hand Surg [Am] 1991;16:438–44.
[67] Bowers WH. Distal radioulnar joint arthroplasty: the hemiresection-interposition technique. J Hand Surg [Am] 1985;10:169–78.
[68] Watson HK, Ryu J, Burgess RC. Matched distal ulnar resection. J Hand Surg [Am] 1986;11:812–6.
[69] Watson Hk, Gabuzda G. Matched distal ulnar resection for posttraumatic disorders of the distal radioulnar joint. J Hand Surg [Am] 1992;17: 724–30.
[70] Bowers WH. Distal radioulnar joint arthroplaty: current concepts. Clin Orthop 1992;275:104–10.
[71] Taleisnik J. The Sauvé–Kapandji procedure. Clin Orthop 1992;275:110–23.
[72] Minami A, Suzuki K, Suenaga N, et al. The Sauvé–Kapandji procedure for osteoarthrritis of the distal radioulnar joint. J Hand Surg [Am] 1995;20:602–8.
[73] McMurty RY, Paley D, Marks P, et al. A critical analysis of Swanson ulnar head replacement arthroplasty: rheumatoid versus nonrheumatoid. J Hand Surg [Am] 1990;15:224–31.
[74] van Schoonhoven J, Herbert TH, Krimmer H. New concepts for endoprostheses of the distal radio-ulnar joint. Hand chir Mikrochir Plast Chir 1998; 30:387–92.
[75] Dingman PVC. Resection of the distal end of the ulna (Darrach operation). An end-result study of twenty-four cases. J Bone Joint Surg Am 1952;34: 893–900.
[76] McKee MD, Richards RR. Dynamic radio-ulnar convergence after the Darrach procedure. J Bone Joint Surg Br 1996;78:413–8.
[77] Bell MJ, Hill RJ, McMurtry RY. Ulnar impingement syndrome. J Bone Joint Surg Br 1985;67: 126–9.
[78] DiBenedetto MR, Lubbers LM, Coleman CR. Long-term results of the minimal resection Darrach procedure. J Hand Surg [Am] 1991;16:445–50.
[79] Field J, Majkowski RJ, Leslie IJ. Poor results of Darrach's procedure after wrist injuries. J Bone Joint Surg Br 1993;75:53–7.
[80] Lees VC, Scheker LR. The radiological demonstration of dynamic ulnar impingement. J Hand Surg [Br] 1997;22:448–50.
[81] Shah M, Klimisch J. Treatment of failed Darrach procedure including the brachioradialis sling. Opin Orthop 2003;14:222–8.
[82] Bowers WH. Instability of the distal radioulnar articulation. Hand Clin 1991;7:311–27.
[83] Graham TJ, Fischer TJ, Hotchkiss RN. Disorders of the forearm axis. Hand Clin 1998;14:305–16.

[84] Lichtman DM, Ganocy TK, Kim DC. The indications for and techniques and outcomes of ablative procedures of the distal ulna: the Darrach resection, hemiresection, matched resection and Sauve-Kapandji procedure. Hand Clin 1988;14:265–77.

[85] Gordon L, Levinsohn DG, Moore SV, et al. The Sauve-Kapandji procedure for the treatment of posttraumatic distal radioulnar joint problems. Hand Clin 1991;7:397–403.

[86] Sanders RA, Frederick HA, Hontas RB. The Sauve-Kapandji procedure: a salvage operation for the distal radioulnar joint. J Hand Surg [Am] 1991;16:1125–9.

[87] Millroy P, Coleman S, Ivers R. The Sauve-Kapandji operation: technique and results. J Hand Surg [Br] 1992;17:411–4.

[88] Carter PB, Stuart PR. The Sauve-Kapandji procedure for post-traumatic disorders of the distal radio-ulnar joint. J Bone Joint Surg Br 2000;82: 1013–8.

[89] Mikkelsen SS, Lindblad BE, Larsen ER, et al. Sauve-Kapandji operation for disorders of the distal radioulnar joint after Colles' fracture. Acta Orthop Scand 1997;68:64–6.

[90] Nakamura R, Tsunoda K, Watanabe K, et al. The Sauve-Kapandji procedure for chronic dislocation of the distal radioulnar joint with destruction of the articular surface. J Hand Surg [Br] 1992;17: 127–32.

[91] van Schoonhoven J, Fernandez DL, Bowers WH, et al. Salvage of failed resection arthroplasties of the distal radioulnar joint using a new ulnar head prosthesis. J Hand Surg [Am] 2000;25: 438–46.

[92] Wnorowski DC, Palmer AK, Werner FW, et al. Anatomic and biomechanical analysis of the arthroscopic wafer procedure. Arthroscopy 1992; 8(2):204–12.

[93] Wagner WF, Tencer AF, Kiser P, et al. Effects of intra-articular distal radius depression on wrist joint contact characteristics. J Hand Surg [Am] 1996;21:554–60.

[94] Anderson DD, Bell AL, Gaffney MB, et al. Stress distributions in malreduced intraarticular distal radius fractures. J Orthop Trauma 1996;10(5):331–7.

[95] Kreder HJ, Hanel DP, Agel J, et al. Indirect reduction and percutaneous fixation versus open reduction and internal fixation for displaced intra-articular fractures of the distal radius: a randomized, controlled trial. J Bone Joint Surg Br 2005;87(6):829–36.

[96] Hastings H, Leibovic SJ. Indications and techniques of open reduction. Orthop Clin North Am 1993;24:309–26.

[97] Bradway JK, Amadio PC, Cooney WP. Open reduction and internal fixation of displaced, comminuted intra-articular fractures of the distal end of the radius. J Bone Joint Surg Am 1989;71: 839–47.

[98] Fernandez DL, Geissler WB. Treatment of displaced articular fractures of the radius. J Hand Surg [Am] 1991;16:375–84.

[99] Knirk JL, Jupiter JB. Intra-articular fractures of the distal end of the radius in young adults. J Bone Joint Surg Am 1986;68:647–59.

[100] Trumble TE, Schmitt SR, Vedder NB. Factors affecting functional outcome of displaced intra-articular distal radius fractures. J Hand Surg [Am] 1994; 19:325–40.

[101] Jupiter JB, Ruder J, Roth D. Computer-generated bone models in the planning of osteotomy of multidirectional distal radius malunions. J Hand Surg [Am] 1992;17:406–15.

[102] Catalano LW, Cole RJ, Gelberman RH, et al. Displaced intra-articular fractures of the distal aspect of the radius. J Bone Joint Surg Am 1997;79(9): 1290–302.

[103] McKay SD, MacDermid JC, Roth JH, et al. Assessment of complications of distal radius fractures and development of a complication checklist. J Hand Surg [Am] 2001;26:916–22.

[104] Prommersberger KJ, Ring D, Del Pino JG, et al. Corrective osteotomy for intra-articular malunion of the distal part of the radius. Surgical technique. J Bone Joint Surg Am 2006;88(Suppl 1 Pt 2): 202–11.

[105] Ring D, Prommersberger KJ, Del Pino JG, et al. Corrective osteotomy for intra-articular malunion of the distal part of the radius. J Bone Joint Surg Am 2005;87:1503–9.

[106] Catalano LW III, Barron OA, Glickel SZ. Assessment of articular displacement of distal radius fractures. Clin Orthop 2004;423:79–84.

[107] Kreder HJ, Hanel DP, McKee M, et al. X-ray film measurements for healed distal radius fractures. J Hand Surg [Am] 1996;21(1):31–9.

[108] Cole RJ, Bindra RR, Evanoff BA, et al. Radiographic evaluation of osseous displacement following intra-articular fractures of the distal radius: reliability of plain radiography versus computed tomography. J Hand Surg [Am] 1997;22(5): 792–800.

[109] Cooney WP, Bussey R, Dobyns JH, et al. Difficult wrist fractures. Perilunate fracture-dislocations of the wrist. Clin Orthop 1987;214:136–47.

[110] Saffar P. Radio-lunate arthrodesis for distal radial intraarticular malunion. J Hand Surg [Br] 1996;21: 14–20.

[111] Bilic R, Zdravkovic V. Planning corrective osteotomy of the distal end of the radius 1. Improved method. Unfallchirurg 1988;91:571–4.

[112] Bilic R, Zdravkovic V. Planning corrective osteotomy of the distal end of the radius 2. Computer-aided planning and follow-up. Unfallchirurg 1988;91:575–80.

[113] Bilic R, Zdravkovic V, Boljevic Z. Osteotomy for deformity of the radius. J Bone Joint Surg Br 1994;76:150–4.

[114] Weeks PM, Vannier MW, Stevens WG, et al. Three-dimensional imaging of the wrist. J Hand Surg [Am] 1985;10:32–9.
[115] Trumble TE, Culp RW, Hanel DP, et al. Intra-articular fractures of the distal aspect of the radius. Instr Course Lect 1999;48:465–80.
[116] Athwal GS, Ellis RE, Small CF, et al. Computer-assisted distal radius osteotomy. J Hand Surg [Am] 2003;28:951–8.
[117] Rieger M, Gabl M, Gruber H, et al. CT virtual reality in the preoperative workup of malunited distal radius fractures: preliminary results. Eur Radiol 2005;15:792–7.
[118] Vasarhelyi EM, Athwal GS, Ellis RE, et al. Multiple bone fragment correction in computer-assisted osteotomy to restore the radial bow of a malunion of the distal radius. Presented at the Adrian E. Flatt Residents and Fellows Conference, American Society for Surgery of the Hand. New York, September 8, 2004.
[119] Orbay JL. The treatment of unstable distal radius fractures with volar fixation. Hand Surg 2000;5:103–12.
[120] Orbay JL, Touhami A. Current concepts in volar fixed-angle fixation of unstable distal radius fractures. Clin Orthop 2006;445:58–67.
[121] Orbay JL, Badia A, Indriago IR. The extended flexor carpi radialis approach: a new perspective for the distal radius fracture. Tech Hand Up Extrem Surg 2001;5:204–11.
[122] Henry MH, Griggs SM, Levaro F, et al. Volar approach to dorsal displaced fractures of the radius. Tech Hand Up Extrem Surg 2001;5:31–41.
[123] Smith DW, Henry MH. Volar fixed-angle plating of the distal radius. J Am Acad Orthop Surg 2005;13:28–36.
[124] McGriry BJ, Amadio PC. Malunion of the distal radius. In: Cooney WP, Linscheid Rl, Dobyns JH, editors. The wrist. St. Louis (MO): Mosby; 1998. p. 356–84.
[125] Fernandez DL, Jubiter JB. Fracture of the distal radius. A practical approach to management. New York: Springer Verlag; 1995. p. 263–315.
[126] Ring D, Roberge C, Morgan T, et al. Osteotomy for malunited fractures of the distal radius: a comparison of structural and nonstructural autogenous bone grafts. J Hand Surg [Am] 2002;27:216–22.
[127] Wieland A, Dekkers G, Brink P. Open wedge osteotomy for malunited extraarticular distal radius fractures with plate osteosynthesis without bone grafting. European Journal Trauma 2005;2:148–53.
[128] Ladd AL, Pliam NB. Use of bone graft substitutes in distal radius fractures. J Am Acad Orthop Surg 1999;7:279–90.
[129] Luchetti R. Corrective osteotomy of malunited distal radius fractures using carbonated hydroxyapatite as an alternative to autogenous bone grafting. J Hand Surg [Am] 2004;29:825–34.
[130] Yasuda M, Masada K, Kentaro I, et al. Early corrective osteotomy for a malunited Colles' fracture using volar approach and calcium phosphate bone cement: a case report. J Hand Surg [Am] 2004;29:1139–42.
[131] Kopylov P, Jonsson K, Thorngren KG, et al. Injectable calcium phosphate in the treatment of distal radius fracture. J Hand Surg [Br] 1996;21:768–71.
[132] Kopylov P. Injectable calcium phosphate bone substitute in distal radius fractures [thesis]. Lund: Wallin&Dalhoim AB; 2001. p. 3–29.
[133] Yetkinler DN, Ladd Al, Poser RD, et al. Biomechanical evaluation of fixation of intraarticular fractures of the distal part of the radius in cadavers: Kirshner wires compared with calcium phosphate bone cement. J Bone Joint Surg Am 1999;81:391–9.

Complications of Distal Radius Fractures

Robert G. Turner, MB, BCh, FRCS,
Kenneth J. Faber, MD, MHPE, FRCSC,
George S. Athwal, MD, FRCSC*

Hand and Upper Limb Centre, St Joseph's Health Care, University of Western Ontario, 268 Grosvenor Street, London, Ontario, Canada N6A 4L6

Fractures occur at the distal end of the radius more frequently than at any other location [1]. The reported complication rates of distal radius fractures in the literature vary from 6% to 80% [2–4]. Complications may occur from the fracture or its treatment.

McKay and colleagues [4] reviewed the overall incidence of complications after distal radius fractures in the literature (Table 1) and subsequently in their series of 250 consecutive patients treated for distal radius factures. They found a physician-reported complication rate of 27% and a patient-reported complication rate of 21%. They also found that patients and physicians report distal radius fractures differently; unsurprisingly, patients focused more on symptoms, whereas physicians were more apt to classify complications into diagnoses. The authors compiled their data and constructed a complication checklist to improve prospective data collection (Table 2).

This article reviews complications caused by distal radius fractures and their treatment. Complications are divided chronologically in to immediate, early (less than 6 weeks), and late (greater than 6 weeks).

Immediate complications

Nerve injury

Distal radius fractures complicated by nerve injury are relatively common, with a reported incidence varying from 0% to 17% [4]. The median nerve is most frequently involved, followed by the radial and ulnar nerves [4]. Acute carpal tunnel syndrome is more common in patients who have more severe and comminuted fractures and also in those undergoing multiple closed reduction attempts [5].

Patients should be carefully examined to rule out neurologic injury. Splinting or casting in extreme wrist flexion should be avoided because this significantly increases carpal tunnel pressures, compromising median nerve function (Fig. 1) [6,7]. Gelberman and colleagues [7] found that mean carpal tunnel pressures were 18 mm Hg in a neutral wrist position, 27 mm Hg in 20° of flexion, and 47 mm Hg in 40° of flexion. In a series of patients who had carpal tunnel syndrome, the pressure was 23 mm Hg in neutral and 38 mm Hg in flexion, but was 8 mm Hg in neutral and 14 mm Hg in flexion for normal control subjects [8].

Mild carpal tunnel symptoms are common and usually related to swelling and contusion around the median nerve. In patients who have significant hand and wrist swelling, splints or bivalved casts should be used rather than circumferential casts. Patients should be encouraged to keep the hand elevated and actively flex and extend their fingers. The symptoms usually diminish as the swelling subsides. A carpal tunnel release should be considered if the symptoms are more severe or progressive, or if surgical intervention is planned that may increase swelling. Patients who undergo early release have a better long-term outcome, because delayed treatment can result in an incomplete or prolonged recovery period [5,9,10].

* Corresponding author.
E-mail address: gathwal@uwo.ca (G.S. Athwal).

Table 1
Incidence of reported complications with distal radius fractures

Complication	Incidence
Loss of motion (marked deformity, decreased ROM, arthrofibrosis, Volkmann's ischemic contracture, finger stiffness.)	0%–31%
Delayed union/nonunion	0.7%–4%
Nerve compression/neuritis	0%–17%
Pain syndromes (RSD, shoulder-hand syndrome, persistent pain)	0.3%–8%
Hardware complications	1.4%–2.6%
Osteomyelitis	4%–9%
Malunion	5%
Tendon (rupture, lag, trigger, tenosynovitis)	0%–5%
Scar (keloids)	3%
Ligament damage	98%
Radioulnar (synostosis, disturbance.)	0%–1.3%
Bone graft hematoma	1%
Dupuytren's contracture (palmar fascia nodules/bands)	2%–9%
Arthritis/arthrosis	7%–65%
Unrecognized injury	2%

Abbreviations: ROM, range of motion; RSD, reflex sympathetic dystrophy.
Data from McKay SD, MacDermid JC, Roth JH, et al. Assessment of complications of distal radius fractures and development of a complication checklist. J Hand Surg Am 2001;26(5):916–22.

Open injury

Open fractures of the distal radius are infrequent. However, open fractures of the distal ulna in association with a distal radius fracture are more common. Gustilo and Anderson type I injuries are the most common and may be easily missed, especially on the volar side of the wrist. The skin around the distal forearm and wrist must be carefully examined before and after manipulation. Intravenous antibiotics should be administered and tetanus status assessed in the emergency department. These injuries require prompt irrigation, debridement, and fracture stabilization.

Patients who have an open fracture should be advised that they have an increased likelihood of a poor outcome. The largest reported series of open fractures included 18 consecutive patients and was collected over 8-years [11]. Type I Gustilo and Anderson injuries were the most common with an incidence of 50%, followed by type II and III injuries with incidences of 17% and 34%, respectively. Most injuries were the result of high-energy trauma. Four patients in this series also had nerve injuries, four patients had tendon injuries, and two had vascular injuries. Patients who had higher Gustilo and Anderson types required a greater number of secondary surgical procedures, because type I injuries required a mean of 0.3 additional procedures, whereas type III fractures required a mean of 4.7 procedures. Eight of the 18 patients developed postoperative infections (five soft tissue and three osteomyelitis) and five patients developed a nonunion.

Skin injury during manipulation

Distal radial fractures are more common in the elderly population [12]. The overlying skin may be thin and can be traumatized during fracture manipulation, converting a closed fracture into a potential open injury.

Compartment syndrome

Compartment syndrome is a rare complication, but can have dramatic consequences. Young male patients are most at risk because they are more likely to have sustained a high-energy injury. In a review of 6395 fractures of the distal radius, 16 patients (0.25%) had an acute compartment syndrome. The mean age was 26 years (range, 14 to 51 years) and 15 of the 16 patients were male. The volar compartment of the forearm was involved in 15 patients, and one also had involvement of the interosseous compartments of the hand. The hand compartments were affected exclusively in only one patient, [13].

Acute injuries should be supported with a noncircumferential splint and bandages. Although a full cast may provide better support to an unstable fracture, it may not accommodate swelling and should be used with caution. If concerns exist about the risk for a developing compartment syndrome, the patient should be admitted for limb elevation and observation.

The onset of compartment syndrome has been reported up to 54 hours after injury [14]. Patients discharged from the emergency department should be counseled to seek prompt medical advice if pain is not controlled with standard analgesia, neurologic changes develop, or color changes occur.

Pain out of proportion to that expected and pain on passive extension of the digits are typical findings in compartment syndrome, whereas neurologic changes or discoloration are late findings in the condition. The threshold for diagnosis of compartment syndrome should be low and, if the condition is suspected, the cast or bandages should be loosened (even if this risks losing the position of a manipulated fracture), the limb elevated, and the patient clinically reassessed. If symptoms persist, compartmental pressures should be measured or prompt fasciotomy performed. In most cases, volar fasciotomy is sufficient; however, one case of a volar and dorsal compartment syndrome has been reported [15].

Missed associated injury

Distal radial fractures in elderly patients are usually caused by a low-energy injury; but are often caused by high-energy forces in young patients. High-energy injuries may be associated with injuries remote to the wrist (eg, elbow, shoulder, spine, lower limb) or local to the wrist (eg, carpal or metacarpal injury). A careful history, thorough physical examination, and appropriate radiographs will identify other sites of injury.

Early complications (<6 weeks)

Although complications may occur with both nonoperative and operative treatment during the first 6 weeks, the spectrum of complications is different for each group.

Cast issues

Applying a full cast on an acute injury will not accommodate subsequent swelling. It may be used for unstable fractures, but patients should be warned of the potential complications of increased pain, nerve compression, and, ultimately, compartment syndrome. A noncircumferential splint provides less support to the fracture, but will accommodate swelling.

Posttrauma swelling reduces in the days and weeks after injury. The cast may become loose and should be changed. If a noncircumferential splint was initially applied, then it may be replaced by a complete cast at 10 to 14 days.

The cast should support the fracture and permit free movement of the fingers and thumb. After application, the cast must be inspected to ensure that it does not compromise finger motion. The patient should be encouraged to exercise the fingers to prevent stiffness and reduce the risk for dystrophy.

Loss of reduction

Charnley's [16] three-point fixation technique is recommended to support the fracture within the cast. If the fracture displaces, then it should be promptly corrected through either closed manipulation or surgery. Many factors have been associated with an increased risk for displacement, including increasing age, dorsal comminution, and degree of dorsal angulation at presentation [17–20]. Mackenney et al. [18] reported that early instability was (1) ten times more common in patients older than 80 years compared with patients younger than 30 years, (2) six times more common in fractures with any form of dorsal comminution, and (3) five times more common in fractures maintaining 5° to 10° of dorsal angulation compared with fractures achieving any degree of volar angulation.

A risk for displacement also exists with operative treatment. With percutaneous K-wires, the risk for displacement is greatest in older individuals and fractures with greater than 50% dorsal comminution [21].

Operative technique is important. A randomized study comparing treatment with two styloid wires and treatment using a single styloid wire with the addition of two dorsal Kapandji wires found that the two-styloid-wire technique was less reliable [22]. A randomized study of external fixators found that an additional pin in the distal radial fragment provided better stability and decreased the pin-track infection rate [23].

Infection

Compound fractures and fractures treated operatively are at risk for infection. The largest reported series of compound fractures reported a 44% infection rate, with 62% of the infections involving the soft tissues and 38% as osteomyelitis [11].

The infection rate with K-wire fixation has been reported to be as high as 33% [24]. Infection may occur within the soft tissues and can be treated with oral antibiotics, or may involve the bone causing an osteomyelitis that requires surgical intervention. Burying the wires beneath the skin reduces the risk for infection. A randomized

Table 2
Distal radius fracture complication checklist and score sheet

Nerve complications
  Median severe compression/carpal tunnel syndrome
    Mild—symptoms only, no specific treatment
    Moderate—diagnostic procedure (EMG) and/or treatment (physiotherapy, splint)
    Severe—surgery required
  Radial nerve compression/neuropathy
    Mild—symptoms only, no specific treatment
    Moderate—diagnostic procedure (EMG) and/or treatment (physiotherapy, splint)
    Severe—surgery required
  Reflex sympathetic dystrophy (including abnormal pain, stiffness and vasomotor syndrome)
    Mild—symptoms only, no specific treatment
    Moderate—symptoms and treatment (physiotherapy, 1–2 stellate ganglion blocks)
    Severe—more than 2 stellate ganglion blocks
  Ulnar nerve compression/neuropathy
    Mild—symptoms only, no specific treatment
    Moderate—diagnostic procedure (EMG) and/or treatment (physiotherapy splint)
    Severe—surgery required
Bone/joint complications
  Arthritis
    Mild—slight joint changes (minute osteophytes)
    Moderate—sclerosis, osteophytic changes, narrowed joint space
    Severe—large cysts, almost obliterated joint space
  Carpal instability/subluxation
    Mild—symptoms only, no specific treatment
    Moderate—treatment (physiotherapy, splint)
    Severe—surgery required
  Delayed union
    Moderate—resolved within 6 months
    Severe—nonunion of fracture
  Distal radioulnar joint problems
    Mild—pain on axial loading, instability with activity, resolved without specific treatment
    Moderate—pain with axial loading/activity, specific diagnosis, resolved with treatment
    Severe—persistent arthritis/instability limiting activity with specific diagnosis
Tendon complications
  Depuytren's contracture
    Mild—nodules present, no contracture
    Moderate—nodules and contracture present, no surgery required
    Severe—contracture surgery required
  Tendon adhesions/scarring
    Mild—symptoms only, no specific treatment
    Moderate—treatment (physiotherapy, injected steroids)
    Severe—surgery required
  Tendon rupture—extensor pollicis longus
    Severe—surgery required
  Tendon rupture tear—other
    Mild—symptoms only, no specific treatment
    Moderate—treatment (physiotherapy, splint)
    Severe—surgery required
  Tendonitis/tenosynovitis
    Mild—symptoms only, no specific treatment
    Moderate—treatment (physiotherapy, injected steroids)
    Severe—surgery required
  Trigger finger
    Mild—symptoms only, no specific treatment
    Moderate—treatment (physiotherapy, injected steroids, surgery)

(continued on next page)

Table 2 (*continued*)

Other complications
  Compartment syndrome
    Severe—surgical fasciotomy required
  Miscellaneous
    Mild—symptoms only, resolved without specific treatment
    Moderate—diagnostic procedure and/or resolved with treatment
    Severe—persistent despite treatment or surgery required
  Pin sites/incisions infections
    Mild—resolved without specific treatment
    Moderate—resolved with treatment
Total number of complications
Total score (sum of all complications scores)

Scoring: Mild = 1, Midvale = 2, Severe = 3.
Abbreviation: EMG, electromyography.
Data from McKay SD, MacDermid JC, Roth JH, et al. Assessment of complication checklist. J Hand Surg Am 2001; 26(5):916–22.

trial reported a 7.5% infection rate with buried K-wires and a 17% infection rate with percutaneous K-wires [24]. If the wires are left in situ for a prolonged period, the risk for infection increases. A review of 137 patients treated with K-wires reported a 7% infection rate overall, with osteomyelitis developing in two patients. The authors reported that infection was more common if the wires were left in situ for 8 weeks or more [25].

An infection rate of 21% has been reported for external fixation (Fig. 2) [26]. A randomized trial of pin tract care compared (1) weekly dry dressing changes without pin-site care, (2) daily pin-site care with a solution of one-half normal saline solution and one-half hydrogen peroxide, and (3) treatment with the placement of chlorhexidine-impregnated discs (Biopatch) around the pins, with weekly changes of the discs by the treating surgeon. An overall infection rate of 19% was seen, with no differences among the pin-care groups. The authors therefore recommend weekly dry dressing changes for simplicity and to minimize expenses [27].

Another study compared two pin-care techniques: (1) daily cleaning with normal saline, crust removal, and simple nonadherent dressings only in the presence of exudates, otherwise left uncovered and (2) the protocol used by the Ilizarov Institute (Immediate pin-site dressings in alcoholic solution of chlorhexidine with pressure to reduce hematoma, changed at completion of the operation if bloodstained; original theater dressings left undisturbed for 48 hours; occlusive pressure dressing after the third day, and pin cleaning and dressing changes repeated every 7 to 10 days using the same technique). The second regime had a significantly lower incidence of infection; however, differences in operative technique were seen between the groups, and smooth thin wires were used instead of threaded half pins or K-wires [28].

Infection with internal fixation is less common. Percutaneous K-wires should not be used to supplement internal fixation, because this can act as a pathway for superficial infection to spread to the deeper tissues and bone (Fig. 3). If infection occurs, then internal fixation should be removed and the fracture treated with cast support or external fixation and antibiotics.

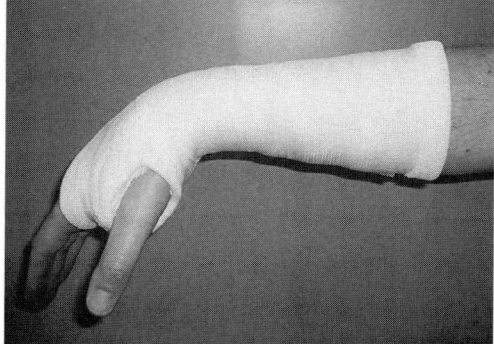

Fig. 1. Casting in extreme wrist flexion and ulnar deviation to maintain a reduction should be avoided because it increases carpal tunnel pressure and the risk for acute carpal tunnel syndrome.

Neurologic

A review of more than 200 patients with displaced Colles' fractures found that 17% had

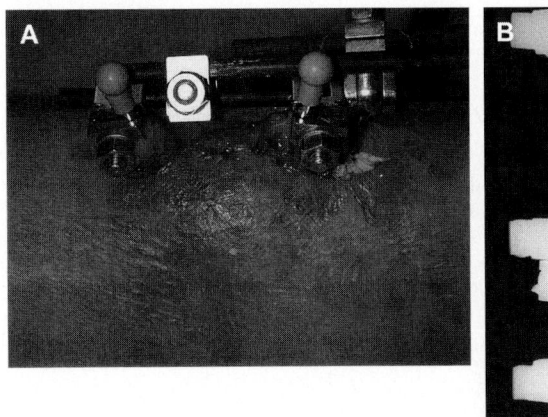
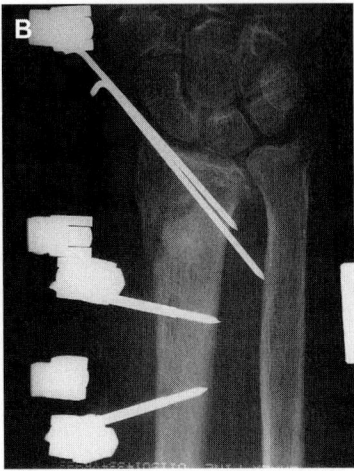

Fig. 2. External fixator pin-tract infection. Note the erythema and purulent exudate (*A*) and the bony lysis around the fixator pins (*B*).

carpal tunnel symptoms at 3 months and 12% had symptoms at 6 months [29]. The patients who had carpal tunnel symptoms were significantly older and their fractures showed significantly greater residual dorsal angulation.

Mackay et al. [4] reported 22% median, 11% radial nerve, and 6% ulnar nerve symptoms complicating distal radius fractures. The radial nerve sensory branch is particularly vulnerable to injury during K-wire fixation. This nerve exits beneath the dense fascia between the tendons of brachioradialis and extensor carpi radialis longus. This anatomy acts as a local tether that prevents excursion of the nerve away from a blindly placed surgical instrument [30]. Care should be taken when inserting K-wires, spreading the overlying tissues, and during blunt dissection to bone before wire insertion. Neuromas in this area are particularly troublesome because they can be irritated by rubbing against shirt cuffs, watches, and bracelets.

Tendon rupture

Tendon ruptures can occur as an early or late complication. The extensor pollicis longus tendon is most commonly ruptured. The incidence in undisplaced distal radius fractures is 3%, with rupture occurring at a mean of 7 weeks (range, 2 weeks to 11 months) [31]. The ruptured tendon usually cannot be directly repaired and function can be well restored by performing an extensor indicis proprius tendon transfer [32].

Extensor tendon ruptures are more common than flexor tendon ruptures in fractures treated nonoperatively [33]. Both flexor and extensor tendon ruptures occur more commonly on the radial side of the wrist. Tendon ruptures have also been reported from multiple passes of K-wires [34] and from volar or dorsal internal fixation [35–37].

Late complications (>6 weeks)

Late complications are not uncommon and may be caused by issues involving the bone, joints, soft tissues, or nerves. This article discusses each of these potential problem areas.

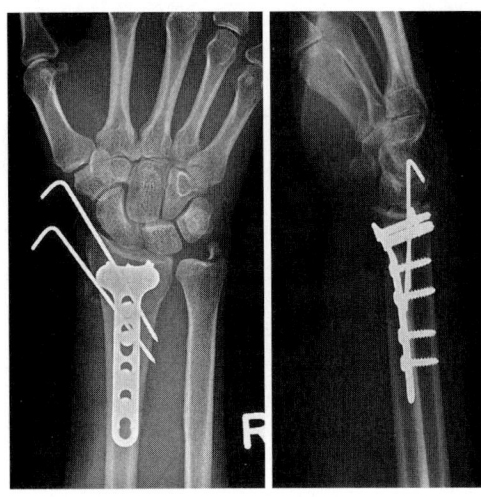

Fig. 3. The use of K-wires in addition to internal plate fixation should be avoided because the wires can act as a conduit for deep infection.

Nerve complications and complex regional pain syndrome

Patients complaining of carpal tunnel symptoms should be advised that their symptoms may settle over the first 6 months [29]. A review of 60 patients reported electrodiagnostically confirmed carpal tunnel syndrome in 20% of patients at a mean of 10 months (range, 1.5 to 27 months) between injury and the onset of symptoms [38]. The authors found a significant correlation between the final clinical results of treatment and the presence of posttraumatic median nerve compression neuropathy, but did not find a correlation with the initial fracture configuration or the final radiographic findings.

Complex Regional Pain Syndrome (CRPS) type 1 was formerly known as reflex sympathetic dystrophy. It refers to a pattern of symptoms and signs that are disproportionate to those usually expected from the degree of trauma. Typical findings include increased pain, swelling, and regional vasomotor instability (changes in color, temperature, and perspiration). CRPS is frequently associated with significant functional impairment of the hand and entire upper extremity.

CRPS type I has been reported to be more common in the elderly, women, and individuals who have a psychologic predisposition [39]. For distal radial fractures, many authors report an increased incidence ($\leq 18\%$) with increased fracture severity [40–43]. For fractures treated nonoperatively, a correlation exists between an increased incidence of CRPS and increased pressure under the cast [44]. Excessive distraction with an external fixator can also raise the risk for developing CRPS [45].

Early recognition of CRPS is important, and patients diagnosed with this condition should be promptly referred for multidisciplinary treatment. For patients who are not improving, sympathetic blocks may be considered.

Arthrosis

A review of patients at a mean of 6.7 years after an intra-articular fracture of the distal radius found that 65% had radiographic evidence of posttraumatic arthrosis. Fractures that healed with residual radiocarpal incongruity had a higher rate of radiographic arthrosis (91%) versus fractures that healed with a congruous joint (11%). The authors reported that restoration and maintenance (extra-articular reduction) of the dorsal tilt and radial length were not critical except when severe radial shortening occurred [46]. A step-off of 2 mm or more in the distal radial articular surface at healing has been found to be a significant risk for arthrosis [46,47].

In a young patient, arthrosis is a challenging problem and treatment options include activity modification, oral analgesics, splinting, or surgery. Surgical options include partial or complete wrist fusions, with arthroplasty having a limited role in young, active patients.

Nonunion/delayed union

Fractures that show no radiographic signs of bridging trabeculae across the fracture site at 4 months are categorized as delayed unions and as nonunions after 6 months [48]. Nonunion of the distal radius is uncommon. In their study of 2000 distal radial fractures, Bacorn and Kurtzke [49] reported a nonunion rate of 0.2%.

Open fractures, severe comminution, infection, tissue interposition, devascularization of the bone ends, and pathologic lesions predispose to nonunion [50]. Several articles have reported nonunion of the distal radius associated with nonunion of a distal ulna fracture [50,51]. The loss of the intact distal ulna may affect the stability of the distal radial fracture and lead to increased motion at the fracture site, with resultant nonunion. A review of 23 nonunions found that 9 had an associated distal ulna fracture [50]. Treatment factors may also predispose to nonunion, including overdistraction of the fracture and inadequate stabilization of the fracture [50]. Medical factors have also been implicated, including diabetes, peripheral vascular disease, peripheral neuropathy [52], alcoholism, and smoking [53].

The diagnosis may be confirmed through mobility of the fracture noted on lateral radiographs of the wrist in dorsiflexion and volar flexion. CT may be used to confirm the diagnosis and is also useful in surgical planning to assess the characteristics of the associated deformity and whether the distal articular fragment is of sufficient size to accommodate internal fixation (Fig. 4).

Surgical treatment options include wrist arthrodesis or bone grafting and stabilization with internal fixation as a single-stage procedure, or primary distraction lengthening (with tenotomy of the brachioradialis) with secondary stabilization and bone grafting [54]. The radius is often shortened and malaligned, requiring correction and lengthening with bone graft augmentation. This

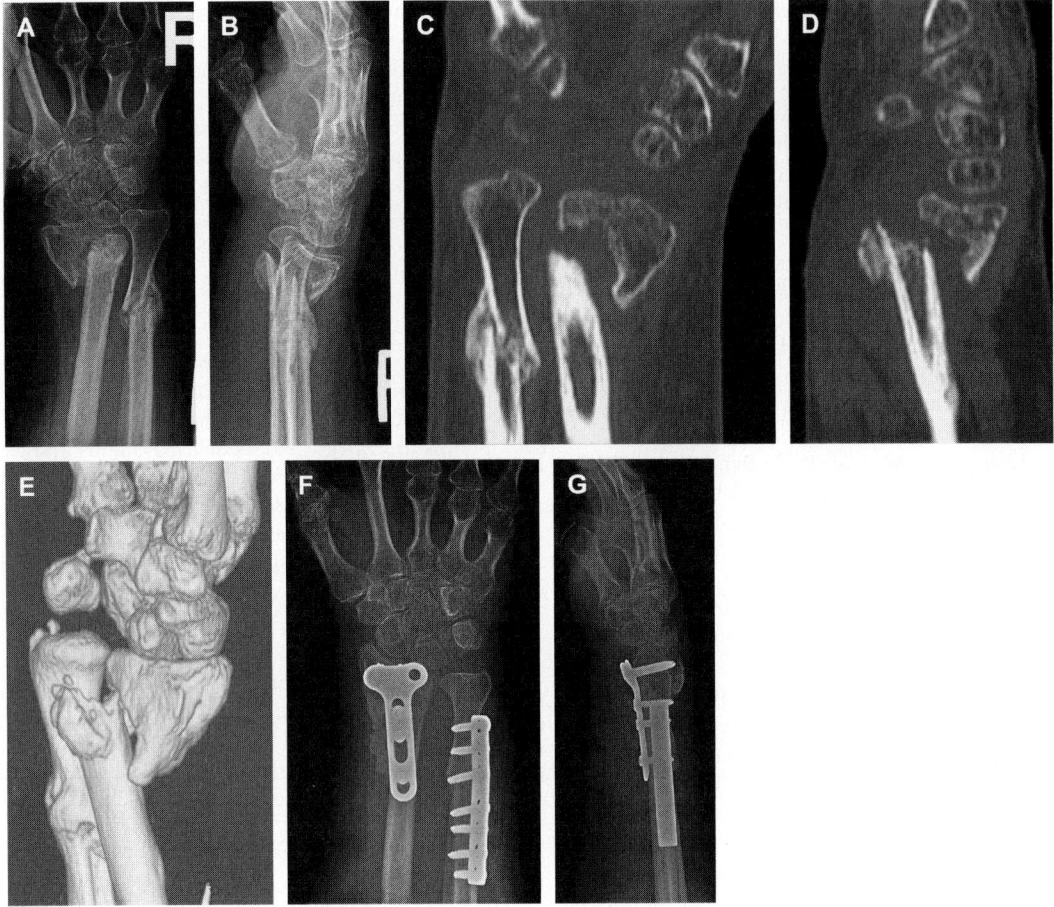

Fig. 4. Posteroanterior (*A*) and lateral (*B*) radiographs of a 49-year-old woman who has a distal radius nonunion and an ulnar malunion. A CT scan (*C*, *D*) with three-dimensional reconstructions (*E*) illustrates the deformity. CT scans assist with preoperative planning to accurately determine the angular and rotational deformities and may be used to assess the available bone stock. This patient underwent bonegrafting with internal fixation for the radial nonunion and corrective osteotomy of the ulnar malunion. Three-month follow-up radiographs (*F*, *G*) show restored alignment with clinical union.

procedure will often restore any associated instability at the distal radioulnar joint, although distal ulna excision may be considered if instability continues. An associated nonunion of the distal ulna may be treated with excision of the distal fragment or open reduction and internal fixation with bone grafting. Locking plates may be help gain sufficient bone purchase in a small distal ulnar fragment.

Malunion

Although malunion may not cause significant problems in low-demand elderly patients [55], a weak, deformed, and painful wrist may result in young, active patients [56]. Malunion of the distal radius is a complex problem and many factors must be considered when planning surgical correction.

Shortening of the distal radius may lead to ulnar abutment, resulting in impaction of the ulnar head against the carpus and gradual development of triangular fibrocartilage complex lesions and ulnocarpal arthrosis. Extra-articular malunion of the distal radius or ulna can result in abnormal alignment of the distal radioulnar joint (DRUJ) surfaces. Symptoms of pain and diminished forearm rotation are recognized

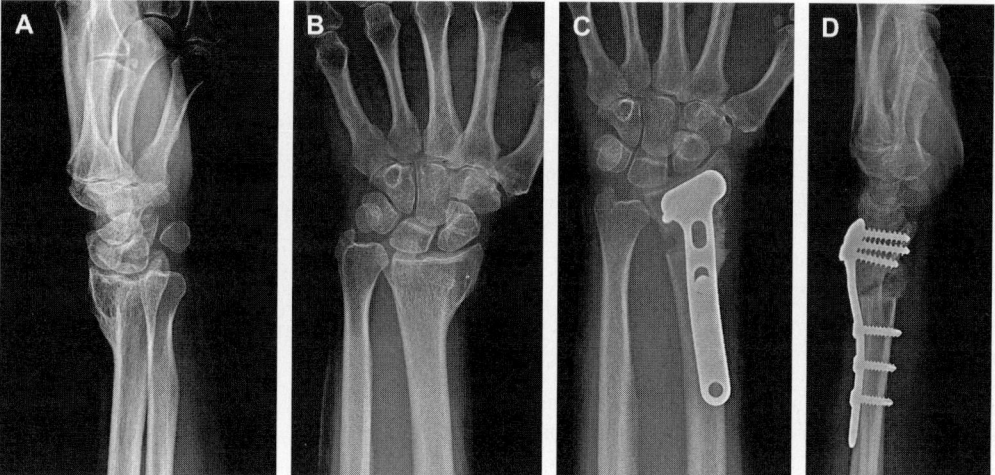

Fig. 5. Radiographs (*A, B*) of a 56-year-old male patient who has malunion of the distal radius with resulting radial shortening, dorsal angulation, and decreased inclination. Three-month follow-up radiographs after correction osteotomy and bone grafting show restoration of alignment and length.

consequences of DRUJ arthrosis and malalignment. CT scanning is an excellent imaging modality to assess DRUJ alignment.

Malunion symptoms may be caused by midcarpal malalignment, which has been classified as adaptive (type I) or fixed (type II) [57]. A lateral wrist radiograph will show that an adaptive malalignment will correct if the wrist is placed in the same amount of dorsal angulation as the distal radius malunion [57,58]. Adaptive malunions may benefit from a corrective distal radius osteotomy to restore carpal alignment, but a nonadaptive or fixed carpal deformity will not correct with osteotomy and may benefit from treatment by fusion [57].

Delaying surgical correction of distal radius malunions has shown a less satisfactory outcome [59]. Several different surgical options exist to treat distal radius malunions and their sequelae. Each case must be approached meticulously,

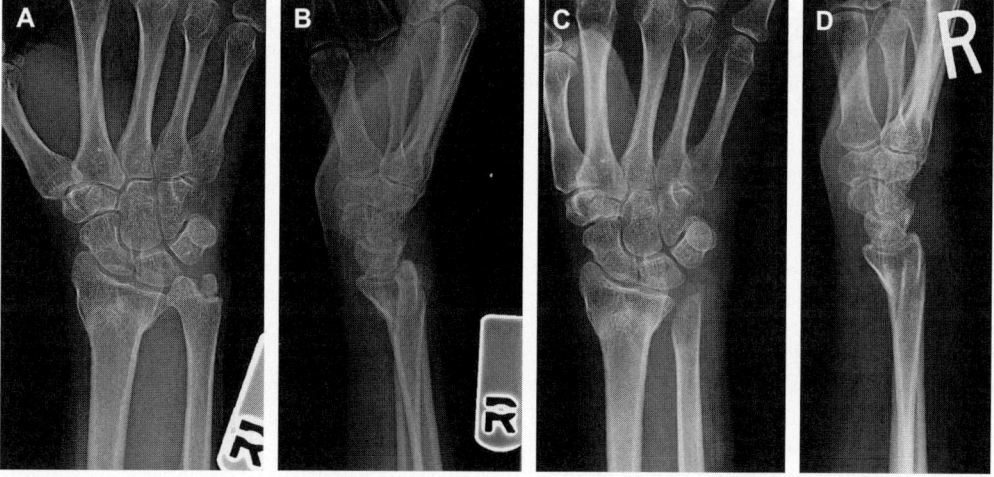

Fig. 6. A 68-year-old woman presented with ulnar impaction-type symptoms after a distal radius fracture. Radiographs (*A, B*) show radial shortening with associated distal radioulnar joint subluxation and ulnocarpal arthrosis. Postoperative radiographs (*C, D*) after ulnar hemiresection show decompression of the ulnocarpal joint.

with treatment individualized to the deformity. Operative treatments options include:

Correction of the distal radius length (Fig. 5)
Correction of dorsal angulation of the radius (See Fig. 5)
Shortening/excision of the distal ulna (Fig. 6)
Osteotomy to realign the DRUJ or ligament reconstruction of the DRUJ
Wrist fusion/arthroplasty

Tendon complications

Tendon rupture, tenosynovitis, adhesions, and trigger finger can all occur as late complications [3,29,60]. Tendon rupture occurs at a mean of 7 weeks, but can occur within the first few weeks after injury [31].

Tendonitis is most commonly found on the dorsum of the wrist. It has been related to dorsal plating [61,62] and is usually relieved by removing the metalwork. Dorsal tenosynovitis is uncommon after volar plating, although an overlong screw from a volar plate may produce dorsal symptoms [63]. Trigger finger has been reported in 2% of cases after distal radius fractures, although an exact origin has not been defined [4].

Tendon adhesions may form at the site of injury. Adhesions that limit motion may benefit from subsequent tenolysis to regain motion [64].

Dupuytren's disease

A review of 235 patients who had displaced Colles' fractures found that 11% of patients developed Dupuytren's nodules between 3 and 6 months post-injury. The disease and related contracture was usually mild, and no patients experienced significant progression when reviewed at a mean of 21 months [19].

Summary

Early identification and prompt treatment can reduce the long-term effects of some complications of distal radius fractures. However, numerous complications may occur and some may go unrecognized if not actively sought. For this reason, McKay and colleagues [4] developed a complication checklist (see Table 2) based on data collected from a literature review of all distal radius complications and from examining 250 of their own patients. This checklist grades individual complications as mild, moderate, or severe, and provides an overall score for the complications encountered. It considers complications under the categories of tendon-related, bone/joint-related, and nerve-related. This framework is useful when reviewing patients and the checklist may be used as a research tool for methodically assessing complications.

Distal radial fractures are common injuries and complications may develop at many stages in the treatment process. The treating surgeon should be aware of all the potential complications and the appropriate management.

References

[1] Larsen CF, Lauritsen J. Epidemiology of acute wrist trauma. Int J Epidemiol 1993;22(5):911–6.
[2] Becton JL, Colborn GL, Goodrich JA. Use of an external fixator to treat comminuted fractures of the distal radius: report of a technique. Am J Orthop 1998;27:619–23.
[3] Chapman DR, Bennett JB, Bryan WJ, et al. Complications of distal radius fractures: pins and plaster treatment. J Hand Surg [Am] 1982;7:509–12.
[4] McKay SD, MacDermid JC, Roth JH, et al. Assessment of complications of distal radius fractures and development of a complication checklist. J Hand Surg [Am] 2001;26(5):916–22.
[5] Bruske J, Niedzwiedz Z, Bednarski M, et al. Acute carpal tunnel syndrome after distal radius fractures—long term results of surgical treatment with decompression and external fixator application. Chir Narzadow Ruchu Ortop Pol 2002;67(1):47–53 [Polish].
[6] Kongsholm J, Olerud C. Carpal tunnel pressure in the acute phase after Colles' fracture. Arch Orthop Trauma Surg 1986;105(3):183–6.
[7] Gelberman RH, Szabo RM, Mortensen WW. Carpal tunnel pressures and wrist position in patients with Colles' fractures. J Trauma 1984;24(8):747–9.
[8] Sanz J, Lizaur A, Sanchez Del Campo F. Postoperative changes of carpal canal pressure in carpal tunnel syndrome: a prospective study with follow-up of 1 year. J Hand Surg [Br] 2005;30(6):611–4.
[9] Mack GR, McPherson SA, Lutz RB. Acute median neuropathy after wrist trauma. The role of emergent carpal tunnel release. Clin Orthop Relat Res 1994; 300:141–6.
[10] Ford DJ, Ali MS. Acute carpal tunnel syndrome. Complications of delayed decompression. J Bone Joint Surg [Br] 1986;68(5):758–9.
[11] Rozental TD, Beredjiklian PK, Steinberg DR, et al. Open fractures of the distal radius. J Hand Surg [Am] 2002;27(1):77–85.
[12] Falch JA. Epidemiology of fractures of the distal forearm in Oslo, Norway. Acta Orthop Scand 1983;54:291–5.

[13] McQueen MM, Gaston P, Court-Brown CM. Acute compartment syndrome. Who is at risk? J Bone Joint Surg [Br] 2000;82(2):200–3.

[14] Simpson NS, Jupiter JB. Delayed onset of forearm compartment syndrome: a complication of distal radius fracture in young adults. J Orthop Trauma 1995;9(5):411–8.

[15] Kupersmith LM, Weinfeld SB. Acute volar and dorsal compartment syndrome after a distal radius fracture: a case report. J Orthop Trauma 2003;17(5): 382–6.

[16] Charnley J. The mechanics of conservative treatment. In: The closed treatment of common fractures. London: Greenwich Medical Media; 2003. p. 43–59.

[17] Nesbitt KS, Failla JM, Les C. Assessment of instability factors in adult distal radius fractures. J Hand Surg [Am] 2004;29(6):1128–38.

[18] Mackenney PJ, McQueen MM, Elton R. Prediction of instability in distal radial fractures. J Bone Joint Surg [Am] 2006;88(9):1944–51.

[19] Hove LM, Solheim E, Skjeie R, et al. Prediction of secondary displacement in Colles' fracture. J Hand Surg [Br] 1994;19:731–6.

[20] Lafontaine M, Hardy D, Delince P. Stability assessment of distal radial fractures. Injury 1989;20: 208–10.

[21] Trumble TE, Wagner W, Hanel DP, et al. Intrafocal (Kapandji) pinning of distal radius fractures with and without external fixation. J Hand Surg [Am] 1998;23(3):381–94.

[22] Strohm PC, Muller CA, Boll T, et al. Two procedures for Kirschner wire osteosynthesis of distal radial fractures. A randomized trial. J Bone Joint Surg [Am] 2004;86(12):2621–8.

[23] Werber KD, Raeder F, Brauer RB, et al. External fixation of distal radial fractures: four compared with five pins: a randomized prospective study. J Bone Joint Surg [Am] 2003;85(4):660–6.

[24] Hargreaves DG, Drew SJ, Eckersley R. Kirschner wire pin tract infection rates: a randomized controlled trial between percutaneous and buried wires. J Hand Surg [Br] 2004;29(4):374–6.

[25] Botte MJ, Davis JL, Rose BA, et al. Complications of smooth pin fixation of fractures and dislocations in the hand and wrist. Clin Orthop Relat Res 1992; 276:194–201.

[26] Ahlborg HG, Josefsson PO. Pin-tract complications in external fixation of fractures of the distal radius. Acta Orthop Scand 1999;70(2):116–8.

[27] Egol KA, Paksima N, Puopolo S, et al. Treatment of external fixation pins about the wrist: a prospective, randomized trial. J Bone Joint Surg [Am] 2006;88(2): 349–54.

[28] Davies R, Holt N, Nayagam S. The care of pin sites with external fixation. J Bone Joint Surg [Br] 2005; 87:716–9.

[29] Stewart HD, Innes AR, Burke FD. The hand complications of Colles' fractures. J Hand Surg [Br] 1985;10(1):103–6.

[30] Dellon AL, Mackinnon SE. Susceptibility of the superficial sensory branch of the radial nerve to form painful neuromas. J Hand Surg [Br] 1984;9(1): 42–5.

[31] Bonatz E, Kramer TD, Masear VR. Rupture of the extensor pollicis longus tendon. Am J Orthop 1996; 25(2):118–22.

[32] Gelb RI. Tendon transfer for rupture of the extensor pollicis longus. Hand Clin 1995;11(3):411–22.

[33] Murase T, Hiroshima K. Rupture of the flexor tendon after malunited Colles' fracture. Scand J Plast Reconstr Surg Hand Surg 2003;37(3):188–91.

[34] Stahl S, Schwartz O. Complications of K-wire fixation of fractures and dislocations in the hand and wrist. Arch Orthop Trauma Surg 2001;121(9):527–30.

[35] Schnur DP, Chang B. Extensor tendon rupture after internal fixation of a distal radius fracture using a dorsally placed AO/ASIF titanium pi plate. Arbeitsgemeinschaft fur Osteosynthesefragen/Association for the Study of Internal Fixation. Ann Plast Surg 2000;44(5):564–6.

[36] Lowry KJ, Gainor BJ, Hoskins JS. Extensor tendon rupture secondary to the AO/ASIF titanium distal radius plate without associated plate failure: a case report. Am J Orthop 2000;29(10):789–91.

[37] Nunley JA, Rowan PR. Delayed rupture of the flexor pollicis longus tendon after inappropriate placement of the pi plate on the volar surface of the distal radius. J Hand Surg [Am] 1999;24(6): 1279–80.

[38] Bienek T, Kusz D, Cielinski L. Peripheral nerve compression neuropathy after fractures of the distal radius. J Hand Surg [Br] 2006;31(3):256–60.

[39] Zyluk A. Complex regional pain syndrome type I. Risk factors, prevention and risk of recurrence. J Hand Surg [Br] 2004;29(4):334–7.

[40] Lidström A. Fractures of the distal radius: a clinical and statistical study of end results. Acta Orthop Scand 1959;41(Suppl):79–81 123–7.

[41] Atkins RM, Duckworth T, Kanis JA. Features of algodystrophy after Colles' fracture. J Bone Joint Surg [Br] 1990;72:105–10.

[42] Bickerstaff DR, Kanis JA. Algodystrophy: an under-recognized complication of minor trauma. Br J Rheumatology 1994;33:240–8.

[43] Zyluk A. Algodystrophy after fractures of the distal radius. Chir Narzadow Ruchu Ortop Pol 1996;61: 349–55 [Polish].

[44] Field J, Protheroe DL, Atkins RM. Algodystrophy after Colles fractures is associated with secondary tightness of casts. J Bone Joint Surg [Br] 1994;76: 901–5.

[45] Combalia A. Over-distraction of the radiocarpal and midcarpal joints with external fixation of comminuted distal radial fractures. J Hand Surg [Br] 1996;21(2):289.

[46] Knirk JL, Jupiter JB. Intra-articular fractures of the distal end of the radius in young adults. J Bone Joint Surg [Am] 1986;68(5):647–59.

[47] Bradway JK, Amadio PC, Cooney WP. Open reduction and internal fixation of displaced, comminuted intra-articular fractures of the distal end of the radius. J Bone Joint Surg [Am] 1989;71(6): 839–47.

[48] Fernandez DL, Ring D, Jupiter JB. Surgical management of delayed union and nonunion of distal radius fractures. J Hand Surg [Am] 2001;26(2): 201–9.

[49] Bacorn RW, Kurtzke JF. Colle's fracture: a study of two thousand cases from the New York State Workmen's Compensation Board. J Bone Joint Surg [Am] 1953;35:643–58.

[50] Prommersberger KJ, Fernandez DL. Non union of distal radius fractures. Clin Orthop Relat Res 2004;419:51–6.

[51] Mckee MD, Waddell JP, Yoo D, et al. Nonunion of distal radius fractures associated with distal ulnar shaft fractures: a report of four cases. J Orthop Trauma 1997;11:49–53.

[52] Segalman KA, Clark GL. Un-united fractures of the distal radius: a report of 12 cases. J Hand Surg [Am] 1998;23:914–9.

[53] Smith VA, Wright TW. Non-union of the distal radius. J Hand Surg [Br] 1999;24:601–4.

[54] Ring D. Nonunion of the distal radius. Hand Clin 2005;21(3):443–7.

[55] Beumer A, McQueen MM. Fractures of the distal radius in low-demand elderly patients: closed reduction of no value in 53 of 60 wrists. Acta Orthop Scand 2003;74(1):98–100.

[56] McQueen M, Caspers J. Colles fracture: does the anatomical result affect the final function? J Bone Joint Surg [Br] 1988;70(4):649–51.

[57] Fernandez DL. Reconstructive procedures for malunion and traumatic arthritis. Orthop Clin North Am 1993;24(2):341–63.

[58] Park MJ, Cooney WP, Hahn ME, et al. The effects of dorsally angulated distal radius fractures on carpal kinematics. J Hand Surg [Am] 2002;27:223–32.

[59] Jupiter JB, Ring D. A comparison of early and late reconstruction of malunited fractures of the distal end of the radius. J Bone Joint Surg [Am] 1996; 78(5):739–48.

[60] Cooney WP, Dobyns JH, Lincheid RL. Complications of Colles' fracture. J Bone Joint Surg [Am] 1980;62:613–9.

[61] Hove LM, Nilsen PT, Furnes O, et al. Open reduction and internal fixation of displaced intraarticular fractures of the distal radius. 31 patients followed for 3–7 years. Acta Orthop Scand 1997;68(1):59–63.

[62] Kambouroglou GK, Axelrod TS. Complications of the AO/ASIF titanium distal radius plate system (pi plate) in internal fixation of the distal radius: a brief report. J Hand Surg [Am] 1998;23(4):737–41.

[63] Orbay JL, Fernandez DL. Volar fixation for dorsally displaced fractures of the distal radius: a preliminary report. J Hand Surg [Am] 2002;27(2):205–15.

[64] Krukhaug Y, Hove LM. Experience with the AO Pi-plate for displaced intra-articular fractures of the distal radius. Scand J Plast Reconstr Surg Hand Surg 2004;38(5):293–6.

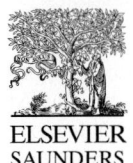

Acute Scaphoid Fractures
Julie E. Adams, MD, Scott P. Steinmann, MD*

The Department of Orthopaedic Surgery, Mayo Clinic, 200 First Street SW, Rochester, MN 55905, USA

Scaphoid fractures often occur as a result of a fall on the outstretched arm or a forced dorsiflexion injury of the wrist [1,2]. The traumatic incident may be minimal and the injury may be mistakenly dismissed as a sprain, especially if a fracture is nondisplaced and radiographs are read as negative. However, the penalty for missing these important injuries is high. The blood supply to the scaphoid is tenuous and, if disrupted by the fracture, healing may be compromised. Avascular necrosis occurs in an estimated 13% to 50% of scaphoid fractures, and the incidence is even higher in fractures involving the proximal one fifth of the scaphoid [2–5].

The scaphoid receives its blood supply primarily from the artery to the dorsal ridge of the scaphoid, a branch of the radial artery. The branches of this vessel enter the nonarticular portion of the scaphoid through foramina at the dorsal ridge at the level of the waist of the scaphoid [4,6]. Subsequently, these vessels divide and run proximally and palmarly to supply the proximal pole of the scaphoid [4,6]. Other branches provide 20% to 30% of the blood flow and arise from the distal palmar area of the scaphoid, originating either directly from the radial artery or the superficial palmar branch [1,2]. Thus, the vascularity of the proximal pole depends entirely on intraosseous blood flow. Because of the limited blood supply, fractures have a prolonged healing period, with an acute proximal pole fracture averaging 3 to 6 months. Nonunion may occur (in 5% to 10% of all cases, with an even higher incidence in displaced fractures), and numerous series document progression of nonunion to collapse and arthritis [1,2]. Because treating the established nonunion can be challenging, especially in the setting of progression to degenerative arthritis, diagnosing and appropriately treating the acute fracture and the possible sequelae of nonunion is essential.

Diagnosis of acute scaphoid fractures

Because early radiographs are normal for many patients, diagnosing a scaphoid fracture can sometimes be difficult. Most patients will experience tenderness to palpation over the anatomic snuff box or the distal scaphoid tubercle, pain with longitudinal compression of the thumb, and limited range of motion and pain at the end arc of motion, especially with flexion and radial deviation [7–9]. Reduced grip strength may be noted [7–9]. However, not all patients will experience pain over the scaphoid, even with a well-defined fracture seen on radiograph [7]. Overall, sensitivity is high for clinical examination, but specificity approaches only 74% to 80% [8,9].

Plain-film radiographs are usually obtained first in the acute setting when a scaphoid fracture is suspected. The lateral radiograph is particularly useful, and a proper study should show a colinear capitate and radius, with the pisiform located between the distal pole of the scaphoid and the body of the capitate. This study allows the carpal alignment and distal radioulnar joint alignment to be evaluated. Classically, patients who had clinical findings of scaphoid fracture but negative initial radiographs were treated with 2 weeks of cast immobilization followed by repeat examination and radiographic studies, with the belief that the delay allows for bony resorption adjacent to the fracture site, making the fracture visible [7,10].

Although this approach remains an accepted option for treatment, it may result in unnecessary

---

* Corresponding author.
E-mail address: steinmann.scott@mayo.edu
(S.P. Steinmann).

immobilization, with adverse effects on return to work and requirement for repeat radiographs, clinical examinations, and splint or cast changes [11–13]. Most patients who have a suspected scaphoid fracture have not actually injured the scaphoid, and casting for no fracture just to present a conservative treatment modality results in overtreatment at the expense of office visits, radiographs, and lost work.

Other options may include use of alternative imaging techniques. Bone scan is sensitive but not specific for diagnosing scaphoid fracture [14]. Bone scintigraphy has shown 100% sensitivity and 98% specificity for a scaphoid fracture compared with approximately 65% to 70% sensitivity for plain-film radiographs [15–20]. MRI is superior to repeat radiographs for detecting occult scaphoid fracture [21] and is considered by many the gold standard for detecting scaphoid fracture, with sensitivity of 95% to 100% and specificity approaching 100% [22–24]. Furthermore, the value of an MRI includes the ability to identify and diagnose other causes of wrist pain if a scaphoid fracture is not present. If a scaphoid fracture is identified, vascularity of the proximal pole can be determined preoperatively with MRI. Acute fractures may show normal or decreased T1 and increased T2 intensity [7]. Nonunion and impaired vascularity is often seen with low T1 and T2 marrow signal intensity, which may correlate with poor healing [25,26].

The importance of missed diagnosis is highlighted by the risk for nonunion in up to 12% of patients if an occult scaphoid fracture is not identified and immobilized. Therefore, many authorities recommend a highly conservative strategy to immobilize patients who have a history suggestive of scaphoid fracture but negative plain films. However, this treatment using splinting and casting can lead to loss of work and economic implications [11,12,14]. Cost of time off from work and serial casting and office visits easily exceeds the cost of an MRI or CT scan for definitive diagnosis [12].

In a randomized control trial of 28 patients who had suspected scaphoid fracture, Brooks and colleagues [13] investigated the cost-effectiveness of MRI for diagnosing suspected scaphoid fractures. Patients were randomized to undergo MRI scan or conservative treatment with immobilization and serial clinical and radiographic evaluation. Those who underwent MRI had a shorter duration of immobilization and decreased use of health care resources but increased cost to treat compared with patients randomized to the non-MRI group, who were immobilized and evaluated with serial clinical and radiographic examination. Cost per day of unnecessary immobilization between the groups was $44.37. However, these costs do not consider absenteeism from work and leisure activities [13]. Pillai and Jain [11] reported a rate of more than 80% of unnecessary immobilization when all clinically suspected scaphoid fractures with negative radiographs were immobilized in the traditional treatment algorithm. In this series, 6.7% of 90 initially radiographic-negative wrists were found to have a scaphoid fracture, whereas 10 additional patients had other injuries of the wrist not involving the scaphoid [11]. The findings suggest that the cost of needless immobilization, with further clinical and radiographic studies, would have exceeded early alternative investigations, such as MRI or bone scan, which were frequently required anyway [11].

Thorpe and colleagues [27] reported a series of 59 patients who had clinical symptoms suggesting scaphoid fracture but negative radiographs. All underwent MRI, bone scintigraphy, and clinical follow-up, with clinical follow-up deemed the gold standard for diagnosis. Clinically, 4 scaphoid fractures, 10 other fractures, and 3 significant ligamentous injuries were identified. Although all scaphoid fractures were identified with both MRI and bone scan, MRI was noted to have better interobserver agreement and fewer false-positives. Likewise, other causes of wrist pain, including ligamentous injury or carpal instability, could be identified with MRI, whereas these findings could not be diagnosed with bone scan. These investigators further noted that costs were similar [27].

In a study comparing sensitivity and specificity of MRI and bone scintigraphy in diagnosing occult scaphoid fractures, 43 patients who had wrist trauma and normal radiographs underwent MRI and bone scan an average of 19 days after injury. Of these, 6 patients (14%) ultimately were diagnosed with a scaphoid waist fracture. Patients were followed up for more than 1 year after injury. MRI was noted to be more sensitive in detecting occult scaphoid fracture, with fewer false-positives than bone scan [28]. Dorsay and colleagues [12] investigated the cost-effectiveness of early MRI for detecting occult scaphoid fractures. They noted that 75% of patients who had clinical evidence of scaphoid fracture would be immobilized unnecessarily if they underwent standard treatment with repeat radiographs after immobilization. The cost differential between standard follow-up and MRI was small [12].

In practice, although MRI can detect a fracture within 4 to 6 hours, this specialized study cannot always be obtained in the emergency department. However, obtaining an MRI at 36 to 48 hours is a reasonable goal. Occasionally, MRI may show a false-positive result, but false-negative examinations are rare. Thus, an early MRI can reliably exclude patients who do not have a scaphoid fracture and in whom immobilization may safely be discontinued. Although CT scans can also identify fractures and are useful for defining incomplete or nonunions and for preoperative planning with respect to intrascaphoid angles and scaphoid collapse, they are not as accurate as MRI for identifying acute occult scaphoid fractures and may not reveal alternative diagnoses, such as ligamentous injury.

Technetium bone scan is sensitive, but false-positives may occur in patients who have arthrosis or prior or concurrent injury. Likewise, bone scans require a delay in performing the test and often do not adequately elucidate alternative diagnoses. MRI is at least as sensitive and more specific, involves less radiation exposure, and may allow alternative problems to be diagnosed [13].

The authors' algorithm in a patient who has wrist trauma is to obtain anteroposterior, lateral, and oblique radiographic views of the wrist. If a scaphoid fracture is identified on the radiographs, then a CT scan can be obtained for surgical planning if necessary. If the radiographs are negative or equivocal, then a limited MRI of the wrist is then obtained to determine the presence or absence of a scaphoid fracture. If needed, a CT scan can also be obtained after the MRI to help plan for surgical treatment.

Classification

Classification of scaphoid fractures has been well described in the literature. Three common classifications used for scaphoid fracture are the Mayo classification, Russe classification, and Herbert classification (Fig. 1).

Some series have shown limited prognostic value and poor inter- and intraobserver reliability of scaphoid fracture classification schemes [29]; nevertheless, the Mayo, Russe, and Herbert classifications are commonly used in clinical practice and many authorities feel they may be helpful in determining treatment options and providing prognostic information. The first two classifications are based on anatomic planes of the scaphoid. However, the Herbert classification defines stable and unstable fractures [1,2,7] and therefore may be particularly helpful in determining treatment options. The type A Herbert [2] classification fracture is a stable acute fracture and type B is an unstable acute fracture. Stable fractures include fractures of the tubercle (A1) and an incomplete fracture of the waist (A2). These fractures can potentially be treated nonoperatively. The other types of fractures in the Herbert classification usually require surgical treatment. Type B fractures (acute unstable fractures) include subtypes B1 (oblique fractures of the distal third), B2 (displaced or mobile fractures of the waist), B3 (proximal pole fractures), B4 (fracture dislocations), and B5 (comminuted fractures). Type C fractures show delayed union after more than 6 weeks of plaster immobilization, whereas type D fractures are established nonunions, either fibrous (D1) or sclerotic (D2).

Treatment of acute scaphoid fractures

Differences of opinion exist on indications for operative therapy in the setting of acute scaphoid fractures. Nonoperative therapy often requires prolonged immobilization of at least 12 weeks, and much longer for more proximal fractures [3,7,30,31]. Although few studies exist in the literature documenting consequences of long-term cast immobilization, clearly this treatment can result in significant stiffness that may require a protracted rehabilitation period, and some series suggest a poorer outcome after prolonged immobilization [30,32,33]. In addition, union rates are higher with operative management, approaching 95% or higher in most series of all types of scaphoid fractures [30,34–36]. Multiple studies of percutaneous fixation of scaphoid fractures have documented satisfactory outcomes and minimal complications [2,30,34,37–44]. Comparative studies of surgery versus casting for acute fractures have documented better range of motion at the wrist, earlier healing (7 weeks until union versus 12 weeks with casting), and earlier return to work with surgical management. Furthermore, minimal differences were seen in these groups with respect to outcomes and satisfaction at final follow-up and, importantly, no increased complication rate related to surgical treatment was observed [30,45,46]. Therefore, percutaneous treatment of acute scaphoid fracture

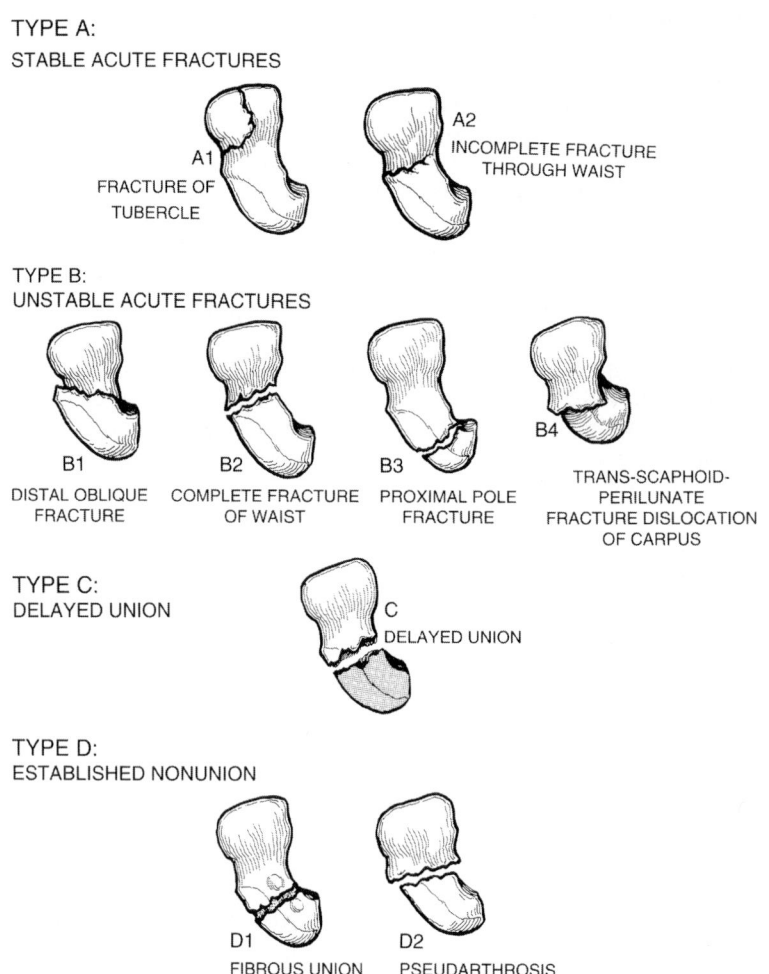

Fig. 1. Herbert classification of scaphoid fractures. (*From* Herbert TJ. The fractured scaphoid. St. Louis (MO): Quality Medical Publishing;1990; with permission.)

seems to have a low morbidity level and, in the hands of an experienced surgeon, will not result in a higher complication rate than nonsurgical treatment [2]. Furthermore, up to one third of proximal pole fractures may result in a nonunion even with appropriate immobilization. Several studies showed good results with early surgical intervention, and a careful dorsal approach does not seem to injure the blood supply.

Authors' preferred approach to acute scaphoid fractures

In considering overall treatment options, perhaps all proximal pole and displaced scaphoid fractures are best treated with surgery (Figs. 2 and 3). Percutaneous screw fixation is preferred. The scaphoid is reduced and preliminarily pinned dorsally to volarly, and then a screw introduced volarly, unless the fracture is of the proximal pole, in which case the opposite approach is taken.

Scaphoid nonunions

Despite optimal therapy, nonunion or malunion may ensue. Patient and nonunion characteristics must be considered when treating the established scaphoid nonunion. Because the bony attachments of the dorsal intercarpal ligament and dorsal scapholunate ligament are maintained in the setting of a fracture of the proximal one third of the scaphoid, these fractures rarely show instability patterns, such as dorsal intercalated segmental instability. Nonunion of a scaphoid fracture,

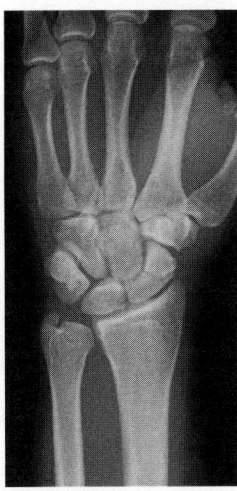

Fig. 2. This acute scaphoid fracture was identified in a 29-year-old man who fell from a ladder injuring his nondominant hand.

however, can result in carpal malalignment and progressive radiocarpal arthrosis [5,7,47,48], but the real effect of a malunion is less clearly defined. In a series of 160 scaphoid nonunions treated with internal fixation and bone grafting in which 90% healed, failure to achieve union was related to a proximal fracture location, avascularity of the proximal pole, instability of the fracture, and delay to surgery. Residual flexion deformity of the scaphoid did not affect the outcome, and therefore malunion was not believed to contribute to a poor result. This study, however, showed that the length of immobilization negatively affects the functional outcome [33].

Summary

Operative fixation is the authors' preferred treatment for acute fractures in which the fracture is clearly visible on plain film radiographs. We believe that a clearly visible fracture line is evidence of a displaced fracture that should be treated operatively. Several authors have shown low morbidity and satisfactory outcomes after operative fixation [2,30,34,37–44]. Surgical time and morbidity are minimal and complications are infrequent. In addition, acute treatment may result in decreased risk for nonunion.

When a patient presents with clinical symptoms suggesting scaphoid fracture, initial radiographs are obtained. A scaphoid fracture readily identified on plain films represents displacement, and acute operative treatment is recommended, with the authors preferring percutaneous placement of a cannulated screw. If no fracture is seen and clinical findings suggest scaphoid fracture, an MRI should be obtained. If the MRI shows a fracture, nonoperative treatment may be undertaken with a short-arm thumb spica cast, with the wrist in neutral position immobilizing the thumb to the interphalangeal joint, unless the fracture is at the proximal pole. This cast is maintained for 6 weeks and then a CT scan is obtained. If the CT still suggests unhealed fracture, cast immobilization is maintained for another 6 weeks, except when a fracture of the proximal pole is identified on MRI. In these cases, percutaneous operative fixation should be undertaken to lessen the chance of nonunion. After operative fixation, the patient is placed in a volarly based thumb spica splint. If the patient is unlikely to comply with postoperative activity restrictions, then a short-arm thumb spica cast is placed. If the patient is reliable, a removable splint may be provided. Activity is restricted to lifting no more than 2 lb, no repetitive use, and using the hand only for activities of daily living and personal hygiene. At 6 weeks, a CT scan is obtained to evaluate for evidence of union. If evidence of healing is present, such as disappearance of the fracture line, spot welding between fragments, or callous formation, then immobilization is discontinued and the patient allowed a gradual return to activities. The literature suggests that partial

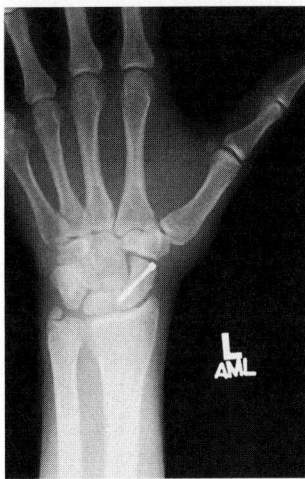

Fig. 3. Treatment consisted of percutaneous screw placement. No treatment was indicated for his chronic ulnar styloid nonunion.

union is often present but usually progresses to full union without the need for additional immobilization [49]. If no evidence of healing is noted, immobilization is continued and another CT scan obtained 4 to 6 weeks later.

References

[1] Russe O. Fracture of the carpal navicular. Diagnosis, non-operative treatment, and operative treatment. J Bone Joint Surg Am 1960;42:759–68.

[2] Herbert TJ, Fisher WE. Management of the fractured scaphoid using a new bone screw. J Bone Joint Surg Br 1984;66(1):114–23.

[3] Cooney WP, Dobyns JH, Linscheid RL. Fractures of the scaphoid: a rational approach to management. Clin Orthop Relat Res 1980;(149):90–7.

[4] Freedman DM, Botte MJ, Gelberman RH. Vascularity of the carpus. Clin Orthop Relat Res 2001;(383):47–59.

[5] Szabo RM, Manske D. Displaced fractures of the scaphoid. Clin Orthop Relat Res 1988;(230):30–8.

[6] Gelberman RH, Menon J. The vascularity of the scaphoid bone. J Hand Surg Am 1980;5(5):508–13.

[7] Linscheid RL, Weber ER. Scaphoid fractures and nonunion. In: Cooney WP, Linscheid RL, Dobyns JH, editors. The wrist: diagnosis and operative treatment. St Louis (MO): Mosby; 1998. p. 385–430.

[8] Parvizi J, Wayman J, Kelly P, et al. Combining the clinical signs improves diagnosis of scaphoid fractures. A prospective study with follow-up. J Hand Surg Br 1998;23(3):324–7.

[9] Grover R. Clinical assessment of scaphoid injuries and the detection of fractures. J Hand Surg Br 1996;21(3):341–3.

[10] Watson-Jones R. Fractures and joint injuries. 4th edition. Baltimore (MD): Williams & Wilkins; 1952–5, vols1–2, p. 86–9, 606–28.

[11] Pillai A, Jain M. Management of clinical fractures of the scaphoid: results of an audit and literature review. Eur J Emerg Med 2005;12(2):47–51.

[12] Dorsay TA, Major NM, Helms CA. Cost-effectiveness of immediate MR imaging versus traditional follow-up for revealing radiographically occult scaphoid fractures. AJR Am J Roentgenol 2001;177(6):1257–63.

[13] Brooks S, Cicuttini FM, Lim S, et al. Cost effectiveness of adding magnetic resonance imaging to the usual management of suspected scaphoid fractures. Br J Sports Med 2005;39(2):75–9.

[14] Nielsen PT, Hedeboe J, Thommesen P. Bone scintigraphy in the evaluation of fracture of the carpal scaphoid bone. Acta Orthop Scand 1983;54(2):303–6.

[15] Brydie A, Raby N. Early MRI in the management of clinical scaphoid fracture. Br J Radiol 2003;76(905):296–300.

[16] Mittal RL, Dargan SK. Occult scaphoid fracture: a diagnostic enigma. J Orthop Trauma 1989;3(4):306–8.

[17] Gabler C, Kukla C, Breitenseher MJ, et al. Diagnosis of occult scaphoid fractures and other wrist injuries. Are repeated clinical examinations and plain radiographs still state of the art? Langenbecks Arch Surg 2001;386(2):150–4.

[18] Brondum V, Larsen CF, Skov O. Fracture of the carpal scaphoid: frequency and distribution in a well-defined population. Eur J Radiol 1992;15(2):118–22.

[19] Leslie IJ, Dickson RA. The fractured carpal scaphoid. Natural history and factors influencing outcome. J Bone Joint Surg Br 1981;63(2):225–30.

[20] Brismar J. Skeletal scintigraphy of the wrist in suggested scaphoid fracture. Acta Radiol 1988;29(1):101–7.

[21] Kukla C, Gaebler C, Breitenseher MJ, et al. Occult fractures of the scaphoid. The diagnostic usefulness and indirect economic repercussions of radiography versus magnetic resonance scanning. J Hand Surg Br 1997;22(6):810–3.

[22] Raby N. Magnetic resonance imaging of suspected scaphoid fractures using a low field dedicated extremity MR system. Clin Radiol 2001;56(4):316–20.

[23] Amrani KK. Diagnosing radiographically occult scaphoid fractures: what's the best second test? Journal of the American Society for Surgery of the Hand 2005;5(3):134–8.

[24] Breitenseher MJ, Metz VM, Gilula LA, et al. Radiographically occult scaphoid fractures: value of MR imaging in detection. Radiology 1997;203(1):245–50.

[25] Perlik PC, Guilford WB. Magnetic resonance imaging to assess vascularity of scaphoid nonunions. J Hand Surg Am 1991;16(3):479–84.

[26] Trumble TE. Avascular necrosis after scaphoid fracture: a correlation of magnetic resonance imaging and histology. J Hand Surg Am 1990;15(4):557–64.

[27] Thorpe AP, Murray AD, Smith FW, et al. Clinically suspected scaphoid fracture: a comparison of magnetic resonance imaging and bone scintigraphy. Br J Radiol 1996;69(818):109–13.

[28] Fowler C, Sullivan B, Williams LA, et al. A comparison of bone scintigraphy and MRI in the early diagnosis of the occult scaphoid waist fracture. Skeletal Radiol 1998;27(12):683–7.

[29] Desai VV, Davis TR, Barton NJ. The prognostic value and reproducibility of the radiological features of the fractured scaphoid. J Hand Surg Br 1999;24(5):586–90.

[30] Bond CD, Shin AY, McBride MT, et al. Percutaneous screw fixation or cast immobilization for nondisplaced scaphoid fractures. J Bone Joint Surg Am 2001;83(4):483–8.

[31] Gellman H, Caputo RJ, Carter V, et al. Comparison of short and long thumb-spica casts for non-displaced fractures of the carpal scaphoid. J Bone Joint Surg Am 1989;71(3):354–7.

[32] Skirven T, Trope J. Complications of immobilization. Hand Clin 1994;10(1):53–61.
[33] Inoue G, Shionoya K, Kuwahata Y. Herbert screw fixation for scaphoid nonunions. An analysis of factors influencing outcome. Clin Orthop Relat Res 1997;(343):99–106.
[34] Saeden B, Tornkvist H, Ponzer S, et al. Fracture of the carpal scaphoid. A prospective, randomized 12-year follow-up comparing operative and conservative treatment. J Bone Joint Surg Br 2001;83(2):230–4.
[35] Rettig ME, Kozin SH, Cooney WP. Open reduction and internal fixation of acute displaced scaphoid waist fractures. J Hand Surg Am 2001;26(2):271–6.
[36] Dias JJ, Wildin CJ, Bhowal B, et al. Should acute scaphoid fractures be fixed? A randomized controlled trial. J Bone Joint Surg Am 2005;87(10):2160–8.
[37] Trumble TE, Gilbert M, Murray LW, et al. Displaced scaphoid fractures treated with open reduction and internal fixation with a cannulated screw. J Bone Joint Surg Am 2000;82(5):633–41.
[38] Chen AC, Chao EK, Hung SS, et al. Percutaneous screw fixation for unstable scaphoid fractures. J Trauma 2005;59(1):184–7.
[39] Herbert TJ. Use of the Herbert bone screw in surgery of the wrist. Clin Orthop Relat Res 1986;(202):79–92.
[40] Herbert TJ. Experience with the Herbert screw in the treatment of scaphoid fractures. J Hand Surg Br 1989;14(4):463.
[41] Filan SL, Herbert TJ. Herbert screw fixation of scaphoid fractures. J Bone Joint Surg Br 1996;78(4):519–29.
[42] Wu WC. Percutaneous cannulated screw fixation of acute scaphoid fractures. Hand Surg 2002;7(2):271–8.
[43] Haddad FS, Goddard NJ. Acute percutaneous scaphoid fixation using a cannulated screw. Chir Main 1998;17(2):119–26.
[44] Haddad FS, Goddard NJ. Acute percutaneous scaphoid fixation. A pilot study. J Bone Joint Surg Br 1998;80(1):95–9.
[45] Drac P, Manak P, Labonek I. Percutaneous osteosynthesis versus cast immobilization for the treatment of minimally and non-displaced scaphoid fractures. Functional outcomes after a follow-up of at least 12 month. Biomed Pap Med Fac Univ Palacky Olomouc Czech Repub 2005;149(1):149–51.
[46] Adolfsson L, Lindau T, Arner M. Acutrak screw fixation versus cast immobilization for undisplaced scaphoid waist fractures. J Hand Surg Br 2001;26(3):192–5.
[47] Mack GR, Bosse MJ, Gelberman RH, et al. The natural history of scaphoid non-union. J Bone Joint Surg Am 1984;66(4):504–9.
[48] Ruby LK, Leslie BM. Wrist arthritis associated with scaphoid nonunion. Hand Clin 1987;3(4):529–37.
[49] Singh HP, Forward D, Davis TR, et al. Partial union of acute scaphoid fractures. J Hand Surg Br 2005;30(5):440–5.

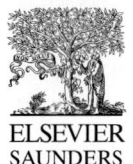

Management of Scaphoid Nonunions

Thanapong Waitayawinyu, MD, H. James Pfaeffle, MD, PhD,
Wren V. McCallister, MD, Nicholas M. Nemechek,
Thomas E. Trumble, MD*

*Department of Orthopaedics and Sports Medicine, University of Washington,
4245 Roosevelt Way NE, Box 354743, Seattle, WA 98195-4743, USA*

Scaphoid nonunions present a challenging problem because of the geometry of the fracture and vascular pattern of the scaphoid. Fractures that are proximal to the perforating vessels on the dorsal radial surface of the scaphoid can cause significant bone ischemia of the proximal pole. A delay in diagnosis, inadequate initial treatment, proximal location, avascular necrosis, and associated carpal instability with acute scaphoid fractures can lead to either nonunions of the scaphoid waist or the proximal pole [1]. Nonunion can exist with or without avascular necrosis (AVN) of the proximal fragment. AVN of the proximal pole can occur with a scaphoid waist nonunion, but there is almost always a loss of blood supply in proximal pole nonunions. Nonunions involving the scaphoid waist usually have significant bone loss and carpal collapse, with palmar rotation of the distal pole to produce an apex dorsal humpback deformity. If left untreated, scaphoid nonunions can progress to carpal collapse, AVN, and a predictable pattern of radiocarpal arthrosis [2]. The goals of surgery for a scaphoid nonunion include not only uniting the fracture but also restoring alignment. Evidence suggests that operative treatment provides better results when care is taken to correct any deformity and address the vascularity of the scaphoid.

Cast immobilization, with or without adjunctive treatments such as pulsed electromagnetic fields, is not as effective as surgical intervention, and is typically not recommended to treat scaphoid nonunions [3]. Immobilization with long-arm casts for prolonged periods of time (longer than 6 months) can have a significant impact on a patient's wrist and elbow motion, as well as quality of life. Because union rates with pulsed electromagnetic fields are inferior to those with surgery, electromagnetic fields should only be used as an adjunct to surgery, or in cases in which surgery is not possible. Several reports indicate that few nonunions remain stable or nondisplaced and free of arthritis after 10 years [2,4]. Because of the evidence linking nonunions with osteoarthritis, surgery is recommended for most young, healthy patients, even if they are free of symptoms and have normal wrist mobility. Most hand surgeons recommend open reduction and internal fixation of the nonunion combined with a bone graft [5–8].

Surgical treatment for correction of scaphoid nonunions with bone grafting and internal fixation is contraindicated in cases of progressive arthrosis. Relative contraindications include chronicity of the nonunion [9], smoking [10,11], and patient age [12], all of which are important to consider when evaluating the potential for success after treatment of a nonunion.

Approach to treatment

Determining the location of the nonunion, the degree of collapse, and viability of the proximal fragment are important steps in approaching the

---

* Corresponding author.
  E-mail address: tnm3@u.washington.edu
  (T.E. Trumble).

treatment of scaphoid nonunions. Without AVN, waist fractures are best treated via a volar approach, and proximal pole fractures via a dorsal approach. Fractures with AVN of the proximal pole are best served by a dorsal approach with a vascularized bone graft.

Plain radiographs are helpful, but not foolproof, in determining whether or not the scaphoid fracture involves the proximal pole. The fracture often angles from distal volar to proximal dorsal, which can make the plain radiographs deceiving. CT can help differentiate nonunions in the waist from those in the proximal pole, especially when there is substantial bone resorption (Fig. 1).

CT scans provide the most precise definition of the osseous anatomy. The sagittal images, parallel to the long axis of the scaphoid, obtained from CT scans provide the best view to determine the extent of collapse (the so-called "humpback deformity"), and assist in planning for bone grafting procedures. The lateral intrascaphoid angle (Fig. 2A) described by Amadio and colleagues [13], and the height-to-length ratio of the scaphoid (Fig. 2B) described by Bain and colleagues [14] can be accurately measured with a CT scan. These measurements, obtained from sagittal images parallel to the long axis of the scaphoid, can help to accurately identify the magnitude of collapse and angulation of the scaphoid.

The classic radiographic signs of sclerosis, cystic changes, and areas of significant bone resorption are not always reliable indicators of the presence of avascular necrosis in scaphoid nonunion. Recent studies have established the value of MRI in assessing vascularity of the proximal pole [15–18]. Low signal on both T1- and T2-weighted images appears to be associated with the greatest compromise of vascular supply and poor healing rates when traditional nonvascularized grafts are used. Proximal fragments with an absence of T1-weighted marrow signal (Fig. 3) have demonstrated osteonecrosis, empty bone lacunae, and poor uptake of fluorescent bone labels on biopsy [18]. In contrast, retention of some proximal pole signal has been associated with viable bone when examined histologically, and normal uptake of fluorescent labels. When the MRI demonstrates avascular necrosis of the proximal pole, the authors recommend a vascularized bone graft.

The recommended techniques for surgical correction of a scaphoid nonunion with bone graft and internal fixation are as follows:

Scaphoid waist nonunion with a viable proximal pole: palmar approach
Proximal pole scaphoid nonunion with a viable proximal pole: dorsal approach
Proximal pole scaphoid nonunion with an avascular proximal pole: dorsal-radial approach with vascularized graft
Scaphoid waist nonunion with an avascular proximal pole: volar-radial approach with vascularized graft

Scaphoid waist nonunion with a viable proximal pole: palmar approach

The palmar approach is widely used for bone grafting and internal fixation of nonunions of the scaphoid waist. It allows access to the distal pole and waist for nonvascularized bone grafting, retrograde internal fixation, and correction of the humpback deformity that can result after scaphoid collapse. The palmar approach is used for scaphoid waist nonunions with a viable proximal pole, so as to preserve the remaining dorsal blood supply. The palmar approach is not recommended for nonunions of the proximal pole. Nonunions of the proximal pole of the scaphoid, with or without avascular necrosis, should be addressed via a dorsal approach. If the nonunion extends into the proximal pole and a palmar approach is used in contrast to a dorsal approach, adequate fixation in the small proximal pole fragment may not be achieved. A preoperative CT scan can help to avoid this problem if there is any doubt based upon plain films. A preoperative

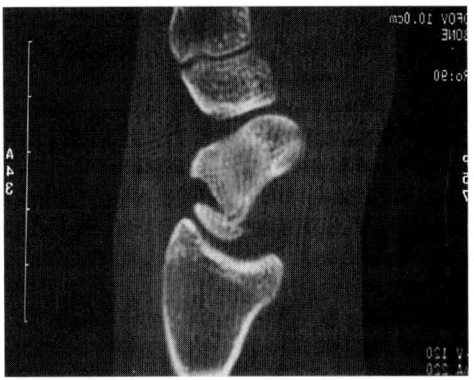

Fig. 1. Sagittal CT scan shows the location of nonunion site over proximal pole of scaphoid, which helps in determining the surgical approach.

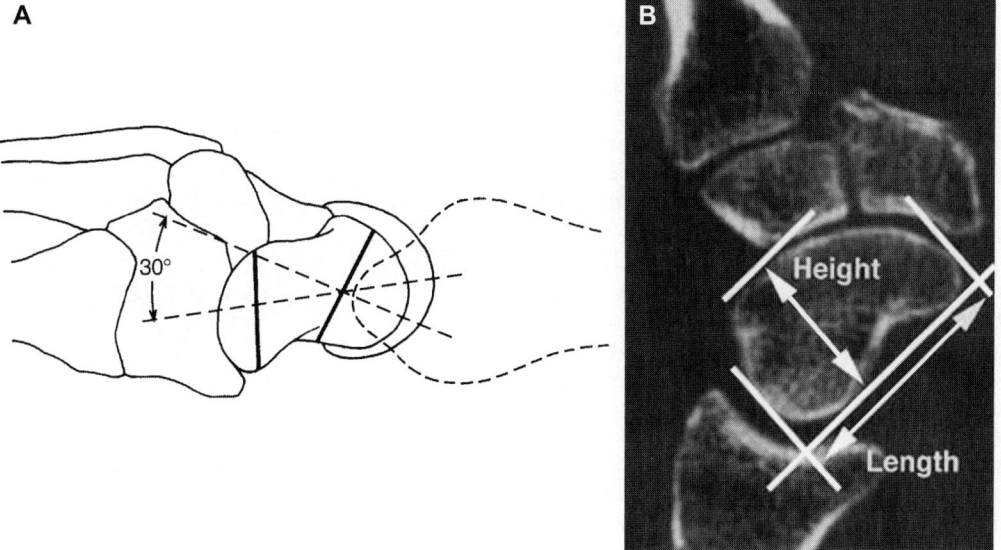

Fig. 2. (*A*) The lateral intrascaphoid angle measured from a sagittal CT image helps to identify the magnitude of collapse and angulation of the scaphoid. (*From* Trumble TE. Principles of hand surgery and therapy, fractures and dislocations of the carpus. Philadelphia: Elsevier Saunders; 2000. p. 94; with permission.) (*B*) The extent of collapse and angulation of scaphoid nonunion can be defined by measuring the height-to-length ratio from the CT scan. (*From* Trumble TE, Gilbert M, Murray LW, et al. Displaced scaphoid fractures treated with open reduction and internal fixation with a cannulated screw. J Bone Joint Surg 2000;82A:633–41; with permission.)

MRI can help identify AVN that is not seen on plain radiographs, so that a vascularized bone graft (best placed via a dorsal approach) can be considered during surgical planning [18].

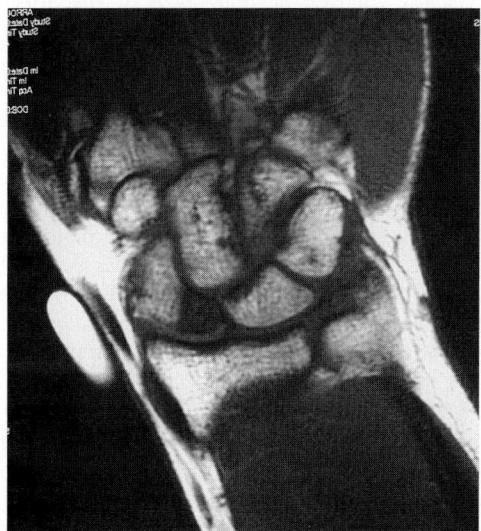

Fig. 3. Decreased signal seen in the proximal pole fragment on T1-weighted MRI indicates avascular necrosis of proximal pole.

General anesthesia is used routinely, and is necessary if one plans to harvest bone graft from the iliac crest. The patient is positioned supine with the operative extremity on a radiolucent arm table. The arm is cleansed with antimicrobial solution and draped sterilely. Exsanguination is performed with an Esmarch's bandage and an upper arm tourniquet inflated. Standard screw fixation is used, which provides significant stable internal fixation for bone graft and fracture. Dental picks are favored over Kirschner wire joysticks to avoid propagation or comminution in the fracture fragments while reducing the scaphoid nonunion. Small osteotomes are used to wedge the collapsed scaphoid into its correct alignment. Kirchner wires can be used to prevent rotation of fragments during drilling. A high-speed burr and fine curettes are used to complete a full excavation of the nonunion site and removal of sclerotic portions of the proximal pole. A fluoroscopy unit is used to monitor the accuracy of fracture reduction and to confirm the position of the guide wire and screw.

To expose the fracture, a standard Russe incision is made along the course of the flexor carpi radialis (FCR) tendon and extending distally along the border of the glabrous skin of the thenar eminence. The distal incision is limited to the level of the scaphotrapezial joint in preparation for screw fixation starting in the distal pole of the scaphoid (Fig. 4). Splitting the sheath of the FCR allows it to be retracted ulnarly, and protects the palmar cutaneous branch of the median nerve. The deep branch of the radial artery to the palmar arch is retracted radially. The floor of the FCR sheath is incised longitudinally to expose the distal pole and waist of the scaphoid (Fig. 5). The fracture is evident at the proximal margin of this incision. Preservation of as much of the radioscaphocapitate (RSC) ligament as possible is crucial, because it helps to contain the proximal pole and prevent it from translating or subluxating volarly [19,20]. If cannulated screws are used, it is not necessary to release the RSC ligament to facilitate placement of the guide jig. In case of nascent nonunions, a volar limited approach can be used as an alternative approach. The limited Russe approach is used to expose the scaphotrapezial trapezoid (STT) joint. The volar beak of the trapezium is removed, and percutaneous screw fixation with bone grafting is performed through this approach.

The humpback deformity must be corrected to allow for stable screw fixation in the long axis of the scaphoid, and to prevent arthrosis [13,19]. Correction of the collapsed scaphoid to obtain acceptable alignment is achieved using small osteotomes. Failure to correct the volar collapse of the scaphoid results in an increased incidence of arthritis and decreased wrist motion [13,20]. Care must be taken not to disrupt the dorsal cortex of the scaphoid, which could damage any remaining blood supply to the proximal pole, and

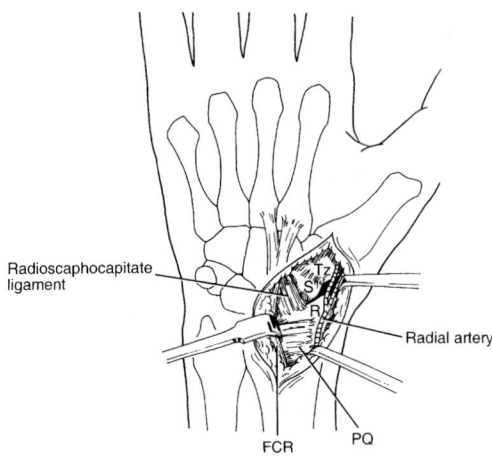

Fig. 5. The palmar approach to the scaphoid. The waist, distal pole of the scaphoid, and STT joint have been exposed through the floor of FCR sheath after the tendon is retracted ulnarly and deep branch of radial artery is retracted radially. PQ, pronator quadratus; R, radius; S, scaphoid; Tz, Trapezium. (*From* Trumble TE. Principles of hand surgery and therapy, fractures and dislocations of the carpus. Philadelphia: WB Saunders; 2000. p. 98; with permission.)

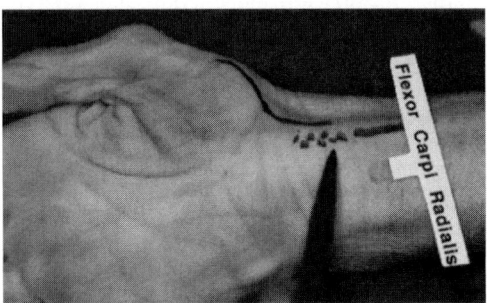

Fig. 4. A standard Russe incision has been drawn out along the course of the FCR, extending along the border of the thenar eminence distally to the scaphotrapezial trapezoid (STT) joint. (*From* Trumble TE. Principles of hand surgery and therapy, fractures and dislocations of the carpus. Philadelphia: WB Saunders; 2000. p. 98; with permission.)

make the fracture highly unstable. Full excavation of the nonunion site and removal of sclerotic portions of the proximal pole are accomplished through the use of fine curettes and a high-speed burr with saline irrigation. Reduction of the nonunion is achieved using dental picks. When approached volarly, the inner wall of the dorsal cortex can be notched to accommodate a wedge graft. A wedge-shaped graft can correct the scaphoid alignment and allow for stable screw placement without cutting out volarly. Great care should be taken, however, to avoid complete penetration of the dorsal cortex. The continuity of the dorsal cortex serves as a hinge around which the distal fragment can be rotated as it is reduced with wrist dorsiflexion. Complete disruption of the dorsal cartilage and fibrous tissue can make the nonunion extremely unstable and allow the graft to be displaced dorsally. Because screw fixation offers significant stability, the authors often use a cancellous bone graft rather than a corticocancellous one. When large segments of the volar cortex are missing, the corticocancellous graft actually improves stability, especially if it can be compressed with a scaphoid screw.

Screw fixation proceeds by first removing the small volar beak or foot process of the trapezium with a small ronguer. The prominent volar lip of the trapezium forces the surgeon to place the screw too dorsal in the proximal pole of the scaphoid. Removing this lip before placing the guide wire provides accurate access for insertion of a screw into the long axis of the scaphoid, so that the proximal screw threads are centered in the central one third of the proximal pole. Failure to do so can result in a screw that is placed too dorsal near the fracture line (Fig. 6). Insert the guide wire into the central axis of scaphoid up to the limits of the subchondral bone of proximal pole to measure the length of the screw. Next, the guide wire is driven into the radius to prevent it from dislodging (Fig. 7A, B).

Placing the screw in the center of the proximal pole helps to provide the most stable fixation of the nonunion. Failure to achieve accurate screw placement can result in an unstable construct and the potential for a lower rate of union [19]. Next, the cannulated drill and tap are used to prepare the path for the screw while monitoring the progress using fluoroscopy. Once the screw is inserted, the guide wire is removed and plain radiographs are obtained to confirm the position of the screw. The volar capsule is repaired with interrupted sutures, especially if any portion of the RSC ligament has been incised. The subcutaneous layer and skin are closed in separate layers.

Postoperatively, patients are splinted for 2 weeks. Sutures are removed and patients are then put into a short-arm cast for 1 month. Subsequently, the patient is placed in a custom molded removable splint until the radiographs confirm union. Once the patient is in the removable splint, protected range-of-motion exercises are begun.

Recent reports of bone grafting and internal fixation of scaphoid nonunions describe greater than 90% union rates, with fairly rapid healing that reduces the need for prolonged immobilization. In the authors' series, patients regained 80% of the motion of the contralateral wrist and more than 70% of the strength of the contralateral hand. Ninety percent of the patients who had painful scaphoid nonunions noted a significant decrease in wrist pain [19,21–23].

Proximal pole scaphoid nonunion with a viable proximal pole: dorsal approach

A proximal pole scaphoid nonunion in which the proximal pole is viable is a rare entity, and an MRI should be obtained to confirm vascularity. These are usually treated by nonvascularized bone grafting, with internal fixation from a dorsal approach. The principle of the dorsal approach is to remove the avascular bone from the proximal pole, and to achieve stable screw fixation without displacing the small proximal fragment or compromising the remaining vascular supply. Realizing that a proximal fragment's vascular supply has already been significantly compromised by a fracture mitigates, but does not eliminate, concerns that a dorsal approach might further threaten its vascularity. The fracture line of a nonunion frequently occurs from distal volar to proximal dorsal; thus a screw placed from a volar approach may not cross the nonunion, and can displace the proximal pole fragment [24]. The dorsal approach allows the screw to be placed into the central portion of the proximal pole fragment (Fig. 8) [25,26]. When avascular necrosis of the proximal pole exists, a vascularized bone graft should be used.

Exposure of the fracture begins with a small longitudinal incision made in the midline of the wrist, centered over the radiocarpal joint. The sheath of the extensor pollicis longus (EPL) tendon is released. The capsule and fourth dorsal compartment are sharply dissected off the dorsal lip of the radius. A longitudinal incision over the radiocarpal joint capsule is made to expose the scapholunate articulation. By flexing the wrist, the entry site for the screw appears just adjacent to the scapholunate interosseous ligament (SLIL), which is exposed. Care should be taken to

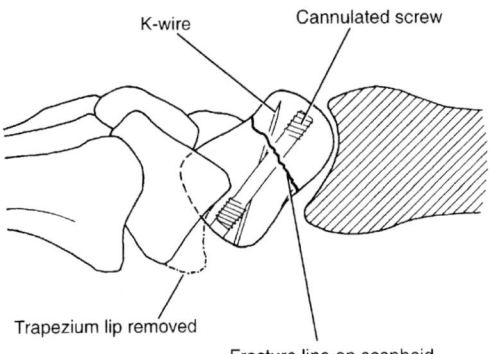

Fig. 6. To expose the distal pole of the scaphoid for accurate insertion of a screw into the long and central axis of the scaphoid, the small volar beak of trapezium needs to be removed. K-wire, Kirschner wire. (*From* Trumble TE. Principles of hand surgery and therapy, fractures and dislocations of the carpus. Philadelphia: WB Saunders; 2000. p. 98; with permission.)

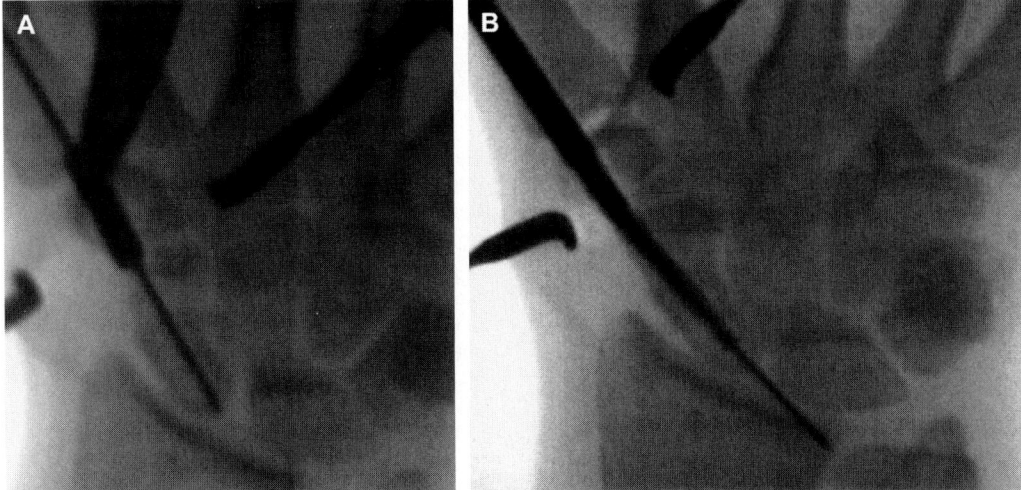

Fig. 7. (*A*) The guide wire is inserted through central axis of the scaphoid to the subchondral bone of the proximal pole, and allows measurement of screw length. (*From* Trumble TE. Principles of hand surgery and therapy, fractures and dislocations of the carpus. Philadelphia: WB Saunders; 2000. p. 98; with permission.) (*B*) To prevent dislodging of guide wire while preparing the screw hole by drilling, the guide pin is driven into the distal radius after determining the screw length. (*From* Trumble TE. Principles of hand surgery and therapy, fractures and dislocations of the carpus. Philadelphia: WB Saunders; 2000. p. 98; with permission.)

preserve the tissue on the dorsal ridge of the scaphoid, in an attempt to preserve as much of the remaining blood supply as possible, which is already significantly compromised by the fracture.

The next step is locating the nonunion, removal of fibrous tissue and necrotic bone, and reduction of the fracture. A small needle may be used to help locate the plane of nonunion. Fine curettes and a high-speed burr are used to remove the necrotic bone. The fracture is reduced and a guide wire for a cannulated screw is inserted via an insertion point that is close to the SLIL's attachment to the scaphoid. The screw should be targeted toward the scaphoid tubercle and inserted to the level of the subchondral bone of the distal pole. It is important to confirm its position with fluoroscopy.

Screw length is then measured. It is imperative that the screw be countersunk adequately, because insertion is performed in the center of the articular surface of the proximal pole. It is therefore important to undersize the screw by 3 to 4 mm to avoid problems countersinking the screw. After determining the screw length with a depth gauge, the guide wire is driven into the trapezium to prevent it from being dislodged during drilling and tapping (Fig. 9A, B). Frequently, a second Kirschner wire is placed to prevent rotation or displacement of the proximal pole fragment during screw insertion. Failure to control the proximal fragment during drilling, tapping, or inserting the screw can result in further displacement of the fracture and lead to inaccurate fixation.

After the guide wire is driven up into the trapezium, screw preparation begins with drilling

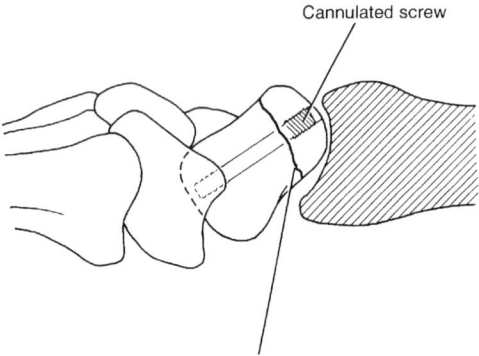

Fig. 8. Because of direction of fracture and size of proximal fragment, the dorsal approach allows proper placement of the screw into the central portion of the proximal pole fragment. (*From* Trumble TE. Principles of hand surgery and therapy, fractures and dislocations of the carpus. Philadelphia: WB Saunders; 2000. p. 101; with permission.)

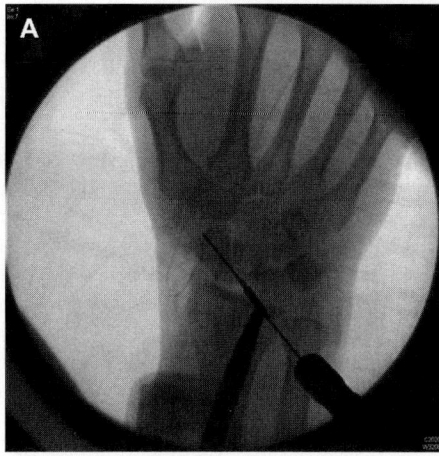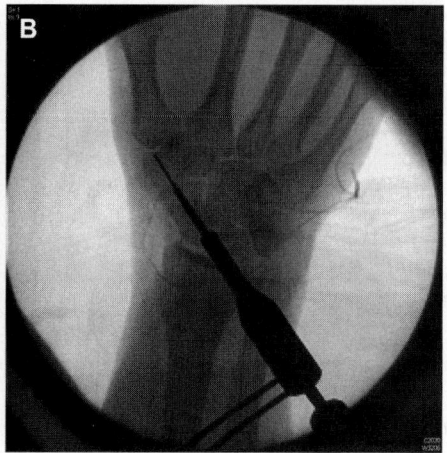

Fig. 9. (A) From dorsal approach to the proximal pole of the scaphoid, a guide wire for a cannulated screw is inserted to the subchondral bone of the distal pole for measurement of screw length; its position can be confirmed with fluoroscopy. (B) The guide wire is driven into the trapezium to prevent it from being dislodged during screw hole preparation.

and tapping. The screw can be inserted either freehand or using a cannulated screw through a guide wire. In small proximal pole fragments, the authors prefer to remove the guide wire and insert a noncannulated Herbert screw, because it leaves a smaller defect or footprint in the cartilage of the proximal pole. The capsule is closed with absorbable sutures. The third dorsal compartment is not repaired and the subcutaneous tissue and skin are closed in subsequent layers.

Postoperatively, the authors use the same postoperative management protocol as the volar approach procedure. Because of the longer times to union and the lower rate of successful healing, a bone stimulator will often be added during the postoperative cast immobilization.

The prognosis for patients who have proximal pole fractures and proximal pole nonunions is more guarded than for those who have fractures and nonunions of the scaphoid waist. The time until union is 2 to 3 months longer for proximal pole nonunions. Healing rates of acute fractures or nonunions of proximal pole are 30% to 50% lower when compared with fractures and nonunions of the scaphoid waist.

Proximal pole scaphoid nonunion with an avascular proximal pole: dorsal-radial approach with vascularized graft

Healing of proximal pole scaphoid nonunions can be achieved with stable internal fixation and bone grafting [22,24], but the rate of healing correlates directly with the vascularity of the proximal pole [27]. Unfortunately, fibrous unions or persistent nonunions tend to develop when osteonecrosis of the proximal pole is present. Such conditions are often refractory to traditional bone grafting methods, even when augmented with internal fixation. The use of pedicled vascularized bone grafts can help revascularize ischemic bone, and thus would theoretically improve the union rate and time to union [28]. A recent meta-analysis [29] reported an 88% union rate when a vascularized bone graft was used for the treatment of scaphoid nonunions with avascular necrosis of the proximal pole, compared with a 47% union rate when a nonvascularized bone graft was used.

Early vascularized grafts were often based on a pedicle from the pronator quadratus insertion on the distal radius [30,31]. Recently, a number of vascularized bone graft sources have been described, including the ulnar artery [32], volar carpal artery [33,34], vascularized periosteal flaps of distal radius [35,36], capsular-based flap vascularized graft [37], implanting the second dorsal intermetacarpal artery into nonunion sites with inlay corticocancellous bone graft [38], and even a free vascularized graft from the iliac crest [39]. At present, the most frequently used donor sites include the dorsoradial aspect of the distal radius, first described by Zaidemberg and colleagues [40], and the second metacarpal graft [25,41].

The vascularized bone graft described by Zaidemberg and colleagues is presented in this article. It relies on the superior irrigating arterial branch of the radial artery that Sheetz and colleagues [7] have defined as the 1,2 intercompartmental supraretinacular artery (1,2 ICSRA). This artery travels in a distal-to-proximal direction along the retinaculum, between the tendons of the first and second dorsal compartment. The 2,3 ICSRA can also be used. These vascularized grafts can be harvested through the same dorsal approach used for internal fixation of the scaphoid nonunion.

Exposure is via a radial extension of the dorsal approach for the viable proximal pole, and allows for harvesting of the graft as well as exposure of the scaphoid nonunion (Fig. 10). A midline incision over the dorsal aspect of the wrist that curves proximally and radially over the interval between the first and second dorsal compartments is created, taking care to protect sensory branches of the radial nerve. The third dorsal compartment is released, and the EPL tendon is retracted radially.

The authors recommend harvesting the vascularized bone graft before debriding the scaphoid. This allows the surgeon to gauge the size of the window in the scaphoid that must be prepared. The 1,2 ICSRA vessel is identified as it takes off from the radial artery and travels proximally and dorsally in the extensor retinaculum to pierce the first dorsal compartment. In 5% or fewer of cases the 1,2 ICRSA is not present, and the second dorsal metacarpal artery graft is used as an alternative [25,41]. The first dorsal compartment is released along its palmar surface, and the tendons are retracted radially with the EPL. The 1,2 ICSRA nutrient vessel is visible as a thin red line in the groove between the first and second dorsal compartments. The ECRB and ECRL are retracted ulnarly, and the arterial pedicle is mobilized by making parallel incisions in the periosteum between the two compartments, tracing the course of the artery from distal to proximal. Once a 2.0 to 2.5 cm pedicle has been prepared, the periosteum around the planned donor site is incised as an ellipse or rectangle, and a fine oscillating saw, with constant irrigation, is used to cut the three sides of the graft, excluding the side under the vascular pedicle. Small osteotomes are then used to complete elevation of the graft (Fig. 11A, B).

To expose the scaphoid fracture, the capsule and fourth dorsal compartment are sharply dissected off the dorsal lip of the radius. A longitudinal incision over the radiocarpal joint capsule is made to expose the scapholunate articulation. By flexing the wrist, the entry site for the screw appears just adjacent to the SLIL, which is exposed. Care should be taken to preserve the tissue on the dorsal ridge of the scaphoid, in an attempt to preserve as much of the remaining blood supply as possible; it is already significantly compromised by the fracture.

Preparation of the scaphoid nonunion site and complete removal of necrotic bone is done next with fine curettes and a high-speed burr, guided by fluoroscopic imaging. After preparation of the nonunion site, the tourniquet is released to observe bleeding from the graft. Additional bone graft is harvested from the bed of the vascularized graft, and is packed into the crevices of the scaphoid defect before tamping in the vascularized graft. The vascularized graft is then rotated into the defect (Fig. 12), and secured with either Kirschner wires or a screw. To improve exposure and decrease tension in the vascular pedicle, a radial styloidectomy is frequently performed. If the graft does not fit into the defect in the scaphoid, the authors' first choice is to enlarge the defect of the scaphoid, rather than risk damaging the vascular pedicle by resizing the graft.

Screw fixation in combination with bone grafting has significantly better union rates when compared with Kirschner-wire fixation in combination with bone grafting [12], and also provides stability, which can reduce the time needed for immobilization. Screw fixation can be performed similar to the technique described above for the dorsal approach (Fig. 13A, B). Care is taken that the screw is countersunk adequately, because

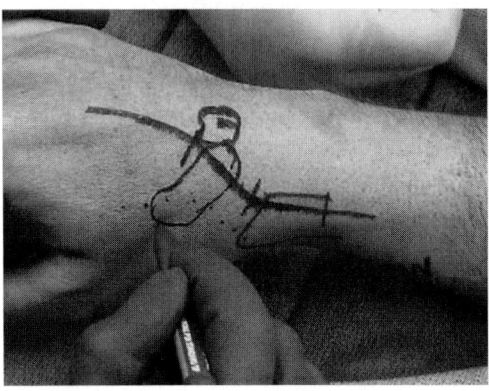

Fig. 10. The dorsal-radial incision to approach an avascular proximal pole nonunion of the scaphoid with harvesting of vascularized bone graft from distal radius has been drawn. Proximal and radial extension of the midline incision over the dorsal aspect of the wrist is shown.

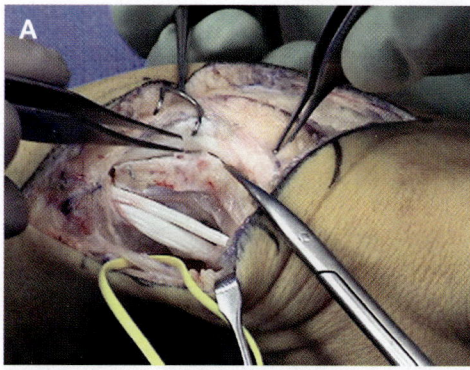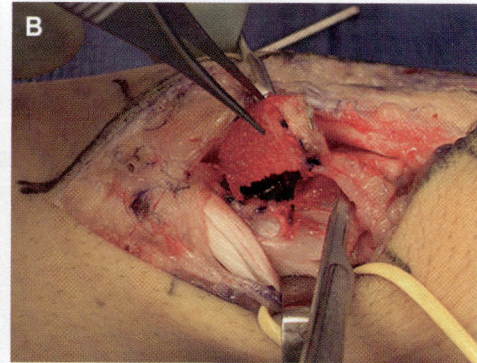

Fig. 11. (*A*) Parallel incisions in the periosteum between the first and second extensor compartments, tracing the course of the 1,2 ICSRA, are created before saw cuts are performed to mobilize the arterial pedicle. (*B*) After the three sides of the graft, excluding the side under the vascular pedicle, are cut by fine oscillating saw and small osteotomes, the graft can be elevated completely.

insertion is performed in the center of the articular surface of the proximal pole. Failure to accurately place screws used for internal fixation of the scaphoid can result decreased rates of union. The capsule is closed loosely to avoid strangulation of the vascular pedicle. The subcutaneous tissues and skin are closed in layers.

Postoperatively, patients are splinted, followed by casting for 2 months after the sutures are removed. Subsequently, the patient is placed in a custom-molded removable splint until the radiographs confirm union. Once the patient is in the removable splint, protected range-of-motion exercises are begun.

Good outcomes are reported following this procedure—union was achieved in all 11 patients included in Zaidemberg's original article [40].

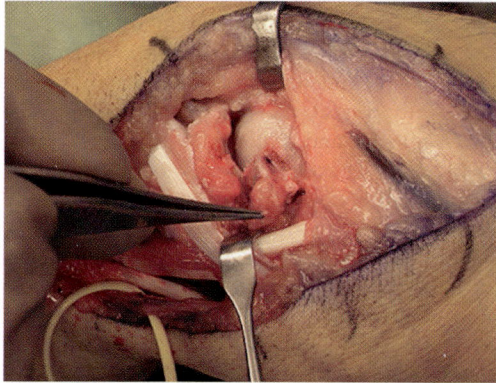

Fig. 12. The vascularized graft is trimmed, mobilized, and rotated into the nonunion site. A screw is placed from dorsal to volar to secure the graft and stabilize the fracture.

Union rates of 100% also have been reported by many researchers [1,42,43], and 72% union rates in large case series were reported by Chang and colleagues [12]. In several of the original cases, a concomitant palmar approach was required to fully address the flexion deformity of the distal scaphoid fragment. This has usually been necessary in waist fractures with a severe humpback deformity. In more recent cases, the authors have rotated the vascular pedicle into a volar defect through a single approach. Vascularized grafting clearly has a role in the treatment of scaphoid nonunions that present with osteonecrosis or prove refractory to traditional grafting.

Scaphoid waist nonunion with an avascular proximal pole: volar-radial approach with vascularized graft

Patients who have significant deformity and collapse from a long-standing scaphoid waist nonunion with AVN may require a more complex procedure, which entails exposure of the scaphoid via a volar-radial approach. The procedure is performed in a similar fashion to that described for waist nonunions and proximal pole nonunions with an avascular proximal pole, except that the graft site is exposed via an extension of the palmar approach.

Exposure is via a Matti-Russe incision extended proximally along the radial margin the distal forearm (Fig. 14). Again, the vascularized graft is identified and mobilized, then the nonunion site is prepared, A radial flap is elevated to expose the first and second dorsal

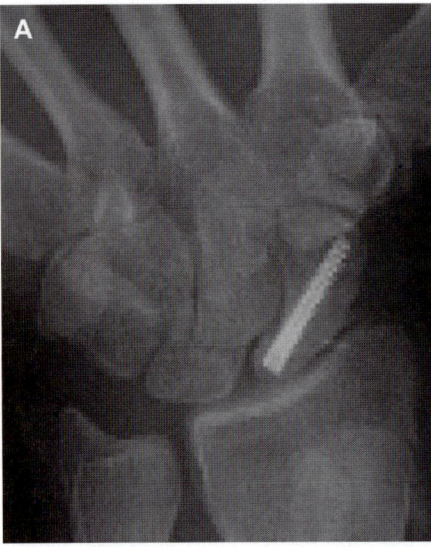
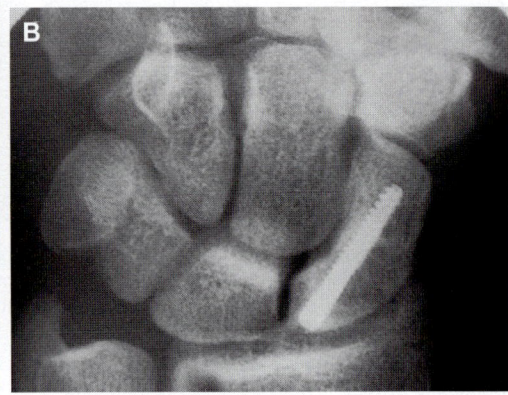

Fig. 13. (*A*) Immediate postoperative radiograph shows the vascularized bone graft fitted into the defect and secured with screw fixation. (*B*) Follow-up radiograph demonstrates smooth connection of trabeculae, indicating union of the scaphoid after vascularized bone grafting with screw fixation.

compartments. The dorsal radial sensory nerve is retracted dorsally. The 1,2 ICSRA vessel is identified longitudinally between the two compartments. The pedicle is mobilized as described in the previous section on avascular proximal pole nonunion.

The scaphoid waist fracture is then exposed by elevation of the ulnar-sided skin flap to expose the FCR sheath. The scaphoid waist is then exposed,

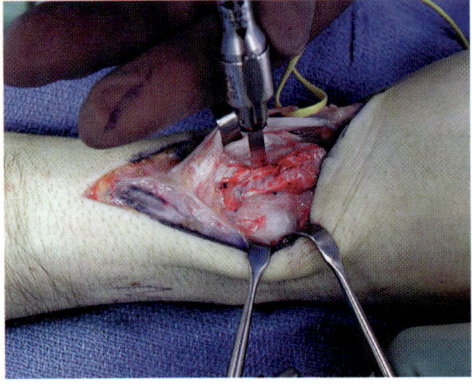

Fig. 14. For scaphoid waist nonunions, the 1,2 ICSRA graft is exposed via a Russe incision that is extended radially. In this picture, the APL is retracted volarly (volar is up and the hand is to the right). Two longitudinal parallel cuts are being made on either side of the artery, which is coming in from a distal direction.

and the nonunion site prepared as described in the section on scaphoid waist nonunion (Fig. 15). Distally, the 1-2 ICSRA arises from a branch of the radial artery that takes off just proximal to the radial styloid and travels under the abductor pollicis longus (APL), before traveling in a retrograde manner between the first and second dorsal compartments. The bone graft and pedicle are passed under the APL and tunneled dorsal to the radial artery, so that the graft can be inserted into the volar defect in the scaphoid (Fig. 16). A radial styloidectomy is usually required. The graft may be trimmed to a wedge shape to correct the humpback deformity. A guide wire followed by a screw is placed from the volar side, as described in the section on scaphoid waist nonunion (Fig. 17). Failure to correct the humpback deformity of the scaphoid, and failure to accurately place screws used for internal fixation of the scaphoid, can result decreased rates of union. The capsule is closed loosely to avoid strangulation of the vascular pedicle. The subcutaneous tissues and skin are closed in layers.

Postoperatively patients are splinted followed by casting for 2 months after the sutures are removed. Subsequently, the patient is placed in a custom-molded removable splint until the radiographs confirm union [Fig. 18]. Once the patient is in the removable splint, protected range-of-motion exercises are begun.

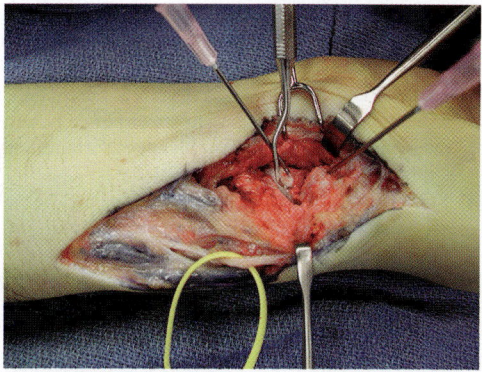

Fig. 15. After mobilizing the 1,2 ICSRA graft, the scaphoid waist nonunion is exposed via dissection through the FCR subsheath. In this picture, the APL is retracted radially and the FCR in an ulnar direction (volar is up and the hand is to the right). The nonunion site is carefully opened to correct the humpback deformity, and a high-speed burr is used to prepare the site for the graft.

Complications following scaphoid nonunion surgery

Persistent nonunion

The persistence of nonunion may require a second bone grafting procedure or a vascularized bone graft (VBG). The collapse of the small proximal fragment can result in degenerative radiocarpal arthritis, requiring salvage surgery.

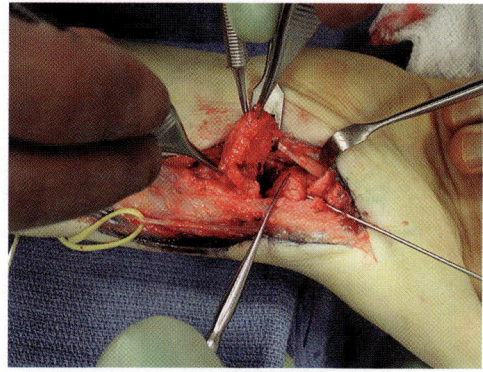

Fig. 16. The 1,2 ICSRA graft is passed underneath the APL and tunneled dorsal to the radial artery. Here the graft was fashioned into a wedge shape with a cortical base. The guide wire for the cannulated screw was placed in the distal scaphoid first, and is advanced to secure the graft after the graft has been placed into the nonunion site.

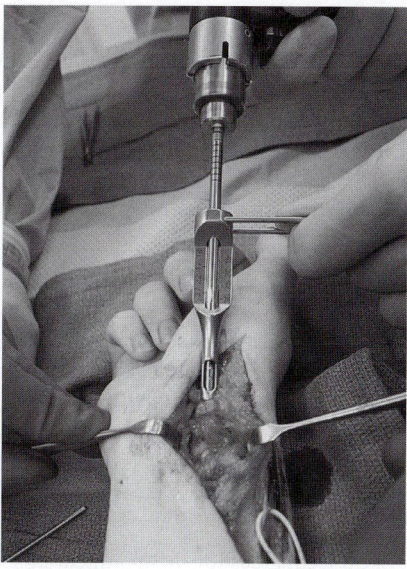

Fig. 17. A volar screw is placed over the guide wire securing the 1,2 ICSRA graft in the scaphoid waist nonunion site.

Hardware malpositioning

Improper positioning of screws in the scaphoid can lead to failure of compression and further delayed healing if the threads do not cross the fracture. Screws that penetrate the articular surface may lead to iatrogenic arthritis.

Stiffness

A further restriction of range of motion of the wrist may be found after bone grafting and internal fixation of scaphoid nonunions.

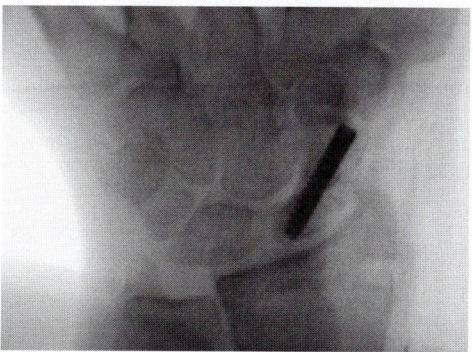

Fig. 18. Postoperative radiograph showing 1,2 ICSRA graft secured in the scaphoid waist nonunion site.

Pain

Postoperative pain is a byproduct of any bony procedure about the wrist; however, these procedures may result in continued postoperative pain at an increased level, particularly when surgery to correct nonunions is performed in relatively asymptomatic patients.

Nerve injury

In the palmar surgical approach, the median nerve and its palmar cutaneous branch are at risk for injury. In a dorsal approach, especially when harvesting a dorsoradial vascularized bone graft, the radial sensory nerve is at risk.

Summary

Surgical techniques for the treatment of scaphoid nonunions are much more demanding than those for acute fracture, because they must address greater bone resorption, carpal collapse, and avascular necrosis. The location of the nonunion site and viability of the proximal fragment are the critical factors in determining the surgical approach. When nonunions are located in the waist and no avascular necrosis is present, the palmar approach is appropriate, and permits correction of the humpback deformity. The dorsal approach is used for accurate screw placement in nonunions of the proximal pole of the scaphoid. For proximal pole nonunions with avascular necrosis of the proximal pole, the addition of a vascularized bone graft from the distal radius using a dorsal-radial approach is considered. When a scaphoid waist nonunion exists with avascular necrosis of the proximal pole, correction of the humpback deformity and vascularized bone grafting from the distal radius using a volar-radial approach are recommended. Screw fixation is always recommended. Salvage procedures, such as proximal row carpectomy, scaphoidectomy with or without limited intercarpal arthrodesis, and total wrist fusion, are reserved for cases with severe carpal collapse and arthrosis.

References

[1] Steinmann SP, Bishop AT, Berger RA. Use of the 1,2 intercompartmental supraretinacular artery as a vascularized pedicle bone graft for difficult scaphoid nonunion. J Hand Surg [Am] 2002;27(3): 391–401.

[2] Ruby LK, Stinson J, Belsky MR. The natural history of scaphoid non-union. A review of fifty-five cases. J Bone Joint Surg Am 1985;67(3):428–32.

[3] Adams BD, Frykman GK, Taleisnik J. Treatment of scaphoid nonunion with casting and pulsed electromagnetic fields: a study continuation. J Hand Surg [Am] 1992;17(5):910–4.

[4] Mack GR, Bosse MJ, Gelberman RH, et al. The natural history of scaphoid non-union. J Bone Joint Surg Am 1984;66(4):504–9.

[5] Bunker TD, McNamee PB, Scott TD. The Herbert screw for scaphoid fractures. A multicentre study. J Bone Joint Surg Br 1987;69(4):631–4.

[6] Herbert TJ, Fisher WE, Leicester AW. The Herbert bone screw: a ten year perspective. J Hand Surg [Br] 1992;17(4):415–9.

[7] Sheetz KK, Bishop AT, Berger RA. The arterial blood supply of the distal radius and ulna and its potential use in vascularized pedicled bone grafts. J Hand Surg [Am] 1995;20(6):902–14.

[8] Stark A, Brostrom LA, Svartengren G. Surgical treatment of scaphoid nonunion. Review of the literature and recommendations for treatment. Arch Orthop Trauma Surg 1989;108(4):203–9.

[9] Schuind F, Haentjens P, Van Innis F, et al. Prognostic factors in the treatment of carpal scaphoid nonunions. J Hand Surg [Am] 1999;24(4):761–76.

[10] Little CP, Burston BJ, Hopkinson-Woolley J, et al. Failure of surgery for scaphoid non-union is associated with smoking. J Hand Surg [Br] 2006;31(3): 252–5.

[11] Nolte PA, van der Krans A, Patka P, et al. Low-intensity pulsed ultrasound in the treatment of nonunions. J Trauma 2001;51(4):693–702 [discussion: 702–3].

[12] Chang MA, Bishop AT, Moran SL, et al. The outcomes and complications of 1,2-intercompartmental supraretinacular artery pedicled vascularized bone grafting of scaphoid nonunions. J Hand Surg [Am] 2006;31(3):387–96.

[13] Amadio PC, Berquist TH, Smith DK, et al. Scaphoid malunion. J Hand Surg [Am] 1989;14(4): 679–87.

[14] Bain GI, Bennett JD, MacDermid JC, et al. Measurement of the scaphoid humpback deformity using longitudinal computed tomography: intra- and interobserver variability using various measurement techniques. J Hand Surg [Am] 1998;23(1):76–81.

[15] Morgan WJ, Breen TF, Coumas JM, et al. Role of magnetic resonance imaging in assessing factors affecting healing in scaphoid nonunions. Clin Orthop Relat Res 1997;336:240–6.

[16] Perlik PC, Guilford WB. Magnetic resonance imaging to assess vascularity of scaphoid nonunions. J Hand Surg [Am] 1991;16(3):479–84.

[17] Sakuma M, Nakamura R, Imaeda T. Analysis of proximal fragment sclerosis and surgical outcome of scaphoid non-union by magnetic resonance imaging. J Hand Surg [Br] 1995;20(2):201–5.

[18] Trumble TE. Avascular necrosis after scaphoid fracture: a correlation of magnetic resonance imaging and histology. J Hand Surg [Am] 1990;15(4):557–64.

[19] Trumble TE, Clarke T, Kreder HJ. Non-union of the scaphoid. Treatment with cannulated screws compared with treatment with Herbert screws. J Bone Joint Surg Am 1996;78(12):1829–37.

[20] Trumble TE, Gilbert M, Murray LW, et al. Displaced scaphoid fractures treated with open reduction and internal fixation with a cannulated screw. J Bone Joint Surg Am 2000;82(5):633–41.

[21] Herbert TJ, Fisher WE. Management of the fractured scaphoid using a new bone screw. J Bone Joint Surg Br 1984;66(1):114–23.

[22] Inoue G, Shionoya K. Herbert screw fixation by limited access for acute fractures of the scaphoid. J Bone Joint Surg Br 1997;79(3):418–21.

[23] Tsuyuguchi Y, Murase T, Hidaka N, et al. Anterior wedge-shaped bone graft for old scaphoid fractures or non-unions. An analysis of relevant carpal alignment. J Hand Surg [Br] 1995;20(2):194–200.

[24] Robbins RR, Ridge O, Carter PR. Iliac crest bone grafting and Herbert screw fixation of nonunions of the scaphoid with avascular proximal poles. J Hand Surg [Am] 1995;20(5):818–31.

[25] Mathoulin C, Brunelli F. Further experience with the index metacarpal vascularized bone graft. J Hand Surg [Br] 1998;23(3):311–7.

[26] Yuceturk A, Isiklar ZU, Tuncay C, et al. Treatment of scaphoid nonunions with a vascularized bone graft based on the first dorsal metacarpal artery. J Hand Surg [Br] 1997;22(3):425–7.

[27] Green DP. The effect of avascular necrosis on Russe bone grafting for scaphoid nonunion. J Hand Surg [Am] 1985;10(5):597–605.

[28] Shin AY, Bishop AT. Pedicled vascularized bone grafts for disorders of the carpus: scaphoid nonunion and Kienbock's disease. J Am Acad Orthop Surg 2002;10(3):210–6.

[29] Merrell GA, Wolfe SW, Slade JF 3rd. Treatment of scaphoid nonunions: quantitative meta-analysis of the literature. J Hand Surg [Am] 2002;27(4):685–91.

[30] Kawai H, Yamamoto K. Pronator quadratus pedicled bone graft for old scaphoid fractures. J Bone Joint Surg Br 1988;70(5):829–31.

[31] Leung PC, Hung LK. Use of pronator quadratus bone flap in bony reconstruction around the wrist. J Hand Surg [Am] 1990;15(4):637–40.

[32] Guimberteau JC, Panconi B. Recalcitrant non-union of the scaphoid treated with a vascularized bone graft based on the ulnar artery. J Bone Joint Surg Am 1990;72(1):88–97.

[33] Kuhlmann JN, Mimoun M, Boabighi A, et al. Vascularized bone graft pedicled on the volar carpal artery for non-union of the scaphoid. J Hand Surg [Br] 1987;12(2):203–10.

[34] Mathoulin C, Haerle M. Vascularized bone graft from the palmar carpal artery for treatment of scaphoid nonunion. J Hand Surg [Br] 1998;23(3): 318–23.

[35] Dailiana ZH, Malizos KN, Urbaniak JR. Vascularized periosteal flaps of distal forearm and hand. J Trauma 2005;58(1):76–82.

[36] Dailiana ZH, Malizos KN, Zachos V, et al. Vascularized bone grafts from the palmar radius for the treatment of waist nonunions of the scaphoid. J Hand Surg [Am] 2006;31(3):397–404.

[37] Sotereanos DG, Darlis NA, Dailiana ZH, et al. A capsular-based vascularized distal radius graft for proximal pole scaphoid pseudarthrosis. J Hand Surg [Am] 2006;31(4):580–7.

[38] Fernandez DL, Eggli S. Non-union of the scaphoid: revascularization of the proximal pole with implantation of a vascular bundle and bone-grafting. J Bone Joint Surg Am 1995;77(6):883–93.

[39] Gabl M, Reinhart C, Lutz M, et al. Vascularized bone graft from the iliac crest for the treatment of nonunion of the proximal part of the scaphoid with an avascular fragment. J Bone Joint Surg Am 1999;81(10):1414–28.

[40] Zaidemberg C, Siebert JW, Angrigiani C. A new vascularized bone graft for scaphoid nonunion. J Hand Surg [Am] 1991;16(3):474–8.

[41] Sawaizumi T, Nanno M, Nanbu A, et al. Vascularised bone graft from the base of the second metacarpal for refractory nonunion of the scaphoid. J Bone Joint Surg Br 2004;86(7):1007–12.

[42] Malizos KN, Dailiana ZH, Kirou M, et al. Long-standing nonunions of scaphoid fractures with bone loss: successful reconstruction with vascularized bone grafts. J Hand Surg [Br] 2001;26(4): 330–4.

[43] Uerpairojkit C, Leechavengvongs S, Witoonchart K. Primary vascularized distal radius bone graft for nonunion of the scaphoid. J Hand Surg [Br] 2000;25(3):266–70.

Carpal Bone Fractures

Steven Papp, MD, MSc, FRCS(C)

Department of Orthopaedic Surgery, University of Ottawa, Ottawa Civic Hospital, 1053 Carling Avenue, Ottawa, Ontario, Canada K1Y 4E9

Carpal bone fractures are probably more common than reported. The eight carpal bones vary significantly in shape and size and how they articulate with the other bones of the wrist. These complex articulations make plain radiologic interpretation of the wrist confusing to many physicians, and therefore missed injuries are probably more common than realized. For example, several case reports have been written on the delayed diagnosis of hamate hook fractures and different radiologic projections that would detect the injury [1–4]. Missed hamate fractures often go undiagnosed for months and can leave patients with wrist dysfunction. The complex three-dimensional relationship of the carpal bones makes plain radiographs difficult to use; therefore CT scanning is probably a more accurate test to understand these fractures fully. Taking CT scans of all wrist injuries is probably not a reasonable solution, however.

Because the incidence of carpal bone fractures is probably underreported, the exact incidence of each injury is difficult to quantify. Scaphoid fractures, which account for about 70% of all carpal bone fractures, are a common source of long-term pain, and often require surgery, are discussed elsewhere in this issue. Thirty percent of carpal bone fractures occur to the other seven bones of the wrist, however, and they can cause significant wrist disability (Fig. 1). Prompt diagnosis and appropriate treatment lead to faster recovery and better long-term outcome in many cases.

E-mail address: spapp@Ottawahospital.on.ca

Hamate fractures

Hook fractures

The hook of the hamate protrudes off the hamate into the base of the hypothenar eminence and is palpable 2 cm distal and radial to the pisiform. The relatively thick layer of skin, palmar fibrofatty tissue, and palmaris brevis make palpation more difficult than that of the pisiform. There are multiple attachments to the hook of the hamate including the transverse carpal ligament radially, the pisohamate ligament ulnarly, and the flexor digiti minimi and opponens digiti muscles. The hamate marks the ulnar border of the carpal tunnel and the radial border of Guyon's canal. These attachments may confer some stability to the hook of the hamate, but the intermittent forces also may explain the high rate of nonunion associated with this fracture. The base of the hamate serves as a pulley to the flexor tendons, in particular to the flexor tendons to the fourth and fifth fingers. Demirkan and colleagues [5] showed that with excision of the hook of the hamate, and therefore loss of the hook as a pulley, flexor tendon force decreases significantly, especially with the wrist in extension and ulnar deviation. The deep branch of the ulnar nerve runs just ulnar and in close proximity to the hamate.

Most commonly, fracture of the hook of the hamate occurs in sports involving racquets or clubs. These fractures may occur by direct trauma or indirect mechanisms. During a forceful swing, the base of the club can impinge against the hook of the hamate and cause a fracture (Fig. 2). This fracture would occur most commonly in the left hand of a right-handed golfer at follow-through or when the club head accidentally strikes the

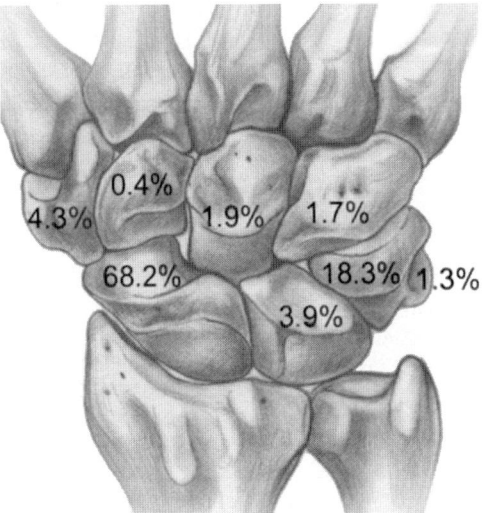

Fig. 1. Relative incidence of carpal bone fractures. (*From* Garcia-Elias M. Carpal bone fractures (excluding scaphoid fractures). In: Watson HK, Weinberg J, editors. The wrist. Philadelphia: Lippincott Williams & Wilkins; 2001. p. 174; with permission.)

ground [6]. It is possible that a strong contraction of the flexor tendons in a wrist position of extension and ulnar deviation or trauma to the pisiform causing tension on the pisohamate ligament could cause an indirect fracture.

Hook of the hamate fractures should be considered in patients presenting with ulnar-sided wrist pain, in particular in patients who play sports that put them at risk. In the acute setting, pain is present with palpation in the hypothenar area. Pain also may be present with resisted flexion of the fourth and fifth finger. These injuries,

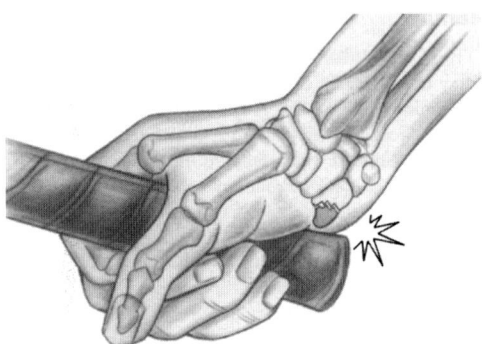

Fig. 2. Mechanism of hook of hamate fracture. (*From* Sennwald GR. Carpal bone fractures other than the scaphoid. In: Berger RA, Weiss AP, editors. Hand surgery. Philadelphia: Lippincott Williams & Wilkins; 2004. p. 418; with permission.)

however, often are missed and are diagnosed as wrist sprains [7]. Therefore, patients may present with more chronic symptoms of pain. Sources of ulnar-sided wrist pain include distal radioulnar joint pathology, triangular fibrocartilaginous complex tears, lunotriquetral (LT) tears, flexor carpi ulnaris tendonitis, pisotriquetral arthritis, and other causes, but hamate fractures should be considered. Pain with resisted small and ring finger flexion, positioning the wrist in ulnar deviation, can suggest hamate nonunion. In fact, hamate nonunion can lead to tendon fraying, and several patients have presented with tendon rupture [8]. Patients who have hook of hamate fracture also may present with symptoms of nerve compression in either the median [9] or ulnar nerve [10].

If a hook of hamate fracture is considered in the differential diagnosis of an acute or chronic wrist problem, appropriate imaging should be ordered. Standard radiographs including posteroanterior, lateral, and pronated oblique views of the wrist may be done. Norman and colleagues [11] proposed three radiologic findings—absence of the hook, sclerosis of the hook, and lack of a cortical density—as signs of hook fractures. Standard views often can be inconclusive, however, and therefore several special views have been proposed. Papilion et al. [12] suggested a lateral radiograph with the thumb maximally opposed (to move it out of the way) and the wrist in ulnar deviation. Having the hand slightly supinated, to bring the hook into greatest profile, can help [2]. A carpal tunnel view is useful also [13]. Any radiograph can miss a hook of hamate fracture if it is not done exactly correctly, especially if the fracture is right at the base. Therefore CT scanning with the hands in a "praying position" remains the criterion for diagnosing this fracture [14].

If the diagnosis of an acute hamate hook fracture is made, and displacement is minimal, cast immobilization can provide consistent healing if treatment is started within 7 days of the fracture [15]. Significantly displaced fractures or fractures that are chronic in nature may not do as well with nonoperative treatment. Boulas et al. [16,17] reported a 14% incidence of flexor tendon rupture in patients who had untreated hook fractures and a low incidence of healing these fractures without treatment. The treatment for these fractures includes fixation with or without bone grafting or hook excision. Success has been reported with bone grafting and fixation. The advantage of this procedure includes good symptom relief and the preservation of the hook as a pulley [18]. Hook excision, however, is the most common procedure and is the one for which there is the greatest experience [10]. Excision involves a carpal tunnel approach, careful dissection of the hook, excision at the base, and soft tissue coverage of the raw bone surface to avoid tendon irritation. Careful dissection is essential to avoid complication such as an injury to the deep motor branch of the ulnar nerve [19].

Body fractures

Hamate body fractures usually occur in association with other injuries, most commonly fracture dislocations of the fourth and fifth carpometacarpal (CMC) joints and fractures to the fourth and fifth metacarpal bases. This injury usually occurs with an axial load injury to a clenched fist. CMC joint anatomy has been studied, and the articular anatomy and ligamentous attachments have been documented in detail [20,21]. The fifth CMC joint, with approximately 30° of motion, is the most mobile; mobility decreases moving radially to the second CMC joint, which has limited motion. The more mobile fourth and fifth CMC joints are more susceptible to injury. Garcia-Elias et al. [22] reported three types of axial dislocations: axial-radial, axial-ulnar, and axial-radial-ulnar. The most common injury is axial-ulnar. Patients present with pain and deformity following an axial load. The injury usually can be identified on plain radiographs. CT scanning can be helpful in preoperative planning.

Hirano and Inou [23] recently classified hamate fractures as type 1 (hook fractures), type 2A (coronal split), and type 2B (transverse split). Coronal split fractures were the most common hamate body fractures in this study. All 2A fractures were associated with CMC dislocations. Because of the motion that occurs at the fourth and fifth CMC joints and the instability associated with fractures in this area, operative treatment is recommended if displacement or subluxation of the joint is evident. In one review in which both the fourth and fifth CMC joints were dislocated, reduction and fixation of the fourth CMC joint always led to spontaneous and stable reduction of the fifth CMC joint because of the ligamentous attachments. Surgery in this series included fixation of the coronal hamate fracture with screw fixation; in addition temporary bridge plate fixation of the fourth CMC joint was done when there was CMC instability despite hamate fixation. Nine of 11 patients in this study had full recovery [24]. A dorsal approach to the CMC joint is used. Treatment involves open reduction and fixation of the hamate body fracture. If the CMC joint remains unstable, temporary bridge plating or Kirschner wire (K-wire) stabilization of the joint should be used (Fig. 3) [25].

Triquetral fractures

The triquetrum is pyramid shaped. It articulates with the hamate distally, the triangular fibrocartilaginous complex proximally, and the lunate medially. Its palmar surface has an almost completely circular cartilaginous articulation with the pisiform. The triquetrum is well protected by ligamentous attachments on both the dorsal and volar side of the wrist. Triquetral fractures, however, make up the most common carpal bone fracture next to scaphoid fractures [26]. Triquetral fractures can involve either the dorsal ridge—the "chip" fracture—or the entire body. Chip fractures are much more common (Fig. 4).

It initially was thought that the chip fracture is an avulsion fracture at the attachment of the strong dorsal ligaments, the radiotriquetral and triquetro-scaphoid ligaments. This fracture would have to occur with the wrist being forced into extreme flexion. Although this may be case in some injuries, it is much more common for chip fractures to occur with the wrist in a position of dorsiflexion and ulnar deviation. The fracture is caused by a shear mechanism with impingement with the proximal hamate, distal ulna, or both. In fact, it has been shown that patients who have dorsal triquetral fractures have a significantly larger ulnar styloid than seen in a control group, suggesting that these patients are at a greater risk of injury from a "chisel" effect from the ulnar styloid [27]. In patients who have wrist injuries and ulnar-sided pain, dorsal ridge triquetral fractures are relatively common and should be considered in the differential diagnosis. Standard anteroposterior, lateral, and oblique radiographs should be obtained. If suspicion remains high, and nothing can be seen on these radiographs, a careful inspection of the oblique radiograph, a repeat radiograph with the hand in slight pronation (bringing the dorsal triquetrum into profile), or even a CT scan should be considered to confirm the diagnosis. With the diagnosis confirmed, rigid immobilization in a cast for a period of 4 to 6 weeks followed by a graded therapy program usually leads to good long-term functional outcomes for isolated injuries of the wrist [26].

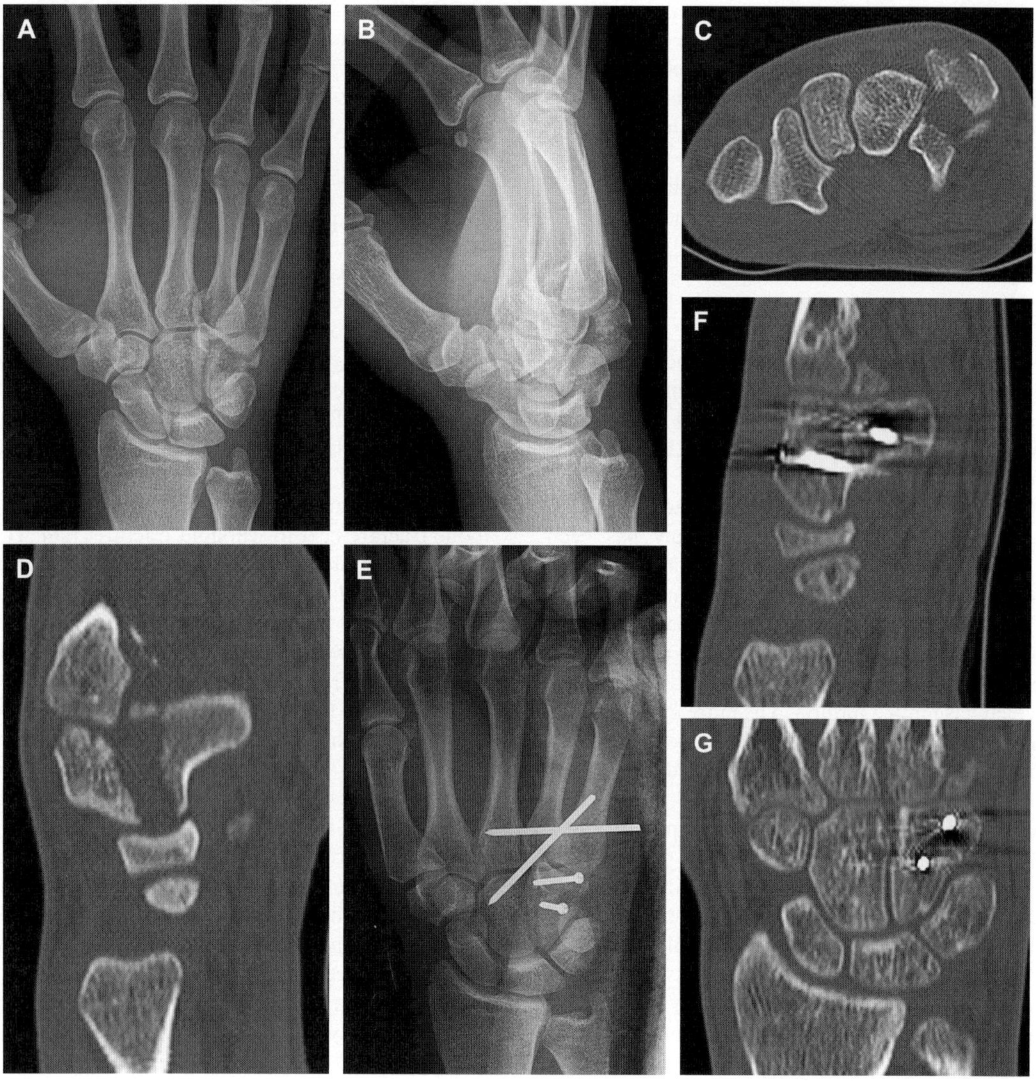

Fig. 3. (*A*) Preoperative radiograph and (*B*) CT scan of a 20-year-old male with an axial load injury and displaced hamate body fracture and associated CMC dislocation. (*E–G*) Postoperative radiograph and CT scan showing reduction of hamate and CMC joints.

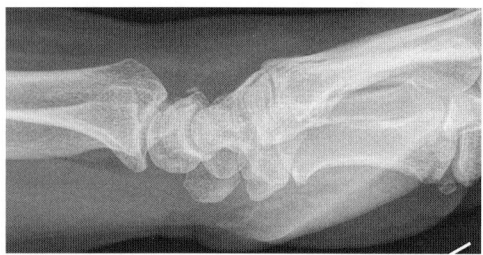

Fig. 4. Lateral radiograph of a patient who had ulnar-sided wrist pain and a diagnosis of a dorsal triquetral fracture.

Triquetral body fractures are not as common. Usually these injuries occur in conjunction with a fracture-dislocation to the wrist such as a perilunate dislocation and therefore are treated as part of a "greater arc" injury [28]. Isolated injuries to the triquetral body can occur, however, and their displacement probably is underappreciated. Porter and Seehra [29] reported a case of triquetral fracture dislocation treated by open reduction and internal fixation. Skelly and colleagues [30] reported a case of a triquetral body fracture in association with a perilunate dislocation. The initial reduction looked acceptable, but at time of surgery the triquetral body fracture was rotated 180°. Aiki and colleagues [31] recently reported a case of persistent ulnar-sided wrist pain that was caused by pisotriquetral arthrosis secondary to a triquetral malunion. This case was treated successfully by pisiform excision. There is not enough evidence to offer good treatment guidelines regarding triquetral body fractures, but fractures in association with perilunate dislocation or those with more than 1 mm of displacement probably should be considered for surgical treatment to maximize long-term wrist function.

Pisiform fractures

The pisiform, like the patella, is a sesamoid bone enclosed in the sheath of the flexor carpi ulnaris tendon. It lies on the volar surface and articulates with the triquetrum. The pisiform is the last bone to ossify between ages 8 and 12 years. There may be multiple centers of ossification, giving it a fragmented appearance. This normal appearance must be distinguished from a fracture [32]. Acute pisiform fractures are reported as a source of ulnar-sided wrist pain [7]. If a fracture is suspected, the pisiform should be imaged appropriately using standard wrist radiographs. Normal radiographs may miss this diagnosis. As with a hamate fracture, a lateral radiograph with the wrist in slight supination will profile the pisiform. Ultimately, CT scanning may be helpful. If the diagnosis is made, initial treatment should include 4 to 6 weeks' immobilization in a cast followed by a graded therapy program. For patients who have persistent problems, pisiform excision offers reliable pain relief [33,34]. Because of the close proximity of the ulnar nerve to the pisiform, ulnar nerve dysfunction can occur in conjunction with a pisiform fracture. This dysfunction is most likely to be caused by a direct blow injury to the nerve itself, but a compressive neuropathy secondary to a displaced pisiform fracture probably should be explored, and the pisiform bone should be excised on a more acute basis [35].

Capitate fractures

The capitate is the largest of the carpal bones and is well protected in the middle column of the wrist where it is surrounded by the other carpal bones and strong wrist ligaments. Fractures of the capitate are relatively rare. In one review, Rand and colleagues [36] found 11 capitate fractures in 978 carpal bone injuries for an incidence of 1.3%. The mechanism of injury of this fracture is debatable. It may involve a direct blow to the wrist, a fall with the wrist in dorsiflexion and ulnar deviation (with the dorsal radius impacting on the waist of the capitate (Fig. 5), or as a part of a greater arc injury in association with a perilunate dislocation. Patients typically present with wrist pain after an acute injury, and a careful examination can pinpoint the area to the capitate. Radiographs can reveal the fracture, and displacement of as much as 180° of the proximal fragment has been reported even with isolated capitate fractures (Fig. 6) [37]. If patients present with pain, and no fracture is seen on initial radiographs, immobilization and close follow-up is warranted. When there is persistent pain in the area of the capitate, MRI should be considered. The relationship of the carpal bones is complex, and radiographs may miss undisplaced fractures [38].

Treatment recommendations for capitate fractures are based on limited experience because of the rarity of the injury. For undisplaced fractures, cast immobilization is sufficient. With displaced fractures, open reduction and internal fixation through a dorsal approach, most commonly with a variable-pitch headless screw or K-wires, is probably best [39]. For unrecognized, untreated fractures that develop nonunion, treatment depends on the chronicity of the problem and the presence or absence of wrist arthritis. Attempting to restore capitate length and normal carpal kinematics by bone grafting and fixation is recommended. As in the scaphoid, the blood supply to the

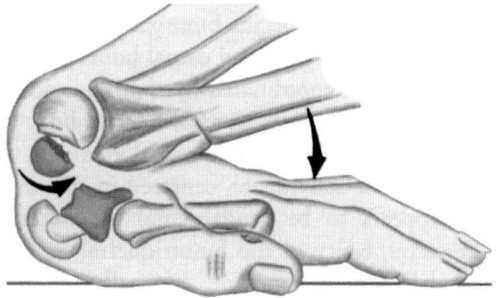

Fig. 5. Potential mechanism of a capitate fracture. (*From* Sennwald GR. Carpal bone fractures other than the scaphoid. In: Berger RA, Weiss AP, editors. Hand surgery. Philadelphia: Lippincott Williams & Wilkins; 2004. p. 410; with permission.)

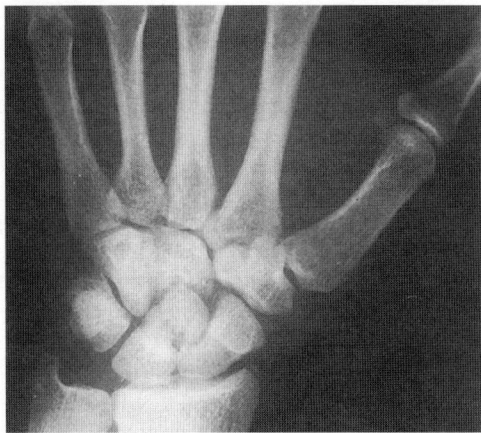

Fig. 6. Capitate body fracture with 180° of displacement of proximal fragment. (*From* Volk AG, Schnall SB, Merkle P, et al. Unusual capitate fracture: a case report. J Hand Surg 1995;20A:581; with permission from The American Society for Surgery of the Hand.)

capitate is retrograde, usually from the volar side, and therefore has been described avascular necrosis in conjunction with a nonunion. This problem may be avoided by prompt diagnosis and treatment of this injury. In one small series reporting five cases of avascular necrosis, four cases were caused by trauma with a nonunion present. Three cases were treated by bone grafting, and two cases were treated by intercarpal fusion [40].

Capitate fractures occur more commonly in association with other injuries. In the study by Rand and colleagues [36], 13 capitate fractures were identified, but only 3 were isolated injuries. The most common associated pattern was transscaphoid transcapitate perilunate dislocation. Other variants, such as transscaphoid, transcapitate, transhamate fractures, have been reported [41]. Each case should be assessed individually to identify the injured bones and ligaments of the wrist and to formulate a treatment plan. Typically, a transscaphoid transcapitate dislocation would be treated by open reduction and internal fixation of both the scaphoid and capitate, and repair of the lunotriquetral ligament should be considered. Results for these complex injuries are more modest, with some loss of motion being the rule and long-term development of arthritis being common.

Lunate fractures

The lunate is shaped like a crescent. Its distal aspect is concave and articulates with the capitate; proximally it articulates with the lunate facet of the distal radius. In a normal situation, the lateral radiographic view shows the capitate, lunate, and distal radius collinear with the wrist in a neutral position. The lunate is integral in the flexion/extension arc and the radial/ulnar deviation arc at both the radiocarpal and midcarpal joints.

Fractures to the lunate are rare. Teisen and Hjarbaek [42] reported on 17 fractures that occurred in more than 3000 carpal bone fractures over a 31-year period. Of these 17 patients, 8 had other fractures to the carpal bones or wrist. Patterns of fracture in this study included fractures of the volar or dorsal pole, osteochondral fractures, and body fractures in both the sagittal and transverse plane. Of all the carpal bones, the lunate bone has proportionally the largest cartilage-covered area. In particular, the proximal portion of the lunate is made up of articular cartilage with no soft tissue attachment and a poor blood supply [43]. Despite this lack of blood supply, the small case series on lunate fractures have reported few cases of avascular necrosis following fracture. The lunate palmar pole fracture may be the most likely to lead to avascular necrosis of the lunate [44].

Treatment recommendations are based on small case series [45]. For minimally displaced fractures, a period of 4 to 6 weeks of immobilization is appropriate. For displaced fractures of the lunate body, open reduction and internal fixation probably is justified [46]. If small avulsion fractures of the dorsal or volar lip are present, and there is carpal subluxation, care must be taken to reduce the fragments accurately to restore carpal congruity (Fig. 7) [47]. Long-term outcomes in these small series are reasonably good, but outcome would be affected by many factors including patient age, related injuries, amount of articular damage, development of avascular necrosis, and other factors.

Trapezium fractures

The trapezium forms a double-saddle articulation with the base of the thumb metacarpal allowing motion in two planes—both flexion/extension and abduction/adduction. The volar "beak" ligament from the metacarpal to the trapezium is a key structure in maintaining joint stability and resisting dorsal radial subluxation during key pinch. The trapezium body articulates

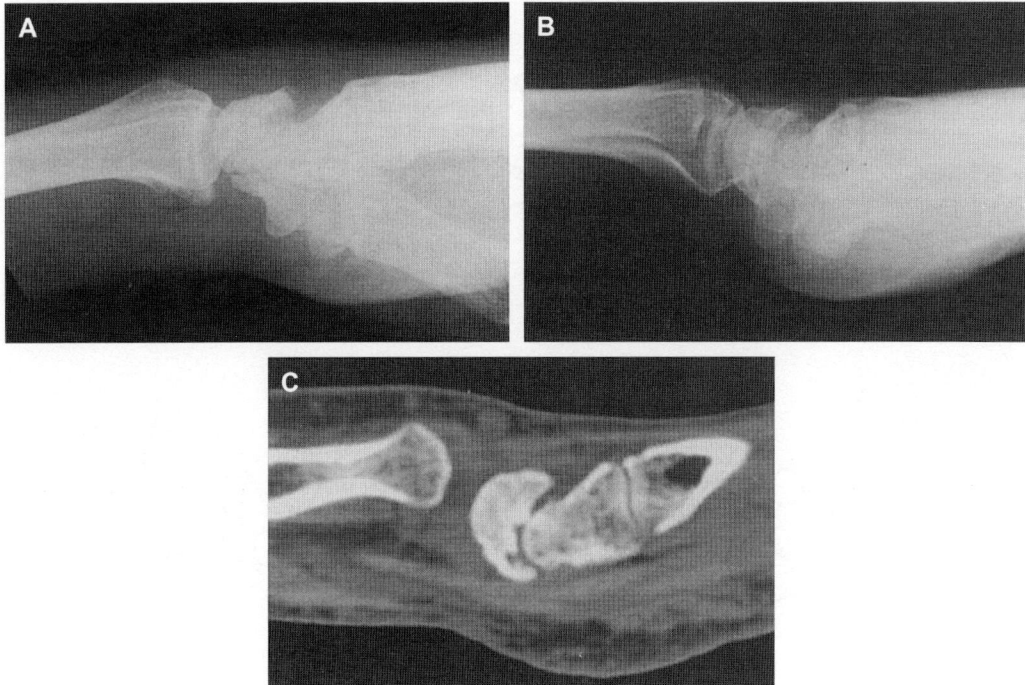

Fig. 7. (*A*) Lateral radiograph of acute volar lip fracture of lunate with associated subluxation. (*B*) Follow-up lateral radiograph with malunion of fracture and subsequent arthrosis. (*C*) CT scan depicting the lunate volar lip malunion with articular incongruity and anthrosis. (*From* Cohen MS. Fractures of the carpal bones. Hand Clinics 1997;13:588; with permission.)

with the carpal bones. The trapezial ridge is a volar structure that serves as a radial attachment for the transverse carpal ligament.

Trapezium fractures include body and ridge fractures. Fractures of the trapezial ridge can result from a direct blow or from an avulsion injury. Pain in the thenar area following a wrist injury should alert surgeons to the possibility of a scaphoid fracture, but trapezial fractures can occur, albeit more rarely. Botte and colleagues [48] reported on an unrecognized trapezial ridge fracture that was a source of longstanding pain for the patient. The fracture was not recognized initially, and a nonunion developed. The patient was offered surgery but refused. She remained unhappy, and litigation was considered because of the delay in diagnosis. Combination injuries including trapezial ridge fractures and hook of hamate fractures secondary to avulsion from the transverse carpal ligament have been reported also [49]. These injuries may be missed on normal radiologic review. Carpal tunnel radiographs should highlight the trapezial ridge. When there is uncertainty, CT scanning can be diagnostic.

Initially, immobilization should be attempted. For ongoing symptoms of trapezial ridge fractures, excision can be considered.

Trapezial body fractures are relatively uncommon but can occur with axially loading or shearing mechanisms across the first CMC joint. Therefore associated fractures of either the base of the first metacarpal [50] or the scaphoid [51] are reported. Walker and colleagues [52] have classified body fractures into five types (Fig. 8). The most common fracture (type IV) involves a sagittal split with a radial and ulnar piece. The fracture line involves both the CMC joint and scaphotrapezial joint. The principles of treatment would be similar to the approach to Bennett's fractures. Because this joint is under great stress during pinching, an anatomic reduction of the joint surface is best. McGuigan and Culp [53] reported on 11 patients who had intra-articular fractures of the trapezium and recommend surgery for patients who have 2 mm of displacement or any subluxation of the first CMC joint. If surgical fixation is chosen, a careful approach is mandatory because of the intimate relationship of the nerves,

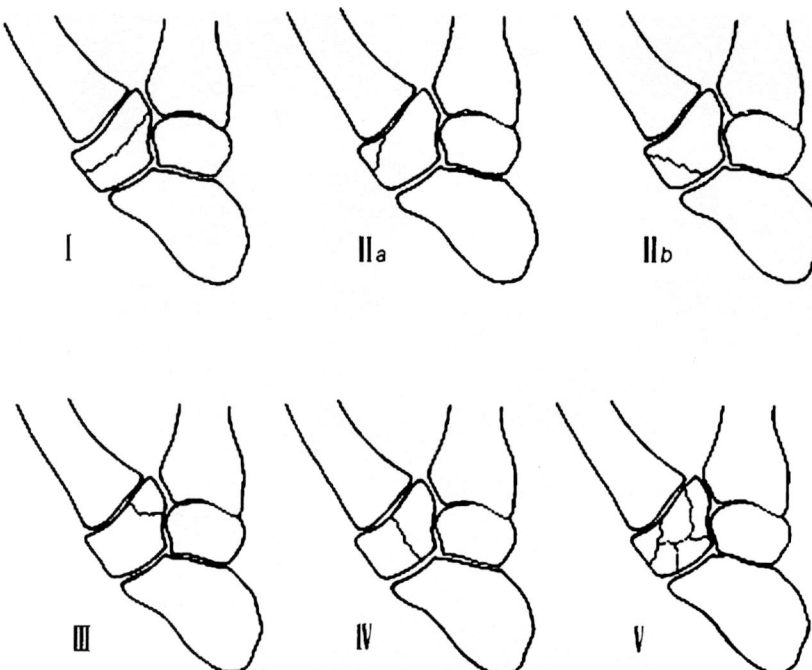

Fig. 8. Classification of trapezial body fractures. (*From* Walker JL, Greene TL, Lunseth PA. Fractures of the body of the trapezium. J Orthop Trauma 1988;2:23; with permission.)

arteries, and tendons in this area. In particular, the radial artery runs between the dorsal radial and dorsal ulnar ridges of the trapezium, and three cases of arterial injury associated with these fractures have been reported [54]. Fixation with K-wires or mini-fragmentary screws usually is sufficient. Unloading of the joint with a mini-external fixator may be necessary for comminuted fractures.

Trapezoid fractures

The trapezoid is tightly positioned between the base of the second metacarpal, capitate, scaphoid, and trapezium with strong intercarpal ligaments. It is wedge shaped, twice as wide dorsally as palmarly, and thereby forms the keystone of the carpal arch. It is the least commonly fractured carpal bone. Because of this position, the more commonly reported injuries include a dorsal dislocation [55]. Axially loading injuries leading to trapezoid fractures can occur [56]. Dislocations can be treated by closed reduction. If closed reduction fails or fracture fragments remain displaced, open reduction is warranted to restore the carpal arch of the hand.

References

[1] Kato H, Nakamura R, Horii E, et al. Diagnostic imaging for fracture of the hook of the hamate. Hand Surg 2000;5(1):19–24.

[2] Akahane M, Onon H, Sada M, et al. Fracture of hamate hook—diagnosis by the hamate hook lateral view. Hand Surg 2000;5(2):131–7.

[3] Andresen R, Radmer S, Sparmann M, et al. Imaging of hamate bone fractures in conventional x-rays and high-resolution computed tomography: an in vitro study. Invest Radiol 1999;34(1):46–50.

[4] Bhalla S, Higgs P, Gilula L. Utility of the radial-deviated, thumb-abducted lateral radiographic view for the diagnosis of hamate hook fractures: case report. Radiology 1998;209(1):203–7.

[5] Demirkan F, Calandruccio JH, DiAngelo D. Biomechanical evaluation of flexor tendon function after hamate hook excision. J Hand Surg Am 2003;28: 138–43.

[6] Parker R, Berkowitz MS, Brahms MA, et al. Hook of the hamate fractures in athletes. Am J Sports Med 1986;14(6):517–23.

[7] Lacey J, Hodge J. Pisiform and hamulus fractures: easily missed wrist fractures diagnosed on a reverse oblique radiograph. J Emerg Med 1998;16(3): 445–52.

[8] Yamazaki H, Kato H, Nakatsuchi Y, et al. Closed rupture of the flexor tendons of the little finger

secondary to nonunion of fractures of the hook of the hamate. J Hand Surg Br 2006;31:337–41.
[9] Sugawara O, Katayama K, Togiya S. Fracture of the hamate hook presenting as median nerve palsy. Arch Orthop Trauma Surg 1998;117:173–4.
[10] Bishp AT, Beckenbaugh RD. Fracture of the hamate hook. J Hand Surg 1988;13:135–9.
[11] Norman A, Nelson J, Green S. Fractures of the hook of the hamate: radiographic signs. Radiology 1985; 154:49–53.
[12] Papilion JK, Dupuy TE, Aulicino PL, et al. Radiographic evaluation of the hook of the hamate: a new technique. J Hand Surg Am 1988;13:437–9.
[13] Hart V, Graynor V. Roentgenographic study of the carpal canal. J Bone Joint Surg 1941;23:382–3.
[14] Egawa M, Asai T. Fracture of the hook of the hamate: report of six cases and the suitability of CT. J Hand Surg 1983;8:393–8.
[15] Whalen JL, Bishop AT, Linscheid RL. Nonoperative treatment of acute hamate hook fractures. J Hand Surg Am 1992;17:507–11.
[16] Boulas JH, Milek MD. Hook of hamate fractures: diagnosis, treatment and complications. Orthop Rev 1990;29:518–28.
[17] Scheufler O, Andersen R, Radmer S, et al. Hook of hamate fractures: critical evaluation of different therapeutic procedures. Plast Reconstr Surg 2005; 115:488–97.
[18] Watson HK, Rogers WD. Nonunion of the hook of the hamate: an argument for bone grafting the nonunion. J Hand Surg Am 1989;14:486–90.
[19] Fredericson M, Kim B, Date E, et al. Injury to the deep motor branch of the ulnar nerve during hook of hamate excision. Orthopedics 2006;29:456–8.
[20] Yoshida R, Shah M, Patteson R, et al. Anatomy and pathomechanics of ring and small finger CMC joint injuries. J Hand Surg Am 2003;28:1035–43.
[21] Nakamura K, Patterson R, Viegas S. The ligament and skeletal anatomy of the second through fifth carpometacarpal joints and adjacent structures. J Hand Surg Am 2001;26:1016–29.
[22] Garcia-Elias M, Dobyns JH, Cooney WP, et al. Traumatic axial dislocations of the carpus. J Hand Surg Am 1989;14:446–57.
[23] Hirano K, Inoue G. Classification and treatment of hamate fractures. Hand Surg 2005;10:151–7.
[24] Schortinghuis J, Kasen H. Open reduction and internal fixation of combined fourth and fifth carpometacarpal dislocations. J Trauma 1997;42(6):1052–5.
[25] Fakih R, Fraser A, Pimpalnerkar A. Hamate fracture with dislocation of the ring and little finger metacarpals. Journal of Hand Surgery 1998;23B:96–7.
[26] Hocker K, Mensschik A. Chip fractures of the triquetrum. J Hand Surg Br 1994;19:584–8.
[27] Garcia-Elias M. Dorsal fractures of the triquetrum—avulsion or compression fractures? J Hand Surg Am 1987;12:266–8.
[28] Soejima O, Iida H, Naito M. Transscaphoid-transtriquetral perilunate fracture dislocation: report of a case and review of the literature. Arch Orthop Trauma Surg 2003;123:305–7.
[29] Porter ML, Seehra K. Fracture-dislocation of the triquetrum treated with a Herbert screw. J Bone Joint Surg Br 1991;73:347–8.
[30] Skelly WJ, Nahigian S, Hidvegi E. Palmar lunate transtriquetral fracture dislocation. J Hand Surg Am 1991;16:536–9.
[31] Aiki H, Wada T, Yamashita T. Pisotriquetral arthrosis after triquetral malunion: a case report. J Hand Surg Am 2006;31:1157–9.
[32] Fleege MA, Jebsen PJ, Renfrew DL, et al. Pisiform fractures. Skeletal Radiol 1991;20:169–72.
[33] Carroll RE, Coyle MP Jr. Dysfunction of the pisotriquetral joint: treatment by excision of the pisiform. J Hand Surg Am 1985;10:703–7.
[34] Arner M, Hagberg L. Wrist flexion strength after excision of the pisiform bone. Scand J Plast Reconstr Surg 1984;18:241–5.
[35] Matsunaga D, Uchiyama S, Nakagawa H, et al. Lower ulnar nerve palsy related to fracture of the pisiform bone in patients with multiple injuries. J Trauma 2002;53:364–8.
[36] Rand JA, Linscheid RL, Dobyns JH. Capitate fractures: a long-term follow-up. Clin Orthop Rel Res 1982;165:209–16.
[37] Volk AG, Schnall SB, Merkle P, et al. Unusual capitate fracture: a case report. J Hand Surg 1995;20(4): 581–2.
[38] Calandruccio JII, Duncan SF. Isolated nondisplaced capitate waist fracture diagnosed by magnetic resonance imaging. J Hand Surg Am 1999; 24:856–9.
[39] Richards RR, Paitich B, Bell RS. Internal fixation of a capitate fracture with Herbert screws. J Hand Surg Am 1990;15:885–7.
[40] Vander Grend R, Dell PC, Glowczewskie F, et al. Intraosseous blood supply of the capitate and its correlation with aseptic necrosis. J Hand Surg Am 1984; 9:677–80.
[41] Kuz JE. Trans-scaphoid, transcapitate, transhamate injury: a case report. J Surg Orthop Adv 2005;14(3): 133–5.
[42] Teisen H, Hjarbaek J. Classification of fresh fractures of the lunate. J Hand Surg Br 1988;13:458–62.
[43] Gelberman RH, Buman TD, Menon J, et al. The vascularity of the lunate bone and Kienbock's disease. J Hand Surg 1980;5:272–8.
[44] Beckenbaugh R, Shives TC, Dobyns JH. Kienbock's disease: the natural history and consideration of lunate fractures. Clin Orthop 1980;146:98–106.
[45] Sennwald GR. Carpal bone fractures other than the scaphoid. In: Berger RA, Weiss AP, editors. Hand surgery. Philadelphia: Lippincott Williams & Wilkins; 2004. p. 409–23.
[46] Freeland AE, Ahmad N. Oblique shear fractures of the lunate. Orthopedics 2003;26(8):805–8.
[47] Cohen MS. Fractures of the carpal bones. Hand Clin 1997;13(4):587–99.

[48] Botte MJ, VonSchroeder HP, Gellman H, et al. Fracture of the trapezial ridge. Clin Orthop Relat Res 1992;276:202–5.
[49] Tracy A, Wheeling WV. Transverse carpal ligament disruption associated with simultaneous fractures of the trapezium, trapezial ridge and hook of hamate: a case report. J Hand Surg Am 1999;24:152–5.
[50] Garcia-Elias M, Henriquez-Lluch A, Rossignani P, et al. Bennett's fractures combined with fractures of the trazezium. J Hand Surg Br 1993;18:523–6.
[51] Hodgkinson JP, Parkinson RW, Davies DR. Simultaneous fracture of the carpal scaphoid and trapezium—avery unusual combination of fractures. J Hand Surg Br 1985;10:393–4.
[52] Walker JL, Greene TL, Lunseth PA. Fractures of the body of the trapezium. J Orthop Trauma 1988;2:22–8.
[53] McGuigan FX, Culp RW. Surgical treatment of intra-articular fractures of the trapezium. J Hand Surg Am 2002;27:697–703.
[54] Checroun AJ, Mekhail AO, Ebraheim NA. Radial artery injury in association with fractures of the trapezium. J Hand Surg Br 1997;22:419–22.
[55] Stein AH. Dorsal dislocation of the lesser multangular bone. J Bone Joint Surg Am 1971;53:377–9.
[56] Yasuwaki Y, Nagata Y, Yamamoto T, et al. Fracture of the trapezoid bone: a case report. J Hand Surg Am 1994;19:457–9.

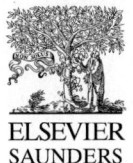

The Diagnosis and Treatment of Scapholunate Instability

Jennifer Manuel, MD[a], Steven L. Moran, MD[a,b],*

[a]Division of Hand Surgery, Department of Orthopedics, Mayo Clinic, 200 First Street, SW, Rochester, MN 55905, USA
[b]Division of Plastic Surgery, Department of Orthopedic Surgery, Mayo Clinic, 200 First Street, SW, Rochester, MN 55905, USA

Scapholunate instability is the most common form of carpal instability. Pain produced by this condition is caused by the wrist's inability to sustain physiologic loads because of an injury to the linkage between the scaphoid and lunate. The term *scapholunate instability* may describe a wide spectrum of clinical conditions ranging from mild wrist dysfunction and partial ligamentous tear to debilitating pain with associated rupture of the scapholunate interosseus ligament (SLIL) complex. This article reviews the pathophysiology of scapholunate instability and its identification and treatment.

History

Scapholunate dissociation (referring to a widening between the scaphoid and lunate as seen on posteroanterior radiographs) was first recognized in 1926 by Destot [1] and published in a description of fracture dislocations of the carpus. However, it was not until 1972 that Linscheid and colleagues [2] detailed traumatic instability of the wrist that the scapholunate instability was widely recognized. These investigators [2] coined the term *scapholunate dissociation* to refer to the loss of mechanical linkage between the scaphoid and lunate. Since then, considerable progress has been made in the pathophysiology and treatment of scapholunate instability.

Pathophysiology

The scaphoid is believed to function as a stabilizer of the midcarpal joint, acting as a bridge between the proximal and distal carpal rows [3]. In the uninjured wrist, the scaphoid is held in a flexed position as it is compressed between the trapezium and radial styloid during radial deviation. This flexion force is balanced by the triquetrum on the ulnar aspect of the proximal row, which has a tendency to extend because of the moment force applied across the hamate–triquetral interface. The lunate is attached to the scaphoid through the SLIL and to the triquetrum through the lunotriquetral interosseus ligament (LTIL). The opposing forces acting through the SLIL and LTIL hold the lunate in a balanced position. Disruption of the SLIL removes the flexion moment arm on the lunate allowing the lunate to assume an extended position under the influence of the triquetrum. The scaphoid in turn falls into further flexion and supination, creating incongruency at the radioscaphoid facet. The loss of scaphoid support to the proximal row was called the *concertina effect* by Fisk [4]. More recently, the term *dorsal intercalated segment instability* (*DISI*) has been used to describe the dorsally extended posture of the lunate seen on lateral radiographs of the wrist, which is highly suggestive of an SLIL injury [2,5]. The term *intercalated segment* refers to the proximal carpal row that has no direct tendinous insertions, and therefore its motion is determined by the muscle forces acting through the distal radius and on the distal carpal row and metacarpals.

The stability of the scapholunate relationship depends on the SLIL and extrinsic capsular ligaments. The SLIL is a C-shaped ligamentous

* Corresponding author.
E-mail address: moran.steven@mayo.edu (S.L. Moran).

structure that connects the dorsal, volar, and proximal surfaces of the lunate to the scaphoid [6]. Between the most proximal portions of the scaphoid and lunate, the SLIL is thin and fibrocartilaginous and blends into the ligament of Testut. No ligamentous attachments exist over the distal portion of the scapholunate joint. This structure is best illustrated as a cleft between the two bones when visualized arthroscopically from the midcarpal joint (Fig. 1).

Each of the three portions (dorsal, volar, proximal) of the SLIL exhibits different structural and mechanical properties. Biomechanical studies of the SLIL found the dorsal portion averaged 3 mm in thickness, whereas the volar portion averaged 1 mm [6]. The dorsal portion of the ligament affords the greatest resistance to traction and torsion between the scaphoid and lunate [7]. The palmar component acts as an additional restraint to rotation. The membranous portion of the ligament is composed mainly of fibrocartilage and provides little mechanical strength [6,8]. The competence of the dorsal and volar components of the SLIL are required for normal kinematics [9,10].

Although the SLIL is important in maintaining the scapholunate interval and relationship, isolated division of the SLIL may not lead to any appreciable change in plain radiographs of the wrist. In 1982, Berger and Blair [8] found few kinematic changes after isolated SLIL sectioning. However, in 1990, Meade et al. [10] published his results on sequential division of the SLIL, showing that division of the palmar SLIL resulted in minimal radiographic change in the assessment of the scapholunate interval. Sectioning the dorsal SLIL resulted in a scapholunate interval of 2.6 mm. Only after the radioscaphocapitate (RSC) ligament was divided did the scapholunate gap substantially widen, as seen on radiograph (average 4.1 mm). Similarly, in 1987, Ruby et al. [7] found that dividing the dorsal capsule and entire SLIL resulted in a scapholunate diastasis of 5 mm. This evidence suggests that scapholunate dissociation involves injury to not only the SLIL but also the dorsal capsule or volar wrist ligaments. The clinical significance of these studies is that considerable alterations in the SLIL may exist despite normal radiographs. When plain radiographs show evidence of scapholunate diastasis, significant injury is already present within the SLIL and secondary constraining ligaments.

Secondary restraints to scaphoid motion include the volar carpal ligaments and dorsal capsule. Major volar constraints include the RSC, long radiolunate, scaphotrapezial ligament, and scaphocapitate ligament. Dorsal constraints include the dorsal intercarpal ligament (DIC) and the dorsal radiocarpal ligament (DRC). The DIC originates from the dorsal ridge of the triquetrum and attaches to both the dorsal distal aspect of the lunate and the dorsal rim of the scaphoid [11]. The DRC ligament originates from the dorsal margin of the distal radius. The ligament extends obliquely with fibers inserting onto the lunate, lunotriquetral ligament, and dorsal ridge of the triquetrum [11]. The DIC and DRC form a V shape over the dorsal wrist capsule and contribute to the stability of the scaphoid and lunate. The dorsal SLIL is intimately intertwined with portions of the dorsal capsule [11].

Building on Ruby's findings, more recent studies have noted the importance of the DIC in maintaining the lunate's position [12]. Division of the SLIL and DIC insertion on the lunate has been shown to result in significant changes in the position of the scaphoid and lunate. Disruption of the SLIL alone does not result in static malrotation of the lunate; however, the lunate assumes a DISI position after it is cut from its connection to the DIC [13]. These findings stress the importance of the secondary stabilizers in supplementing the function of the SLIL. Repetitive motion after SLIL injury may produce attritional

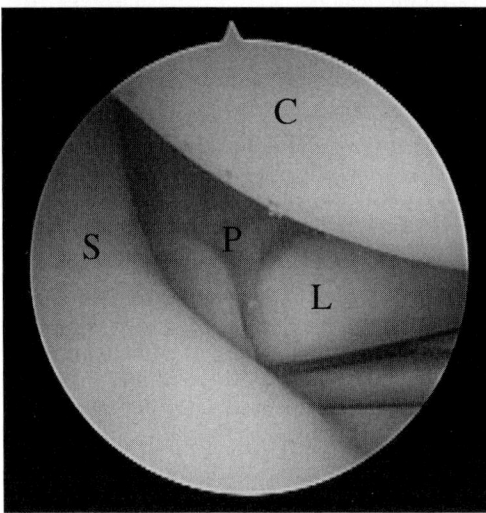

Fig. 1. SLIL as viewed from the radial midcarpal dorsal portal. (P) marks the palmar component of the SLIL ligament. The probe rests in the cleft seen normally between the scaphoids and lunate (L) over the distal aspect of the membranous portion of the ligament. Most tears to the SLIL start palmarly. (C) Capitate.

changes in these secondary stabilizers, leading to eventual failure [12,14]. Thus, radiographic malposition of the lunate and scaphoid suggests injury to not only the SLIL but also additional extrinsic wrist ligaments.

Mechanism

Scapholunate dissociation represents the first stage in the spectrum of perilunate dislocations. In 1980, Mayfield and colleagues [15] reported on their results from loading cadaveric wrists to failure in extension, ulnar deviation, and intercarpal supination. The researchers found that perilunate dislocations occurred in a sequential fashion after specific ligamentous disruption. This pattern of injury was classified into stages according to the degree of perilunar instability. Stage I represents a scapholunate ligament injury and corresponds to the first ligament injured in the Mayfield scheme of carpal dislocation (Fig. 2).

The exact mechanism that produces an injury to the SLIL is still not fully understood. Investigators have suggested that an impact load applied to the base of the hypothenar region of the hand with the wrist in extension, ulnar deviation, and supination is responsible for producing a scapholunate injury

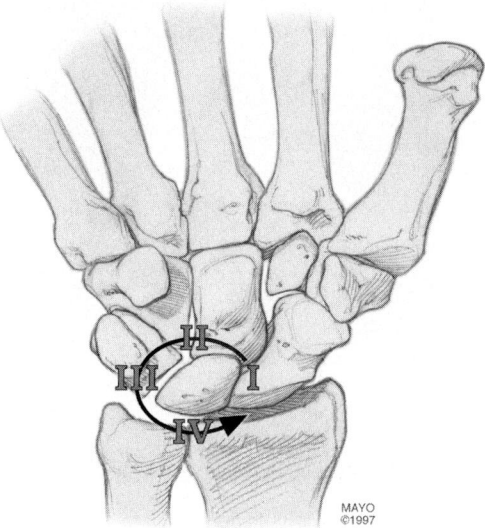

Fig. 2. Progressive perilunar instability of the wrist was defined and presented by Mayfield and colleagues [15]. Illustrated are the stages of progressive perilunar instability of the wrist. The description of each stage is elaborated in text. (By permission of Mayo Foundation for Medical Education and Research. All rights reserved.)

[16–18]. In this model, the capitate is driven proximally between the scaphoid and lunate at its palmar portion of the SLIL, and the scaphoid is driven dorsal and radial, while the lunate is forced ulnar and volar. The scaphoid and lunate are therefore forced in opposite directions. This results in a tear of the SLIL that begins at the volar margin and progresses dorsally [16,19]. Clinically, this point should be remembered during arthroscopy and MRI evaluation of the wrist, because early tears are usually noted at the palmar portion of the SLIL (Fig. 3).

Diagnosis

The diagnosis of scapholunate dissociation relies on a thorough history and physical examination and imaging studies. Early diagnosis offers the best chance for successful surgical outcome. Despite this, scapholunate injury is often not diagnosed until later stages of disease when plain radiographs show clear evidence of abnormality. Occasionally, a patient will seek treatment and report a fall or sudden load applied to the wrist. However, patients often will not seek immediate care, partly because the initial injury seems too trivial or the initial symptoms minimal [20]. Patients may not recall any specific fall, or injuries may result from minor repetitive trauma [21,22]. Scapholunate may also be associated with extracarpal injuries, such a distal radius fracture [23,24] and types of inflammatory synovitis, such as rheumatoid arthritis [25]. In these cases, SLIL injury may go unnoticed because of more obvious radiographic abnormalities, such as a distal radius fracture.

Although symptoms vary widely among patients, most patients will complain of pain or weakness with loading of the wrist. Some patients will complain of swelling, which can often be confused with a dorsal ganglion [26,27]. Often patients complain of a painful click or snapping sensation with motion [28,29]. Limited motion is rarely a complaint in the early phases of the disease, but becomes more common as the disease progresses.

Physical examination will often find mild swelling in the scapholunate region. The scapholunate interval is located by placing the wrist into flexion and palpating the dorsal aspect of the wrist just distal to Lister's tubercle. Pain localized to the site of maximal tenderness often alerts examiners to a possible scapholunate dissociation [26].

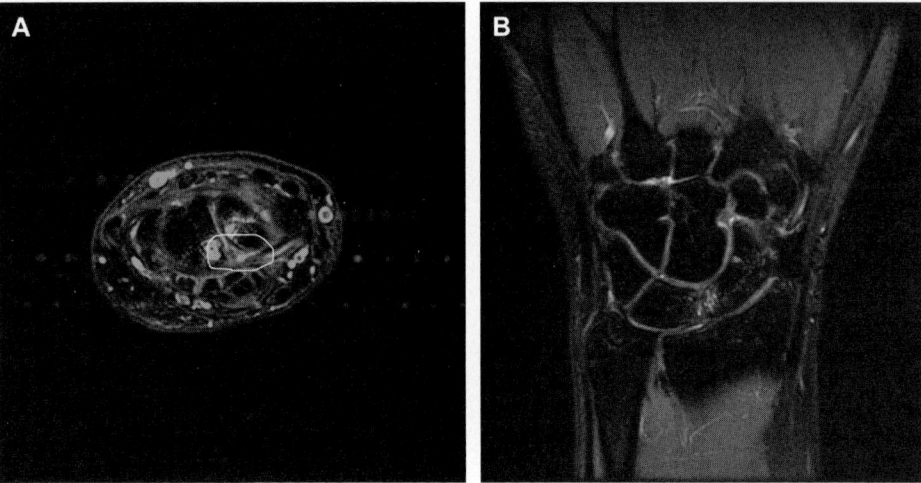

Fig. 3. (*A*) Axial MRI of the wrist in a 28-year-old woman showing a tear of palmar margin of SLIL. (*B*) Posteroanterior view shows area interosseous edema in scaphoid and lunate in area of acute palmar tear.

Additionally, a provocative maneuver, such as Watson's scaphoid shift test [30], will often increase pain and produce a clunk or snap.

Watson's scaphoid shift test is performed by having the patient rest the affected extremity's elbow on the examination table. The examiner places the one hand behind the radius to move the wrist into radial and ulnar deviation, and the opposite thumb on the tuberosity of the scaphoid and applies pressure. This technique prevents palmar flexion of the scaphoid as the wrist is moved from ulnar to radial deviation. When the scapholunate joint is unstable, the proximal pole of the scaphoid will sublux dorsally over the dorsal rim of the radius, producing pain. When the pressure on the scaphoid is released, the scaphoid relocates into the scaphoid fossa and a snapping or clunk is appreciated (Fig. 4) [30].

The scaphoid shift test has been shown to have a low specificity [31]. Pain may be elicited in synovitis, radioscaphoid impingement, or the presence of an occult ganglion. Also, evaluating the normal hand is important for comparison. Although the scaphoid in the uninjured wrist may also elicit a snap or clunk, typically the test will be more painful on the injured side [31,32].

Radiographic examination

Radiographic examination should include at least two views: an anteroposterior projection with the forearm and hand in full supination, and a lateral view with the wrist in neutral flexion/extension. Additional views, including stress radiographs, may be needed for early instabilities in which the anteroposterior and lateral radiographs may be normal.

An anteroposterior radiograph may reveal an increased scapholunate joint space, referred to as *scapholunate diastasis* or the so called "Terry Thomas sign" [33]. Typically, this widening is

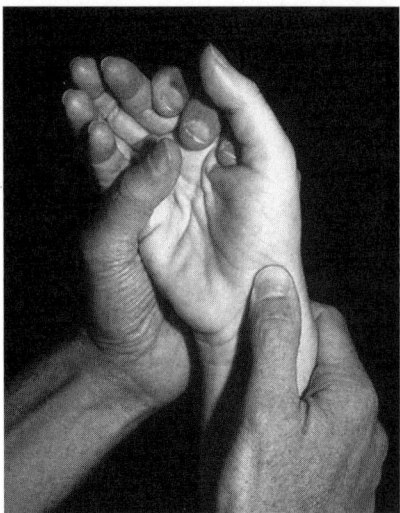

Fig. 4. Watson's test (scaphoid displacement test), for the diagnosis of scapholunate dissociation is performed by pushing upward on the scaphoid tuberosity while the hand is in ulnar deviation. This action tends to cause the scaphoid to ride out of the radial fossa over the dorsal rim, at times producing a painful snap. The test might be positive in loose-jointed individuals and should always be compared with the contralateral side.

more noticeable in the anteroposterior or supinated view than the posteroanterior or pronated view [34]. The scapholunate interval should be measured in the middle of the flat medial facet of the scaphoid. The diastasis is considered abnormal when the gap is greater than 2 mm and increased from the opposite extremity and other intercarpal spaces (Fig. 5) [35].

The anteroposterior radiograph may also show the scaphoid ring sign: when the scaphoid is collapsed into flexion, the end-on projection of the distal pole of the scaphoid looks similar to a ring. This finding together with a shortened distance (<7 mm) between the ring and proximal pole of the scaphoid suggest a rotatory subluxation of the scaphoid (see Fig. 5) [23,36,37].

The lateral radiograph in patients who have scapholunate instability may show rotatory subluxation of the scaphoid; the scaphoid will be abnormally flexed and the lunate may be abnormally extended, where the radiolunate angle exceeds 15°. This positioning leads to an increase in the scapholunate angle as viewed on the lateral radiograph. The scapholunate angle may range from 30° and 60° with an average of 46°. Angles found to be greater than 70° are considered abnormal and of scapholunate dissociation (Fig. 6) [2,38]. Also, in the normal wrist, the long axis of the scaphoid and a line drawn tangential to the volar flare of the distal radius are almost parallel to each other. In the wrist with an abnormally flexed scaphoid, these two lines converge at an acute angle. For the same reason, the palmar cortical outlines of the scaphoid and radial styloid, which normally create a wide C-shaped line, change into a sharp V-shaped line [39].

Additional radiographic views known as *stress views* may show a dynamic instability not appreciated on the static anteroposterior and lateral radiographs [40]. These views consist of posteroanterior views with the wrist in ulnar and radial deviation and a longitudinal compression load view applied to the wrist when the patient makes a tight fist. Maximum ulnar deviation of the wrist will stress the SLIL and exacerbate any preexisting diastasis. A clenched fist view will load the capitate and force it proximally into the scapholunate interval, potentially widening it [41]. Any image found to be abnormal should always be compared with the contralateral wrist.

Additionally, cineradiography or video fluoroscopy may show abnormal movement between

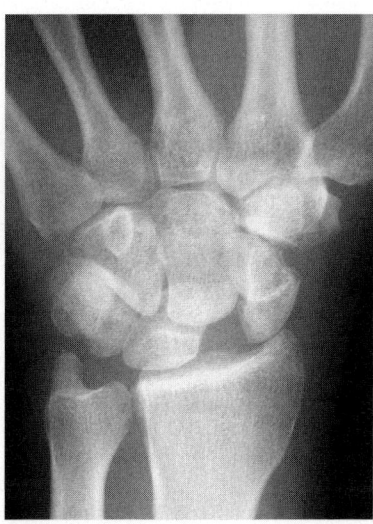

Fig. 5. Posteroanterior radiograph of the wrist depicting severe scapholunate dissociation with increased scapholunate gap, also referred to as a positive Terry-Thomas sign. The scaphoid is foreshortened with respect to the longitudinal axis of the forearm. The scaphoid tuberosity is seen in profile providing the ring sign. The lunate appears to be trapezoidal in shape because the palmar pole is rotated under the capitate.

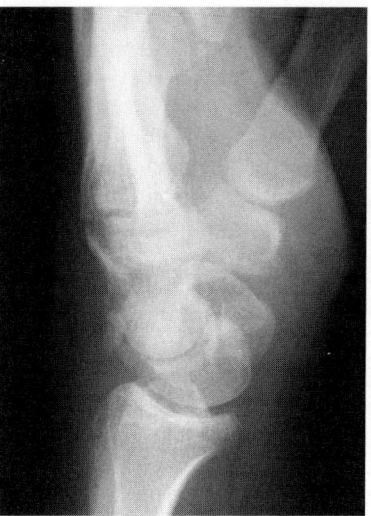

Fig. 6. Lateral radiograph of a wrist in a patient with scapholunate dissociation. The scaphoid is flexed with its dorsal pole subluxed over the dorsal rim of the radius. The capitate and remainder of the distal carpus are subluxed dorsally while the lunate is rotated into extension. The capitolunate angle is approximately 30°. This exact effect has been termed *dorsal intercalated segment instability* or DISI. The angle between the lunate and scaphoid is also increased to more than 90° from the normal values between 40° and 70°.

the scaphoid and lunate. Typically a fluidity of motion occurs between the scaphoid and lunate as the wrist is moved from ulnar to radial deviation. In patients who have scapholunate dissociation, a loss of this synchronous motion occurs and a jump may be visualized as the scaphoid is subluxed dorsally from the radial fossa during radial deviation and then falls back into the radial fossa during ulnar deviation [42].

Bone scintigraphy

Bone scintigraphy uses a radionuclide, usually technitiuum-99, that when injected is transiently taken up by bone. This test is nonspecific, but may be helpful when negative. A positive result simply localizes the site of injury or inflammation. The test is performed in three phases and may distinguish soft tissue from bony injuries.

Arthrography

Arthrography can be useful in defining partial and complete tears of the SLIL. Its use has been primarily replaced with arthroscopy. Comparative studies have found only a 60% sensitivity compared with arthroscopy [43]. The interpretation of wrist arthrography must account for the fact that many ligamentous tears may be degenerative rather than traumatic [44]. With age older than 40 years, degenerative perforations of the SLIL occur more frequently. In addition, many of these findings are bilateral in nature [45]. Therefore, arthrographic findings should be correlated with symptoms, clinical findings, and the results of other tests.

MRI

MRI may not be as useful in defining ligamentous injuries in the wrist as in larger joints [46]. The complex anatomy of the radiocarpal and intercarpal joints makes interpreting the MRI difficult [47]. Schadel-Hopfner et al. [48] performed a prospective study on 103 patients who had suspected tears of the SLIL. Using MRI, 75% of cases were correctly diagnosed, with an overall sensitivity of 63% and a specificity of 86%. Furthermore, no improvement in diagnostic ability was seen with intravenous contract medium. These results and many similar studies have led many authors to conclude that MRI is not reliable for diagnosing SLIL injury [49–51].

Arthroscopy

Arthroscopy has become the gold standard for identifying and grading scapholunate injuries [52]. When compared with other modalities, such as MRI and arthrography, arthroscopy has been shown to be superior at detecting internal derangement of wrist ligaments [43,48,53]. In addition, arthroscopy allows a more accurate appraisal of the extent of tearing and visualization of the articular surfaces. These changes in the articular surfaces, particularly the proximal pole of the scaphoid, may not be appreciated using other imaging methods [54].

An arthroscopic grading system for ligamentous tears has been developed by Geissler et al. [55]. Grade 1 injuries consist of attenuation or hemorrhage of the membranous portion of the scapholunate ligament with a smooth and intact scapholunate interval. Grade II lesions consist of an attenuated fibrocartilaginous membrane. A step-off is present between the scaphoid and lunate and a 1-mm probe may be placed between these bones. Grade III lesions consist of a step-off visualized from both the radiocarpal and midcarpal joints. A 1-mm probe may be inserted into and freely rotated in the scapholunate interval. Grade IV lesions consist of complete disruption of the ligament, allowing a 2.7-mm arthroscope to be passed between the radiocarpal and midcarpal joints (Fig. 7 and Table 1).

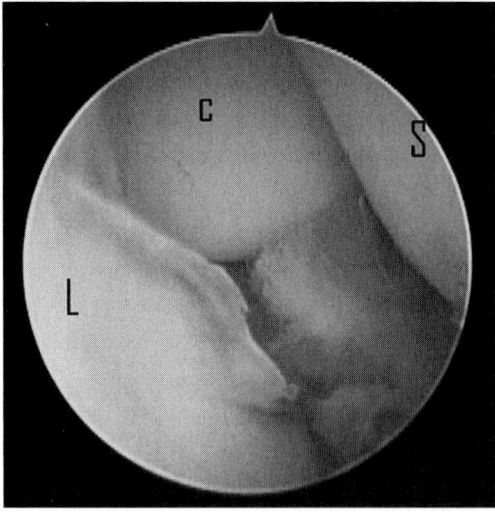

Fig. 7. Grade IV SLIL tear as seen from radiocarpal 3,4 portal. The capitate can be visualized between rent in SLIL from the radiocarpal joint. C, capitate; L, lunate; S, scaphoid.

Table 1
Arthroscopic classification of carpal interosseous ligament tears

Grade	Description
I	Attenuation and hemorrhage of interosseous ligament seen radiocarpal joint, with no step-off present as seen from midcarpal joint
II	Attenuation and hemorrhage of interosseous ligament seen radiocarpal joint, with step-off as seen through midcarpal joint; the probe can be placed between scaphoid and lunate
III	Incongruency or step-off is seen between the scaphoid and the lunate from the radiocarpal and midcarpal portals; the probe can be placed and freely rotated between the scaphoid and lunate
IV	Incongruence or step-off is seen between the scaphoid and lunate from the radiocarpal and midcarpal portals; gross instability is noted, and the 2.7-mm arthroscope may be passed through the gap between the scaphoid and lunate

As with other imaging techniques, arthroscopic findings should be correlated to the patient's history and physical examination to determine the significance of the lesion.

Clinical stages of scapholunate instability

To better describe the severity of the injury to the scapholunate joint, a four-stage classification system has been developed: predynamic instability, dynamic instability, static instability, and scapholunate advanced collapse (SLAC) [56]. Static instability may be further divided into one in which a DISI deformity is present and one in which a DISI deformity is absent. SLAC represents the final-most severe stage of scapholunate dissociation in which arthritic changes are present on plain radiographs.

Predynamic instability consists of the earliest stage of scapholunate injury [56]. This stage is characterized by a partially ruptured or attenuated scapholunate membrane. This partial rupture leads to abnormal motion between the scaphoid and lunate and produces synovitis and subsequent wrist pain. During this stage, plain radiographs and stress radiographs will be normal. Arthroscopy may show attenuation of the scapholunate ligament or hemorrhage within the scapholunate joint. If left untreated, secondary stabilizers of the joint may also become attenuated, leading to further deterioration of the SLIL and progression to dynamic or static instability.

Dynamic instability is characterized by a ligamentous tear of the palmar or dorsal aspect of the SLIL. Again, plain radiographs may be normal. However, stress radiographs may show widening of the scapholunate interval and an arthrogram may show abnormalities within the ligament. Arthroscopy will show evidence of ligamentous disruption with a type II or III Geissler pattern and a step-off between the joint. This stage is considered dynamic because the instability is only apparent radiographically when the wrist is subject to stress-loading.

Static instability consists of an injury to or attenuation of the secondary stabilizers of the wrist [12]. This stage differs from dynamic instability in that the abnormality is apparent on plain radiographs without the application of stress, and the instability or dissociation is static or fixed. Plain radiographs will show a scapholunate diastasis of greater than or equal to 3 mm [27]. The scapholunate angle as viewed on the lateral radiograph is typically greater than 70°. Arthroscopy will show significant instability with a grade IV Geissler injury pattern.

Static instability may be accompanied by a lunate that is rotated into a DISI position. In addition to an abnormal scapholunate angle of greater than 70°, the lateral wrist radiograph will typically show a radiolunate angle greater than 15°. Furthermore, this stage is often accompanied by chronic scarring of the dorsal capsule and volar ligamentous structures that prevents reduction of the scaphoid and lunate, thus limiting the reconstructive options available.

SLAC refers to the final stage of scapholunate dissociation. Over time, as continued loads are applied to a wrist with altered biomechanics secondary to a scapholunate dissociation, stresses lead to progressive deterioration of the articular cartilage and the development of arthritis. Typically this form of arthritis begins in the scaphoid–radial styloid region and may progress to include the lunocapitate joint. The least commonly involved joint is the radiolunate joint [57,58]. This physiology becomes important when considering treatment options for this advanced stage of disease.

Natural history of scapholunate dissociation

The natural progression of untreated isolated SLIL injury is somewhat unclear. Some authors believe that progression to the development of an SLAC wrist is inevitable after an isolated rupture of the SLIL [59]. In 2003, O'Meeghan et al. [60] studied 11 patients who had documented SLIL injury who were treated nonoperatively. At an average of 7 years follow-up, all patients continued to have pain but did not show evidence of an SLAC arthritis. Although the time to development of degenerative arthritis remains unknown, SLIL injury and SLIL dissociation alter the biomechanics within the wrist, setting the stage for the development of degenerative arthritis.

Treatment

Treatment of scapholunate instability represents an ongoing challenge to the hand surgeon and reported results have been less than consistent [61], partly because the injury is often not initially recognized. Traditionally, scapholunate injuries have been described in relation to the time from injury. Acute injuries are defined, arbitrarily, as those that present within 2 to 4 weeks of the initial injury. Subacute injuries are those that present between 4 weeks and 6 months. Chronic injuries are defined as those presenting greater than 6 months from the initial injury. However, not all scapholunate injuries are alike, and the most appropriate treatment for an individual patient depends on many factors other than time from injury.

In 2006, Garcia-Elias et al. [62] published an algorithm for treating scapholunate dissociation based on five criteria or questions: (1) is the dorsal scapholunate ligament partially or completely torn, (2) if complete, can the ligament be repaired and what is the healing potential, (3) what is the status of the secondary scaphoid stabilizers (ie, is the radioscaphoid angle less than 45°, (4) is the carpal malalignment reducible, and (5) are the cartilaginous surfaces normal. Based on the answers, Garcia-Elias et al. [62] proposed six stages of scapholunate dissociation: (1) partial scapholunate injury, (2) complete scapholunate ligament tear with repairable dorsal ligament, (3) complete scapholunate tear with nonrepairable dorsal ligament but a normally aligned scaphoid, (4) complete scapholunate tear with nonrepairable tissue and a reducible rotatory subluxation of the scaphoid, (5) complete scapholunate tear with irreducible malalignment but no evidence of cartilage degeneration, and (6) complete scapholunate tear with irreducible malalignment and cartilage degeneration.

Each stage of scapholunate dissociation represents a different treatment strategy. In general, in wrists without fixed bony deformity, attempts should be made to restore the bony relationships with soft tissue augmentation as needed. In wrists with fixed deformity, soft tissue procedures are more likely to fail and salvage surgical procedures, such as limited fusions, are probably needed to alleviate pain.

Partial scapholunate ligament injury

A partial tear of the scapholunate ligament typically presents with pain over the dorsal scapholunate interval. Patients may have a normal radiographic appearance or show slight widening of the scapholunate interval. Diagnosis is typically made at arthroscopy.

Complete scapholunate ligament injury with repairable dorsal ligament

A repairable ligament is one that possesses good healing potential. Typically it is a ligament that has been acutely torn or is attached to an osteochondral fragment that has been avulsed from the bone. Patients may have intact secondary stabilizers of the scaphoid and therefore a normal radiographic appearance of the scaphoid. Again, patients will experience tenderness over the scapholunate interval and diagnosis is typically made at arthroscopy.

Complete nonrepairable scapholunate ligament injury with normal alignment of the scaphoid

Midsubstance ruptures of the scapholunate ligament have poor healing potential. The ends tend to retract and degenerate quickly, often within the first week after injury [63]. Again, intact secondary stabilizers of the scaphoid will help maintain the normal position of the scaphoid within the carpus.

Complete nonrepairable scapholunate ligament injury with reducible rotatory subluxation of the scaphoid

In patients who have complete nonrepairable scapholunate ligament injuries with reducible rotatory subluxation of the scaphoid, radiographs show injury to the secondary stabilizers of the scaphoid with an abnormal radioscaphoid angle and DISI appearance of the lunate.

The treatment goal of these first four stages of scapholunate dissociation involves reestablishing the link or connection between the scaphoid and lunate and maintaining the reduction of both bones.

Casting/immobilization

Some authors have reported success with manipulation of the scaphoid followed by immobilization of the wrist in plaster for acute scapholunate dissociation [64,65]. These patients were immobilized in the "wine waiter's position" of full supination, ulnar deviation, and mid-dorsiflexion [64]. Despite these reports, most surgeons have found this method of treatment to be unreliable. In 1992, Tang [66] reported on the results of 20 patients treated with casting alone for scapholunate dissociation associated with distal radius fractures. He found that all patients continued to have clinical signs of scapholunate dissociation 1 year after treatment.

The difficulty with closed reduction is in the position of the scaphoid with changes in wrist position. When the wrist is extended, the scaphoid and lunate diastasis is exaggerated, which may delay or prevent healing of the SLIL. When the wrist is flexed, the already flexed scaphoid assumes a posture of exaggerated flexion or a state of presubluxation [15]. Because of the unreliability of closed manipulation and casting, most surgeons have abandoned this treatment in favor of more predictable methods.

Closed reduction and Kirschner wire fixation

Unlike casting and immobilization, excellent results have been obtained with Kirschner wire (K-wire) fixation of the acutely injured scapholunate joint [67]. Pinning and reliable reduction may allow primary healing of the injured SLIL [63,68].

Verification of reduction is aided by intraoperative fluoroscopy or arthroscopy [69,70]. Reduction may be facilitated by the use of two K-wires placed dorsally: one into the scaphoid and one into the lunate. By "joysticking" the scaphoid proximally and ulnarly, and the lunate distally and radially, the abnormally displaced joint is reduced. Additional K-wires are then used to maintain the reduction. In 1995, Whipple [69] reported on his series of 40 patients treated with arthroscopic reduction and pinning of the scapholunate interval. His results showed that 83% of patients who had symptoms for less than 3 months and a small diastasis of less than 3 mm experienced good results; however, only 53% of patients who had more chronic symptoms for longer than 3 months were pain-free and maintained their reduction.

Arthroscopic debridement

Arthroscopic debridement alone has also been recommended for partial acute SLIL tears [71]. The rationale for this procedure is based on the fact that frayed ligaments may lead to synovitis and mechanical irritation within the joint. Reporting on their series of arthroscopic debridement in patients who had complete and partial SLIL tears, Weiss and colleagues [71] showed complete resolution or improved symptomatology in 66% of patients who had complete tears and 85% of patients who had partial tears. If such a treatment plan is performed, these authors would recommend pin reduction in addition to debridement followed by 6 to 8 weeks of immobilization.

Electrothermal collagen shrinkage

Some recent interest has been shown in the use of thermal energy, in the form of electrothermal collagen shrinkage for the treatment of the SLIL laxity or stretch. Electrocautery is capable of denaturing type I collagen, the main constituent of ligaments and joint capsules. The increased temperature of the tissue causes an alteration in the ultrastructural properties of the collagen fibril, resulting in a contracted collagen mass with increased stiffness [72,73].

In 2005, Hirsh et al. [74] studied 10 patients who had attenuation of the SLIL associated with step-off or incongruity of the intercarpal space diagnosed through arthroscopy. These patients all underwent arthroscopy with debridement of the membranous portion of the SLIL and thermal stabilization (maximum temperature 75°C) until the ligament was visualized as being taut. Nine patients experienced complete resolution of their symptoms and remained pain-free at an average of 28 months postoperatively. Additionally, all had no clinical evidence of instability on examination.

Potential complications with the use of thermal shrinkage relate to the heat generated during the procedure. Collagen denatures at a temperature between 65°C to 80°C. Beyond 80°C, collagen necrosis may take place. The proximity of the articular surfaces and periarticular neurovascular bundles also put these structures at risk for severe heat injury.

Open reduction, internal fixation with repair of ligaments

Direct repair of the SLIL is recommended when joints lack arthritis and the secondary stabilizers are intact or capable of repair. Open repair allows not only for direct visualization of the joint during reduction but also for repair of the dorsal component of the SLIL.

Repair of the SLIL with sutures or suture anchors remains a reliable treatment for acute scapholunate dissociation [75,76]. This repair is limited to the dorsal portion of the SLIL. Long-term results have shown that greater than 70% of patients experience significant improvement in pain. Grip strength is approximately 85% of normal, and wrist motion is approximately 78% of normal. Progression to degenerative changes within the carpus occurs in less than one third of patients who undergo repair of the ligament [75,77,78].

Dorsal capsulodesis

Typically the repair of the SLIL is augmented with a dorsal capsulodesis. Capsulodesis involves the imbrication or modification of the dorsal capsule to improve scaphoid stability. It may also be used in cases where the SLIL is inadequate for repair or is intact but attenuated, or when the secondary stabilizers have experienced significant injury.

The capsulodesis procedure, as originally described by Blatt [79], uses a proximally based strip of the dorsal wrist capsule to create a dorsal tether for scaphoid stabilization. The strip of capsule is left attached to the distal radius and inserted distally into a fresh groove on the reduced scaphoid. By inserting the capsule into the scaphoid distal to the axis of rotation, a checkrein effect is created, preventing excessive scaphoid flexion and collapse. This loss of scaphoid flexion corresponds to a loss of wrist flexion, which should be expected after capsulodesis. Wrist flexion has been estimated to be diminished by between 12° and 20°. These results have been verified both clinically and in biomechanical models [79–81].

Blatt's [79] initial results of the capsulodesis procedure found range of motion and grip strength to be adequate and most patients returned to preinjury work status. In 1995, Wintman and colleagues [80] reported results on 17 patients who had scapholunate dissociation with dynamic instability treated with capsulodesis. Results showed significant improvement in pain and functional status. Patients experienced a mean loss of wrist flexion of 12°. Fifteen patients returned to their previous occupation, and 15 stated they would undergo the surgery again if faced with the same choice.

In 2005, Moran et al. [82] published results of dorsal capsulodesis performed in 31 patients who had chronic scapholunate dissociation, which was defined as wrist pain for greater than 3 months. Of these, 18 had dynamic lesions and 13 had static lesions. All patients underwent a dorsal capsulodesis using either a Blatt or Mayo technique [83]. The Mayo technique consists of a ligament-sparing dorsal capsulotomy (Fig. 8). The proximal strip of the DIC is then rotated proximally and attached to the dorsal lunate after reduction of the scapholunate

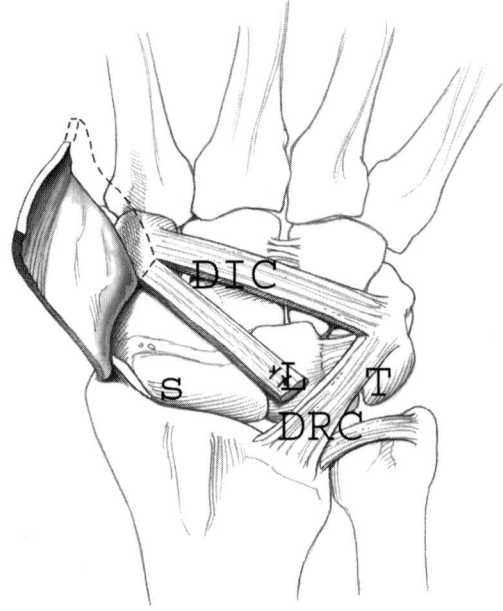

Fig. 8. Mayo capsulodesis (after Berger) in which the dorsal intercarpal ligament (DIC) is detached (50%) from the dorsal aspect of the triquetrum (T), dissected radially to the distal scaphoid (S), where it is firmly attached, and then with the scaphoid extended to a neutral position, the DIC is sutured to the lunate (L) using suture anchors and to the origin of the dorsal radiocarpal ligament (DRC). L, lunate. (By permission of Mayo Foundation for Medical Education and Research. All rights reserved.)

interval, which is held in place with two or three K-wires [8]. Of patients who had static lesions, six underwent concurrent scapholunate ligament repair. At 54-month follow-up, results showed that most patients had some improvement in pain, but only two patients were pain-free. Radiographically, the scapholunate gap increased from 2.7 mm before surgery to 3.9 mm at follow-up. The scapholunate angle increased from 56° before surgery to 62° at follow-up. No significant difference in function was seen between the dynamic and static groups [82].

Bone–retinaculum–bone/bone–ligament–bone

The healing potential of an injured ligament in the subacute or chronic setting may be limited because of attritional changes in the ligament. To recreate the ligamentous connection between the scaphoid and lunate, various bone–ligament–bone composite grafts have been used to reconstruct the dorsal component of the SLIL [84–86]. These grafts have included bone–retinaculum–bone grafts from the wrist extensor retinaculum, tarsometatarsal ligament autograft, dorsal capitohamate ligament graft, dorsal trapeziometacarpal ligament graft, and periosteal flap of iliac crest.

In 2003, Kalb et al. [87] reported on his results in 12 patients who had chronic scapholunate dissociation treated with dorsal trapeziometacarpal ligament autograft. At a mean of 12 months follow-up, results showed that only three patients experienced radiographic correction of the instability. Four patients experienced recurrence of the scapholunate gap, representing failure of the procedure.

In 1998, Weiss [86] published his results in 19 patients who underwent bone–retinaculum–bone reconstruction of the SLIL for both dynamic and static scapholunate dissociation. Of the 14 patients who had dynamic instability evaluated at an average of 3.6 years postoperatively, 12 experienced no pain and 2 experienced pain with heavy activity of the wrist. Of the 5 patients who had static instability, 2 experienced no pain, 1 experienced pain with heavy activity, and 2 experienced constant pain. He concluded that bone–retinaculum–bone reconstruction is a reliable and predictable procedure for dynamic scapholunate instability, but less reliable in the patient who has static instability.

Concerns exist regarding long-term outcomes for bone–ligament–bone grafts, because some results suggest recurrence of a scapholunate diastasis. In 1995, Schuind [88] suggested the use of a vascularized portion of the radioulnar interosseus membrane to recreate the linkage between the scaphoid and lunate. In 2006, Harvey et al. [89] published a technique of using a vascularized pedicled autograft based on the intermetacarpal artery. A vascularized graft is believed to avoid some of the late complications associated with other bone–ligament–bone grafts, such as loss of elasticity and strength of the ligament, preventing recurrence of the diastasis. More long-term studies are needed [88]. The major problem with these reconstructions is their inability to reconstruct the volar component of the SLIL.

Tenodesis

An alternative approach to the reducible subacute or chronic scapholunate dissociation is tenodesis of the scapholunate joint. Initially described by Dobyns et al. in 1975 [41], tenodesis had fallen out of favor until recently. Dobyns et al. [41] original technique consisted of passing a strip of tendon through oblique drill holes in the scaphoid and lunate to recreate the interosseus ligament. Problems included interference in blood supply and resulted in fracture.

Subsequently, in the early 1990s, Almquist et al. [90] reported his results of a four-bone ligament reconstruction. This technique uses the distally based strip of the extensor carpi radialis brevis and weaves it through the capitate, scaphoid, lunate, and radius. In his initial series of 36 patients, 86% returned to work. Grip strength was 73% of the uninjured side. Postoperative scapholunate gaps averaged 3.3 mm radiographically, compared with 10 mm at surgery. No patient in the 4-year follow-up showed evidence of arthritis [90].

Since then, modifications of this procedure have been reported, including one by Brunelli et al. [91] using a strip of flexor carpi radialis to address the proximal and distal aspects of the scaphoid in rotatory subluxation. In this technique, a strip of distally based flexor carpi radialis tendon is passed through the scaphoid tuberosity to the dorsal rim of the scaphoid, where it is sutured to the remnants of the scapholunate ligament. The tendon is then pulled tight and anchored to the dorsal ulnar corner of the distal radius. This technique showed good initial results in a study of 11 patients [91]. Van Den Abeele et al. [92] published early results of 22 patients who underwent the Brunelli procedure, showing that 17 patients experienced pain relief. Grip strength recovered, but flexion/extension motion arcs were reduced from preoperative values. The radiographic appearance of dynamic or static scapholunate was unchanged after the procedure.

These newer techniques have shown improved early results for several reasons. Not only is the proximal scapholunate relationship restored but also the distal component of scaphoid rotatory instability is addressed, preventing excessive flexion of the scaphoid. In addition, the drill holes are placed in regions of the bones where vascularity is improved, theoretically allowing for incorporation of the tendon within the bone and preventing fracture. Long-term follow-up studies are needed to assess for durability.

Reduction and association of the scaphoid and lunate

In 1997, Rosenwasser et al. [93] published his results using a Herbert screw to stabilize the scaphoid and lunate in subacute scapholunate dissociation. In this procedure, the Herbert screw is used as the link between the bones. The goal of the procedure is to recreate an association between the scaphoid and lunate with a bony or fibrous link. However, the procedure is not considered an arthrodesis because it allows a small degree of motion between the bones. In this series, no patients experienced screw breakage or cutout. The scaphoid and lunate remained associated without any diastasis or loss of reduction noted radiographically. Potential problems with this procedure are that in radial and ulnar deviation, the scaphoid and lunate move through three different planes: translating, rotating, and flexion and extension. These three planes of motion will eventually test the longevity of any static metal construct. Further long-term studies are needed with this procedure.

Complete scapholunate ligament injury with irreducible malalignment and normal cartilage

Long-standing malalignment of the scapholunate relationship allows the deformity to become fixed. Typically, fibrosis occurs within the dissociated bones, making reducibility of the deformity difficult. As such, any soft tissue procedure will have a higher rate of failure. More typically, partial fusions can be used to maintain the reduction of the deformity while preserving some motion.

Limited carpal fusion

Thornton [94] reported the first limited wrist arthrodesis in 1924. In 1967, Peterson and Lipscomb [95] described various combinations of intercarpal arthrodeses and concluded that these procedures stabilize while relieving pain and preserving some motion. Various different fusions have been described for scapholunate dissociation, including scaph-trapezial-trapezoidal (STT or triscaphe) fusion, scaphocapitate fusion, scapholunate fusion, and scapholunocapitate (SLC) fusion.

Although a scapholunate fusion seems the most logical solution for scapholunate dissociation, this procedure has been less than reliable. The small articular surface areas in contact between the two bones and the force exerted by the capitate to separate the bones have resulted in high nonunion rates [96]. In 1991, Hom et al. [97] reported the results of seven patients treated with scapholunate fusion. Of these, one showed radiographic evidence of union. Some authors have argued that although a bony union may not occur, a fibrous union forms between the scaphoid and lunate. Some believe this fibrous union is sufficiently strong to reduce complaints of pain [98].

The STT fusion, popularized by Watson et al. [99], realigns the proximal pole of the scaphoid within the scaphoid fossa by linking the proximal and distal carpal rows. This fusion corrects the deformity of the scaphoid, but the DISI deformity of the lunate is not addressed. However, loads across the wrist after STT fusion are transmitted across the radioscaphoid joint. Accordingly, reduction of the lunate deformity should not be critical. As the wrist goes into radial deviation, the distally fused scaphoid can no longer flex, causing increased pressure on the scaphoid fossa. Critics of the STT fusion are concerned about the long-term effects of this increased pressure across the radioscaphoid joint [100]. Some authors, including Watson, now recommend a radial styloidectomy as a routine part of STT fusion to avoid this problem [101]. Watson reported nonunion rates as low as 2%, but those in the literature average approximately 14% [99,102]. Postoperative range of motion is usually diminished by approximately 20% to 30% [103].

An alternative to the STT fusion, the scaphocapitate fusion is also a popular choice for treating irreducible scapholunate dissociation

[104]. The scaphocapitate fusion functions similarly to an STT fusion. Decreases in postoperative wrist motion between the procedures have been shown to be similar [105]. Kinematic behavior of the carpus has also been shown to be similar, with increased load-bearing across the scaphoid fossa and loss of midcarpal motion [96].

By adding the lunate to a scaphocapitate fusion, the SLC fusion allows stabilization between the scaphoid and lunate and across proximal and distal carpal rows, typically resulting in decreased motion of approximately 50% [106]. However, despite this greater loss of motion, proponents note that any limited carpal fusion that controls only the scaphoid, and not the lunate, exaggerates the pattern of increased load on the scaphoid. A biomechanical study published by Viegas et al. [96] in 1990 concluded that fusions incorporating the scaphoid and lunate redistributed load in a more physiologic manner, reestablishing the lunate as a load-bearing bone.

Complete scapholunate ligament injury with irreducible malalignment and cartilage degeneration

The SLAC wrist represents the end stage of scapholunate dissociation. Once the cartilaginous surfaces of the wrist have been compromised, repairing ligamentous structures and restoring the bony architecture of the wrist will probably not alleviate pain.

Scaphoid excision with a four-corner fusion (the SLAC procedure)

The SLAC procedure was popularized by Watson and Ballet and is a reliable procedure for end-stage advanced scapholunate dissociation [57,107]. The procedure consists of excising the scaphoid and fusing the lunate, capitate, hamate, and triquetrum. Load-bearing of the wrist is performed through the preserved radiolunate articulation. Accordingly, degenerative changes at the radiolunate fossa are contraindications to the procedure. The addition of the hamate and triquetrum to the fusion mass increases the surface area and decreases nonunion rates [108].

One of the most common complications after four-corner fusion is dorsal radiocarpal impingement in wrist extension. Ashmead et al. [109] found that dorsal radiocarpal impingement occurred in 13% of his patients. This complication is secondary to inadequate reduction of the capitolunate joint [107] and may be managed with a limited resection of the dorsal distal radius and abutting dorsal capitate.

In 1996, a study by Siegel and Ruby [102] reviewed the literature published between 1924 and 1994 on four-corner fusions and found that the nonunion rate was approximately 4.3%, the lowest of all intercarpal fusions.

Traditionally, the fusion mass is secured with K-wires. However, circular plates have recently become popular and are advocated by some authors [110], although results have been varied. Enna et al. [110] reported a 0% nonunion rate with the use of circular plating. However, Vance et al. [111] reported a major complication rate (nonunion and impingement on the plate) of 48% with the use of a circular plate as opposed to 4% with the use of K-wires.

Proximal row carpectomy

Proximal row carpectomy (PRC) is also an option for the advanced scapholunate dissociation with intact cartilage on the proximal aspect of the capitate. PRC consists of excising the scaphoid, lunate, and triquetrum, allowing the capitate to be seated within the lunate fossa. Carpal impingement may occur on the radial styloid in radial deviation and a styloidectomy may be performed concurrently to prevent this. However, care must be taken not to destabilize the RSC ligament.

In 2001, Cohen and Kozin [112] published a study comparing PRC and scaphoid excision with four-corner fusion. Results showed no significant differences, with arc of motion averaging approximately 80° in both groups. However, patients undergoing four-corner fusion had greater radioulnar deviation motion compared with those undergoing PRC. Grip strength was 71% in the PRC group and 79% in the four-corner fusion group. Pain relief was similar between the groups.

Additional salvage procedures, which are beyond the scope of this article, include total wrist arthrodesis and total wrist arthroplasty. When deciding on the salvage procedure, surgeons must consider patient age, degree of symptomatology, patient occupation, and physical demands on the wrist.

Summary

Scapholunate dissociation remains a complex problem for the treating physician. Its diagnosis in the early phase may be difficult secondary to normal radiographs. A high index of suspicion is needed because early repair offers the best chance at long-term stability.

References

[1] Destot E. Injuries of the wrist: a radiological study. New York; 1926.
[2] Linscheid RL, Dobyns JH, Beabout JW, et al. Traumatic instability of the wrist. Diagnosis, classification, and pathomechanics. J Bone Joint Surg Am 1972;54(8):1612–32.
[3] Weber ER. Concepts governing the rotational shift of the intercalated segment of the carpus. Orthop Clin North Am 1984;15(2):193–207.
[4] Fisk GR. Carpal instability and the fractured scaphoid. Ann R Coll Surg Engl 1970;46(2):63–76.
[5] Linscheid RL, Dobyns JH, Beckenbaugh RD, et al. Instability patterns of the wrist. J Hand Surg [Am] 1983;8(5 Pt 2):682–6.
[6] Berger RA. The gross and histologic anatomy of the scapholunate interosseous ligament. J Hand Surg [Am] 1996;21(2):170–8.
[7] Ruby LK, An KN, Linscheid RL, et al. The effect of scapholunate ligament section on scapholunate motion. J Hand Surg [Am] 1987;12(5 Pt 1):767–71.
[8] Berger RA, Blair WF, Crowninshield RD, et al. The scapholunate ligament. J Hand Surg [Am] 1982;7(1):87–91.
[9] Walsh JJ, Berger RA, Cooney WP. Current status of scapholunate interosseous ligament injuries. J Am Acad Orthop Surg 2002;10(1):32–42.
[10] Meade TD, Schneider LH, Cherry K. Radiographic analysis of selective ligament sectioning at the carpal scaphoid: a cadaver study. J Hand Surg [Am] 1990;15(6):855–62.
[11] Viegas SF, Yamaguchi S, Boyd NL, et al. The dorsal ligaments of the wrist: anatomy, mechanical properties, and function. J Hand Surg [Am] 1999;24(3):456–68.
[12] Short WH, Werner FW, Green JK, et al. Biomechanical evaluation of ligamentous stabilizers of the scaphoid and lunate. J Hand Surg [Am] 2002;27(6):991–1002.
[13] Mitsuyasu H, Patterson RM, Shah MA, et al. The role of the dorsal intercarpal ligament in dynamic and static scapholunate instability. J Hand Surg [Am] 2004;29(2):279–88.
[14] Short WH, Werner FW, Green JK, et al. Biomechanical evaluation of the ligamentous stabilizers of the scaphoid and lunate: part II. J Hand Surg [Am] 2005;30(1):24–34.
[15] Mayfield JK, Johnson RP, Kilcoyne RK. Carpal dislocations: pathomechanics and progressive perilunar instability. J Hand Surg [Am] 1980;5(3):226–41.
[16] Mayfield JK. Mechanism of carpal injuries. Clin Orthop Relat Res Jun 1980;149:45–54.
[17] Johnson RP. The acutely injured wrist and its residuals. Clin Orthop Relat Res. Jun 1980;149:33–44.
[18] Armstrong GW. Rotational subluxation of the scaphoid. Can J Surg 1968;11(3):306–14.
[19] Mayfield JK. Patterns of injury to carpal ligaments. A spectrum. Clin Orthop Relat Res. Jul–Aug 1984(187):36–42.
[20] Demos TC. Radiologic case study: painful wrist. Orthopedics 1978;1(2):151–3.
[21] Hergenroeder PT, Penix AR. Bilateral scapholunate dissociation with degenerative arthritis. J Hand Surg [Am] 1981;6(6):620–2.
[22] Vance RM, Gelberman RH, Braun RM. Chronic bilateral scapholunate dissociation without symptoms. J Hand Surg [Am] 1979;4(2):178–80.
[23] Bjelland JC, Bush JC. Case 21. Secondary rotational subluxation of the carpal navicular associated with a Smith's type fracture. Ariz Med 1977;31(4):267–8.
[24] Rosenthal DI, Schwartz M, Phillips WC, et al. Fracture of the radius with instability of the wrist. AJR Am J Roentgenol 1983;141(1):113–6.
[25] Taleisnik J. Rheumatoid synovitis of the volar compartment of the wrist joint: its radiological signs and its contribution to wrist and hand deformity. J Hand Surg [Am] 1979;4(6):526–35.
[26] Taleisnik J. Current concepts review. Carpal instability. J Bone Joint Surg Am 1988;70(8):1262–8.
[27] Ruby LK. Carpal instability. Instr Course Lect 1996;45:3–13.
[28] Jackson WT, Protas JM. Snapping scapholunate subluxation. J Hand Surg [Am] 1981;6(6):590–4.
[29] Howard FM, Fahey T, Wojcik E. Rotatory subluxation of the navicular. Clin Orthop Relat Res Oct 1974;104:134–9.
[30] Watson HK, Ashmead D, Makhlouf MV. Examination of the scaphoid. J Hand Surg [Am] 1988;13(5):657–60.
[31] Wolfe SW, Crisco JJ. Mechanical evaluation of the scaphoid shift test. J Hand Surg [Am] 1994;19(5):762–8.
[32] Easterling KJ, Wolfe SW. Scaphoid shift in the uninjured wrist. J Hand Surg [Am] 1994;19(4):604–6.
[33] Frankel VH. The Terry-Thomas sign. Clin Orthop Relat Res. Nov–Dec 1977;129:321–2.
[34] Thompson TC, Campbell RD Jr, Arnold WD. Primary and secondary dislocation of the scaphoid bone. J Bone Joint Surg Br 1964;46:73–82.
[35] Kindynis P, Resnick D, Kang HS, et al. Demonstration of the scapholunate space with radiography. Radiology 1990;175(1):278–80.
[36] Cautilli GP, Wehbe MA. Scapho-lunate distance and cortical ring sign. J Hand Surg [Am] 1991;16(3):501–3.

[37] Kleinman WB, Steichen JB, Strickland JW. Management of chronic rotary subluxation of the scaphoid by scapho-trapezio-trapezoid arthrodesis. J Hand Surg [Am] 1982;7(2):125–36.

[38] Sarrafian SK, Melamed JL, Goshgarian GM. Study of wrist motion in flexion and extension. Clin Orthop Relat Res Jul–Aug 1977(126):153–159.

[39] Taleisnik J. Wrist: anatomy, function and injury. Instr Course Lect 1978;27:61–87.

[40] Ozcelik A, Gunal I, Kose N. Stress views in the radiography of scapholunate instability. Eur J Radiol 2005;56(3):358–61.

[41] Dobyns JH, Linscheid RL, Chao EYS, et al. Traumatic instability of the wrist. Instr Course Lect 1975;24:182–99.

[42] Arkless R. Cineradiography in normal and abnormal wrists. Am J Roentgenol Radium Ther Nucl Med 1966;96(4):837–44.

[43] Weiss AP, Akelman E, Lambiase R. Comparison of the findings of triple-injection cinearthrography of the wrist with those of arthroscopy. J Bone Joint Surg Am 1996;78(3):348–56.

[44] Viegas SF, Ballantyne G. Age-related changes in the ligamentous anatomy of the wrist [abstract]. J Hand Surg [Am] 1988;13:303.

[45] Herbert TJ, Faithfull RG, McCann DJ, et al. Bilateral arthrography of the wrist. J Hand Surg [Br] 1990;15(2):233–5.

[46] Totterman SM, Miller RJ. Scapholunate ligament: normal MR appearance on three-dimensional gradient-recalled-echo images. Radiology 1996;200(1): 237–41.

[47] Daunt N. Magnetic resonance imaging of the wrist: anatomy and pathology of interosseous ligaments and the triangular fibrocartilage complex. Curr Probl Diagn Radiol 2002;31(4):158–76.

[48] Schadel-Hopfner M, Iwinska-Zelder J, Braus T, et al. MRI versus arthroscopy in the diagnosis of scapholunate ligament injury. J Hand Surg [Br] 2001;26(1):17–21.

[49] Cooney WP, Dobyns JH, Linscheid RL. Arthroscopy of the wrist: anatomy and classification of carpal instability. Arthroscopy 1990;6(2):133–40.

[50] Abe Y, Katsube K, Tsue K, et al. Arthroscopic diagnosis of partial scapholunate ligament tears as a cause of radial sided wrist pain in patients with inconclusive x-ray and MRI findings. J Hand Surg [Br] 2006;31(4):419–25.

[51] Morley J, Bidwell J, Bransby-Zachary M. A comparison of the findings of wrist arthroscopy and magnetic resonance imaging in the investigation of wrist pain. J Hand Surg [Br] 2001;26(6): 544–6.

[52] Cooney WP. Evaluation of chronic wrist pain by arthrography, arthroscopy, and arthrotomy. J Hand Surg [Am] 1993;18(5):815–22.

[53] Scheck RJ, Kubitzek C, Hierner R, et al. The scapholunate interosseous ligament in MR arthrography of the wrist: correlation with non-enhanced MRI and wrist arthroscopy. Skeletal Radiol 1997; 26(5):263–71.

[54] Adolfsson L. Arthroscopy for the diagnosis of post-traumatic wrist pain. J Hand Surg [Br] 1992; 17(1):46–50.

[55] Geissler WB, Freeland AE, Savoie FH, et al. Intracarpal soft-tissue lesions associated with an intraarticular fracture of the distal end of the radius. J Bone Joint Surg Am 1996;78(3):357–65.

[56] Watson HK, Weinzweig J, Zeppieri J. The natural progression of scaphoid instability. Hand Clin 1997;13(1):39–49.

[57] Watson HK, Ballet FL. The SLAC wrist: scapholunate advanced collapse pattern of degenerative arthritis. J Hand Surg [Am] 1984;9(3):358–65.

[58] Watson HK, Ryu J. Evolution of arthritis of the wrist. Clin Orthop Relat Res Jan 1986;202: 57–67.

[59] Harrington RH, Lichtman DM, Brockmole DM. Common pathways of degenerative arthritis of the wrist. Hand Clin 1987;3(4):507–27.

[60] O'Meeghan CJ, Stuart W, Mamo V, et al. The natural history of an untreated isolated scapholunate interosseus ligament injury. J Hand Surg [Br] 2003;28(4):307–10.

[61] Linscheid RL, Dobyns JH. Treatment of scapholunate dissociation. Rotatory subluxation of the scaphoid. Hand Clin 1992;8(4):645–52.

[62] Garcia-Elias M, Lluch AL, Stanley JK. Three-ligament tenodesis for the treatment of scapholunate dissociation: indications and surgical technique J Hand Surg [Am] 2006;31(1):125–34.

[63] Larsen CF, Amadio PC, Gilula LA, et al. Analysis of carpal instability: I. Description of the scheme J Hand Surg [Am] 1995;20(5):757–64.

[64] King RJ. Scapholunate diastasis associated with a Barton fracture treated by manipulation, or Terry-Thomas and the wine waiter. J R Soc Med 1983;76(5):421–3.

[65] Tang JB, Shi D, Gu YQ, et al. Can cast immobilization successfully treat scapholunate dissociation associated with distal radius fractures? J Hand Surg [Am] 1996;21(4):583–90.

[66] Tang JB. Carpal instability associated with fracture of the distal radius. Incidence, influencing factors and pathomechanics. Chin Med J (Engl) 1992; 105(9):758–65.

[67] O'Brien ET. Acute fractures and dislocations of the carpus. Orthop Clin North Am 1984;15(2): 237–58.

[68] Hodge JC, Gilula LA, Larsen CF, et al. Analysis of carpal instability: II. Clinical applications. J Hand Surg [Am] 1995;20(5):765–76 [discussion: 777].

[69] Whipple TL. The role of arthroscopy in the treatment of scapholunate instability. Hand Clin 1995; 11(1):37–40.

[70] Ruch DS, Poehling GG. Arthroscopic management of partial scapholunate and lunotriquetral

injuries of the wrist. J Hand Surg [Am] 1996;21(3): 412–7.

[71] Weiss AP, Sachar K, Glowacki KA. Arthroscopic debridement alone for intercarpal ligament tears. J Hand Surg [Am] 1997;22(2):344–9.

[72] DeWal H, Ahn A, Raskin KB. Thermal energy in arthroscopic surgery of the wrist. Clin Sports Med 2002;21(4):727–35.

[73] Arnoczky SP, Aksan A. Thermal modification of connective tissues: basic science considerations and clinical implications. J Am Acad Orthop Surg 2000;8(5):305–13.

[74] Hirsh L, Sodha S, Bozentka D, et al. Arthroscopic electrothermal collagen shrinkage for symptomatic laxity of the scapholunate interosseous ligament. J Hand Surg [Br] 2005;30(6):643–7.

[75] Bickert B, Sauerbier M, Germann G. Scapholunate ligament repair using the Mitek bone anchor. J Hand Surg [Br] 2000;25(2):188–92.

[76] Beredjiklian PK, Dugas J, Gerwin M. Primary repair of the scapholunate ligament. Tech Hand Up Extrem Surg 1998;2(4):269–73.

[77] Schweizer A, Steiger R. Long-term results after repair and augmentation ligamentoplasty of rotatory subluxation of the scaphoid. J Hand Surg [Am] 2002;27(4):674–84.

[78] Wyrick JD, Youse BD, Kiefhaber TR. Scapholunate ligament repair and capsulodesis for the treatment of static scapholunate dissociation. J Hand Surg [Br] 1998;23(6):776–80.

[79] Blatt G. Capsulodesis in reconstructive hand surgery: dorsal capsulodesis for the unstable scaphoid and volar capsulodesis following excision of the distal ulna. Hand Clin 1987;3:81–102.

[80] Wintman BI, Gelberman RH, Katz JN. Dynamic scapholunate instability: results of operative treatment with dorsal capsulodesis. J Hand Surg [Am] 1995;20(6):971–9.

[81] Dagum AB, Hurst LC, Finzel KC. Scapholunate dissociation: an experimental kinematic study of two types of indirect soft tissue repairs. J Hand Surg [Am] 1997;22(4):714–9.

[82] Moran SL, Cooney WP, Berger RA, et al. Capsulodesis for the treatment of chronic scapholunate instability. J Hand Surg [Am] 2005;30(1):16–23.

[83] Berger RA, Bishop AT, Bettinger PC. New dorsal capsulotomy for the surgical exposure of the wrist. Ann Plast Surg 1995;35(1):54–9.

[84] Hofstede DJ, Ritt MJ, Bos KE. Tarsal autografts for reconstruction of the scapholunate interosseous ligament: a biomechanical study. J Hand Surg [Am] 1999;24(5):968–76.

[85] Lutz M, Kralinger F, Goldhahn J, et al. Dorsal scapholunate ligament reconstruction using a periosteal flap of the iliac crest. Arch Orthop Trauma Surg 2004;124(3):197–202.

[86] Weiss AP. Scapholunate ligament reconstruction using a bone-retinaculum-bone autograft. J Hand Surg [Am] 1998;23(2):205–15.

[87] Kalb K, Markert S. [Preliminary results with Cuenod's osteoligamentoplasty and capsulodesis for treatment of chronic scapholunate dissociation]. Handchir Mikrochir Plast Chir 2003;35(5): 310–6 [German].

[88] Schuind F. Scapholunate reconstruction using a vascularized flap of the interosseus membrane. Orthopedic Surgical Technology 1995;9:21–6.

[89] Harvey EJ, Sen M, Martineau P. A vascularized technique for bone-tissue-bone repair in scapholunate dissociation. Tech Hand Up Extrem Surg 2006;10(3):166–72.

[90] Almquist EE, Bach AW, Sack JT, et al. Four-bone ligament reconstruction for treatment of chronic complete scapholunate separation. J Hand Surg [Am] 1991;16(2):322–7.

[91] Brunelli GA, Brunelli GR. [A new surgical technique for carpal instability with scapho-lunar dislocation. (Eleven cases)]. Ann Chir Main Memb Super 1995;14(4–5):207–13 [French].

[92] Van Den Abbeele KL, Loh YC, Stanley JK, et al. Early results of a modified Brunelli procedure for scapholunate instability. J Hand Surg [Br] 1998; 23(2):258–61.

[93] Rosenwasser MP, Miyasajsa KC, Strauch RJ. The RASL procedure: reduction and association of the scaphoid and lunate using the Herbert screw. Tech Hand Up Extrem Surg 1997;1(4):263–72.

[94] Thornton L. Old dislocation of os magnum: open reduction and stabilization. South Med J 1924;17: 430.

[95] Peterson HA, Lipscomb PR. Intercarpal arthrodesis. Arch Surg 1967;95(1):127–34.

[96] Viegas SF, Patterson RM, Peterson PD, et al. Evaluation of the biomechanical efficacy of limited intercarpal fusions for the treatment of scapho-lunate dissociation. J Hand Surg [Am] 1990;15(1):120–8.

[97] Hom S, Ruby LK. Attempted scapholunate arthrodesis for chronic scapholunate dissociation. J Hand Surg [Am] 1991;16(2):334–9.

[98] Pettersson K, Wagnsjo P. Arthrodesis for chronic static scapholunate dissociation: a prospective study in 12 patients. Scand J Plast Reconstr Surg Hand Surg 2004;38(3):166–71.

[99] Watson HK, Belniak R, Garcia-Elias M. Treatment of scapholunate dissociation: preferred treatment—STT fusion vs other methods. Orthopedics 1991;14(3):365–8 [discussion: 368–70].

[100] Garcia-Elias M, Cooney WP, An KN, et al. Wrist kinematics after limited intercarpal arthrodesis. J Hand Surg [Am] 1989;14(5):791–9.

[101] Rogers WD, Watson HK. Radial styloid impingement after triscaphe arthrodesis. J Hand Surg [Am] 1989;14(2 Pt 1):297–301.

[102] Siegel JM, Ruby LK. A critical look at intercarpal arthrodesis: review of the literature. J Hand Surg [Am] 1996;21(4):717–23.

[103] Meier R, Prommersberger KJ, Krimmer H. [Scapho-trapezio-trapezoid arthrodesis (triscaphe

arthrodesis)]. Handchir Mikrochir Plast Chir 2003; 35(5):323–7 [German].
[104] Cooney WP, DeBartolo T, Wood MBPost traumatic arthritis of the wrist, vol. 1. St. Louis (MO): Mosby-Year Book; 1998.
[105] Douglas DP, Peimer CA, Koniuch MP. Motion of the wrist after simulated limited intercarpal arthrodeses. An experimental study. J Bone Joint Surg Am 1987;69(9):1413–8.
[106] Siegel JM, Ruby LK. Midcarpal arthrodesis. J Hand Surg [Am] 1996;21(2):179–82.
[107] Tomaino MM, Miller RJ, Cole I, et al. Scapholunate advanced collapse wrist: proximal row carpectomy or limited wrist arthrodesis with scaphoid excision? J Hand Surg [Am] 1994; 19(1):134–42.
[108] Krakauer JD, Bishop AT, Cooney WP. Surgical treatment of scapholunate advanced collapse. J Hand Surg [Am] 1994;19(5):751–9.
[109] Ashmead D, Watson HK, Damon C, et al. Scapholunate advanced collapse wrist salvage. J Hand Surg [Am] 1994;19(5):741–50.
[110] Enna M, Hoepfner P, Weiss AP. Scaphoid excision with four-corner fusion. Hand Clin 2005;21(4):531–8.
[111] Vance MC, Hernandez JD, Didonna ML, et al. Complications and outcome of four-corner arthrodesis: circular plate fixation versus traditional techniques. J Hand Surg [Am] 2005;30(6):1122–7.
[112] Cohen MS, Kozin SH. Degenerative arthritis of the wrist: proximal row carpectomy versus scaphoid excision and four-corner arthrodesis. J Hand Surg [Am] 2001;26(1):94–104.

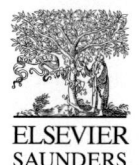

Perilunate Injuries

David J. Sauder, MD, FRCSC, George S. Athwal, MD, FRCSC*,
Kenneth J. Faber, MD, MHPE, FRCSC,
James H. Roth, MD, FRCSC

*Hand and Upper Limb Centre, St. Joseph's Health Care, University of Western Ontario,
268 Grosvenor Street, London, ON, N6A 4L6, Canada*

Perilunate injuries (PLIs) are uncommon, severe disruptions of carpal anatomy. Their defining feature is dislocation of the capitate head from the concavity of the distal lunate. These injuries affect both soft tissues and bony elements of the wrist and present in two common patterns: the perilunate dislocation (PLD) and the transscaphoid perilunate dislocation (TSPLD) [1]. The PLD is a soft tissue circumferential disruption around the lunate. The injury pattern occurs sequentially, starting at the scapholunate joint, then to the lunocapitate and lunotriquetral joints, and finally complete dislocation of the lunate. TSPLDs are more common than PLDs and are different because they involve a scaphoid fracture rather than a scapholunate ligamentous disruption. Carpal dislocations were first described by Etienne Destot in 1926 [2]. Since that time, knowledge about the anatomy of the wrist and pathomechanics of this injury has grown substantially and treatment has evolved. There is now general agreement that these injuries require open reduction and internal fixation.

A PLI is a high-energy injury that commonly is the result of a fall from a height, a motor vehicle or motorcycle accident, or a sporting event. Perilunate injuries usually affect young men with an average age of 30 [1,3]. Patients often have associated injuries that may require more urgent attention. Definitive treatment may need to be delayed, and lifesaving trauma principles should be observed in treating these injuries.

Anatomy

The ligaments of the wrist are categorized as intracapsular or intra-articular [4]. Intracapsular ligaments can be further divided into extrinsic or intrinsic ligaments. An extrinsic ligament originates from the radius or ulna and inserts on the carpus, whereas an intrinsic ligament connects two carpal bones. The ligamentous anatomy of the wrist is complex; however, knowledge of a few important ligaments allows one to understand the pathology of perilunate injuries.

The scapholunate ligament is intra-articular and connects the scaphoid and lunate at the proximal aspect of their articulation (Fig. 1). It has three main parts. The dorsal aspect of the ligament is the strongest and thickest portion [5–8]. This aspect contributes to a dorsal axis of rotation at the scapholunate joint [9]. The volar portion is not as strong as the dorsal portion, and the proximal or membranous portion is made of fibrocartilage and is not truly a ligament. The lunotriquetral ligament is also intra-articular and lies at the proximal aspect of the articulation between the lunate and triquetrum. Unlike the scapholunate ligament, the lunotriquetral ligament's strongest and thickest portion is volar. It also has a dorsal ligamentous portion and a proximal membranous portion.

The critical volar intracapsular ligaments originate on the radius and ulna (Fig. 2). The long and short radiolunate ligaments are strong and often remain intact after a PLD. The radioscaphocapitate (RSC) ligament originates from the radius, runs volar to the waist of the scaphoid, and attaches to the capitate. The ulnocapitate ligament

---

* Corresponding author.
E-mail address: gathwal@uwo.ca (G.S. Athwal).

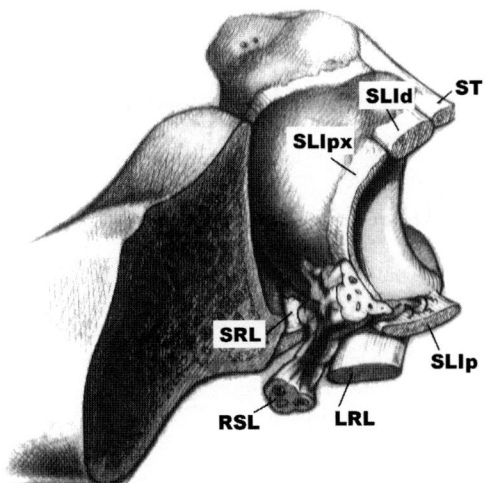

Fig. 1. Interpretive drawing of the scapholunate interosseous (SLI) ligament from the radial perspective with the radial styloid and scaphoid removed. The SLI ligament is made up of dorsal (d), proximal (px), and palmar (p) regions. The palmar ligaments, attaching the lunate to the radius, are the long radiolunate (LRL) and short radiolunate (SRL). The scaphotriquetral (ST) and radioscapholunate (RSL) ligaments are also portrayed. (*From* Berger RA. The gross and histologic anatomy of the scapholunate interosseous ligament. J Hand Surg [Am] 1996;21:172; with permission from The American Society for Surgery of the Hand.)

originates from the ulna, runs volar to the lunotriquetral joint, and interdigitates with the RSC ligament. The ulnolunate ligament originates from the palmar radioulnar ligament and attaches to the lunate. There is weakness in the volar capsule, between the volar ligaments attached to the capitate and those attached to the lunate. This area of weakness is termed the space of Poirier and is the anatomic area through which the lunate dislocates [10,11].

Pathomechanics

Perilunate dislocations are high-energy injuries that occur after a tremendous amount of force is transferred to the wrist in a specific loading pattern. Performing cadaveric studies, Mayfield [9–12] was able to establish the four stages of progressive ligamentous injury (Fig. 3). He placed wrists in hyperextension, ulnar deviation, and carpal supination. When force was administered to the radial aspect of the hand, a reproducible injury pattern occurred.

During a PLD, the ligamentous elements fail in a radial to ulnar direction. In stage I, the RSC and scapholunate ligaments are torn, producing scapholunate instability. Stage II involved dislocation of the lunocapitate joint. Clinically, this is almost always dorsal [1]. Stage III is a disruption of the lunotriquetral joint. In stage IV, the dorsal radiocarpal ligament is torn, allowing the lunate to dislocate volarly. The radiolunate ligaments remain intact throughout this injury and anchor the lunate proximally. During a lunate dislocation, these ligaments cause a 180° rotation of the lunate. Slight alteration in the position of the wrist and the force applied will result in injuries that may involve fracture of the radial styloid, scaphoid, capitate, or triquetrum. Clinically, fractures through the bony elements surrounding the lunate are known as greater arc injuries, and injury through the ligamentous elements are known as lesser arc injuries (Figs. 4 and 5) [13]. Cartilage damage can also occur and is most common on the head of the capitate (Fig. 6) [3].

Other injury patterns, although unusual, do occur. Naviculocapitate syndrome (also known as scaphocapitate syndrome) is a fracture through the scaphoid waist and capitate that rotates the proximal capitate 180° so its proximal articular surface points distally (Fig. 7) [14]. The scaphoid and lunate can also dislocate as a unit [15]. Alternatively, a volar lunate transscaphoid dislocation may occur [16]. Finally, the scaphoid can fracture in conjunction with a scapholunate injury [17].

Diagnosis

Despite the severe disruption of carpal anatomy, diagnosis can be surprisingly difficult. Injuries were missed in 25% of patients in a study of 166 cases [1]. Patients commonly present with pain, swelling, and decreased range of motion. Evidence of median nerve injury is common, and acute carpal tunnel syndrome is present in approximately 25% of patients (range, 16%–46%) [1,18,19].

Posteroanterior and lateral plain radiographs are usually adequate to make the diagnosis, but the findings can be subtle. Traction views may help to define the pattern of injury. The key to diagnosis is recognizing the disruption of the radius–lunate–capitate axis. The dislocated head of the capitate is usually displaced dorsal to the lunate. In stage IV instability, the lunate will be dislocated and rotated volarly, resulting in

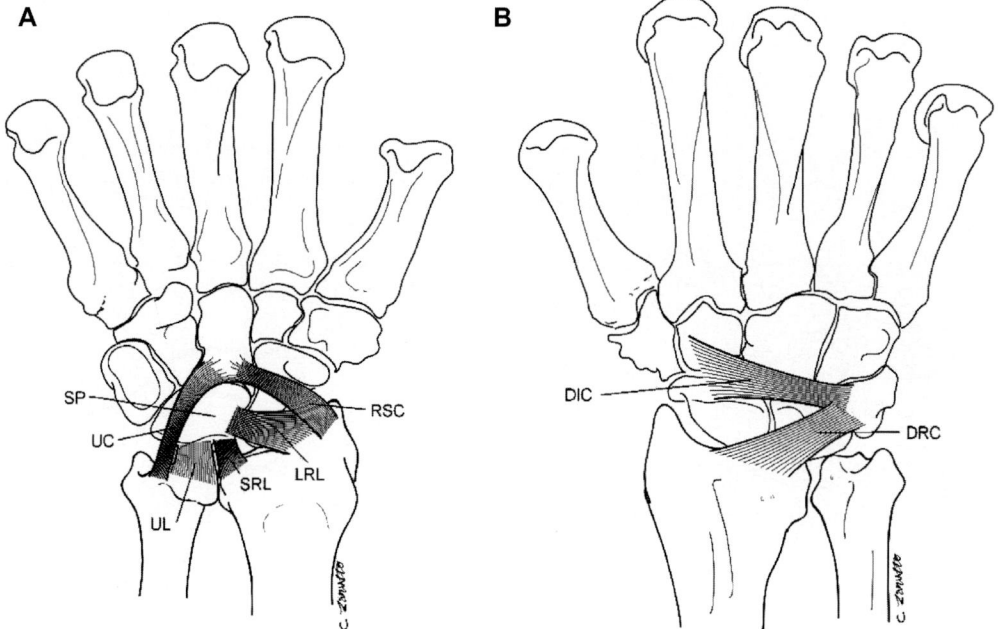

Fig. 2. An illustration of the volar (*A*) and dorsal (*B*) intracapsular ligaments. The radioscaphocapitate (RSC) and ulnocapitate (UC) ligaments connect the capitate to the distal forearm. The long radiolunate (LRL), short radiolunate (SRL), and ulnolunate (UL) ligaments attach the lunate to the distal forearm. In between is the space of Poirier (SP), where the lunate may herniate through the capsule in a lunate dislocation. The main dorsal intracapsular ligaments are the dorsal intercarpal (DIC) and dorsal radiocarpal (DRC) ligaments. (*Adapted from* An KN, Berger RA, Cooney WP III. Biomechanics of the wrist joint. New York: Spinger Verlag; 1991. p. 10; with permission.)

a "spilled tea cup" sign [20]. More subtle findings on plain radiographs include a disruption of Gilula's lines and an increase in carpal joint spaces >2 mm. Gilula's lines are seen as three smooth arcs on the posteroanterior view (Fig. 8) [21,22]. These lines are produced by the proximal and distal surfaces of the proximal carpal row and the proximal aspect of the distal carpal row.

Radiographs need to be examined carefully for bony injury of the distal radius and carpus. The scaphoid waist fracture is the most common bony injury, whereas radial styloid fractures and fractures of the capitate, hamate, and triquetrum are less common [1].

Classification

The accepted nomenclature for PLI requires that the fracture is mentioned first and is indicated by the prefix *trans*. The dislocation portion of the injury is mentioned second. A common TSPLD occurs when the scaphoid is fractured and the capitate is dislocated dorsally. PLD indicates the lunate remains in the lunate fossa of the radius. Lunate dislocation refers to the displacement of the lunate out of the lunate fossa wherein the capitate maintains its axial alignment with the radius. Many classifications of PLI exist [20,23]. The severity of injury was separated by Mayfield into four stages [9–12] and is described in the Pathomechanics section of this article. Herzberg et al. [1] divided PLI into two main groups: PLD and perilunate fracture dislocation.

Initial management

Management begins with an appropriate assessment including a pertinent history and physical examination. A PLI is often associated with other injuries, especially injuries in the ipsilateral forearm and elbow [1]. A careful examination of the median nerve should be performed at every stage of treatment. The greatest insult to the median nerve occurs at the time of injury when the carpus is maximally displaced. Therefore, the only absolute indication for urgent carpal tunnel

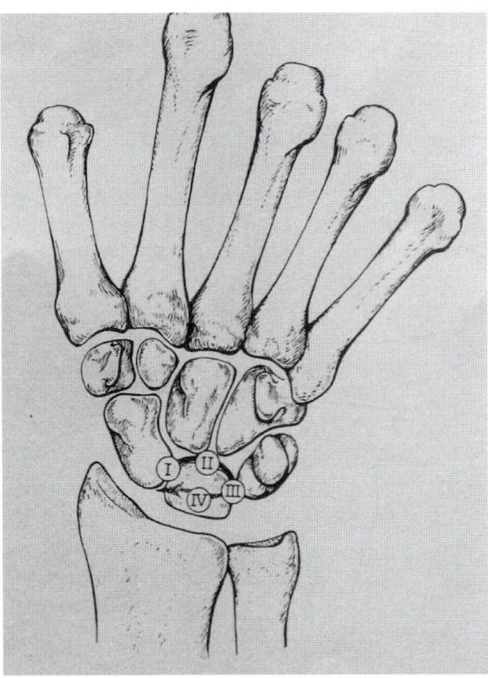

Fig. 3. Mayfield described four stages of perilunate instability. The first stage (I) is disruption of the scapholunate articulation. The second (II) and third (III) stages are separation of the capitolunate and lunotriquetral joints. The fourth (IV) stage is a volar lunate dislocation. (*From* Mayfield JK. Wrist ligamentous anatomy and pathogenesis of carpal instability. Ortho Clin North Am 1984;15(2):214; with permission.)

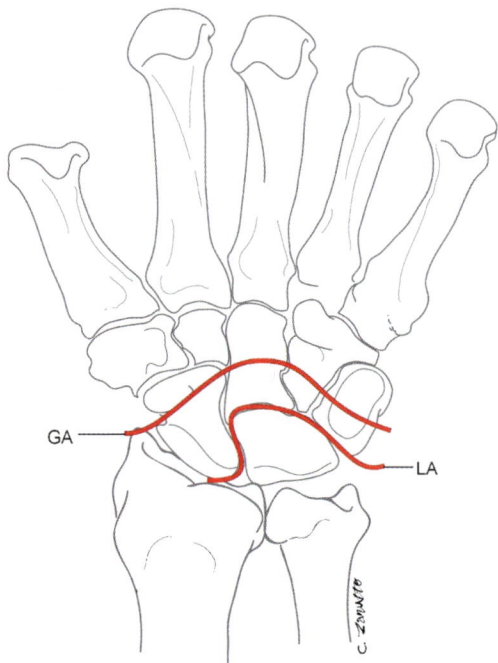

Fig. 4. Lesser arc (LA) injuries occur through the ligamentous structures surrounding the lunate. Greater arc (GA) injuries occur through osseous structures such as the radial styloid, scaphoid, capitate, and triquetrum. Perilunate injuries are often a combination of the two.

release is a progressive median deficit that suggests worsening compression in the carpal tunnel. However, the carpus does need to be reduced, because there is evidence that a perilunate injury left unreduced has a high likelihood of residual median nerve compression [1].

A closed reduction in the emergency room will aid in pain control, reduction of swelling, a decrease of any residual pressure on the median nerve, and a better assessment of the injury. This can be accomplished using a method described by Watson-Jones [24,25]. Ten pounds of traction is applied for 10 minutes through finger traps. Then a closed reduction maneuver is performed. The treating physician maintains traction. A gentle dorsiflexion maneuver followed by volar flexion allows the head of the capitate to slip back into the sulcus of the lunate. Counterpressure must be maintained on the volar surface of the lunate. A palpable "clunk" is felt upon reduction of the carpus. If the injury is a lunate dislocation, the

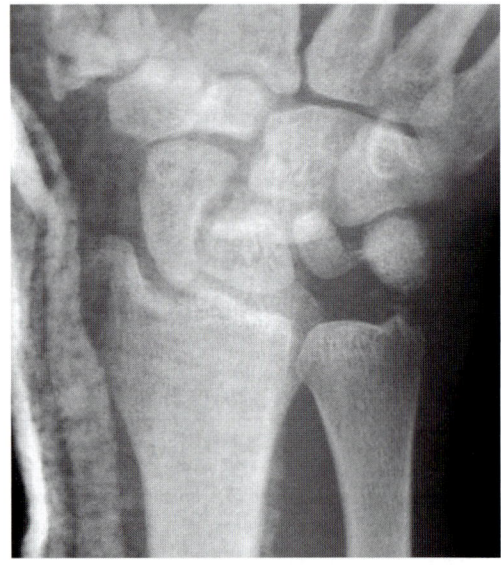

Fig. 5. Posteroanterior radiograph demonstrating a greater arc injury with fractures through the radial styloid and triquetrum.

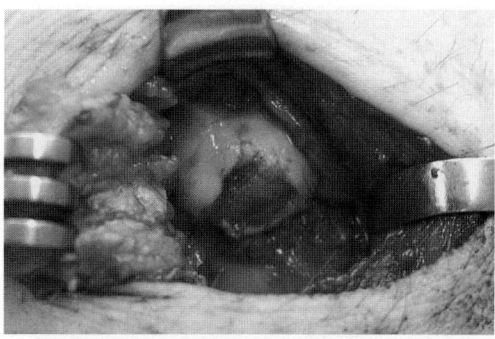

Fig. 6. A clinical photograph showing the loss of cartilage from the head of the capitate during operative management of a perilunate injury by way of a transverse wrist incision.

lunate must first be reduced onto the radius, then followed by the aforementioned procedure. The wrist must be splinted to maintain reduction and postreduction films are obtained. Closed reduction often is not possible. The dorsal capsule may be caught in the midcarpal joint or may be impaled on a spike of scaphoid [26].

Operative management

The recommended treatment for PLD and TSPLD is surgery. They are complex ligament and/or bony injuries that require an accurate open reduction and restoration of anatomy. To maintain reduction, internal fixation must be used. Closed reduction and immobilization cannot reliably maintain normal carpal alignment and has been shown to have poor results [19,27]. If a closed reduction can be achieved, surgery can be delayed for up to a week after the injury [25]. This allows for decreased swelling and easier exposure. If a closed reduction cannot be achieved, operative management should be performed urgently.

There is agreement in the literature that one should perform open reduction and internal fixation of fractures and ligamentous repair. Restoration of the function of the scapholunate ligament is important to decrease the rate of late dorsal intercalated segment instability (DISI) deformity [28]. Even with good repair techniques, an increase in the scapholunate angle occurs over time. In a study of 22 people, Trumble and Verheyden [18] maintained postoperative scapholunate angle over the course of 4 years by placing an intraosseous cerclage wire between the scaphoid and lunate with a combined approach. Despite this excellent radiographic outcome, the clinical outcomes were similar to other studies in the literature with only 10 patients returning to the same job. Also, 16 patients required hardware removal because of cerclage wire breakage.

Many different approaches to PLD and TSPLD have been described. There are supporters of the isolated dorsal approach [25,29–31], the isolated volar approach [32,33], and the combination of both approaches [3,18,27,34–37]. The authors' varying beliefs illustrate this controversy. One author (GSA) believes that the dorsal approach alone is adequate for visualization and accurate reduction of the carpus in neurologically intact patients. He believes it affords good exposure of the scaphoid for anatomic reduction and fixation. To him, the most critical part of the scapholunate ligament (the dorsal portion) is most readily repaired with the dorsal approach. However, the senior author (JHR) believes that the volar ulnar approach is necessary in addition to the dorsal approach. He believes the combination of these approaches repairs the disrupted volar capsule and allows decompression of the median nerve in the carpal tunnel and the ulnar nerve in Guyon's canal [38]. A Russe approach to the volar scaphoid also can be helpful in anatomic restoration of the scaphoid. A more recent development is the use of arthroscopic techniques for reduction and fixation [39–41].

Surgical technique

The patient is brought to the operating room, and a general or regional anesthetic is administered. A tourniquet is placed on the arm and used throughout the case. The approach begins with a midline longitudinal dorsal incision; however, a short transverse incision centered over the carpus may be used as well (see Fig. 6). The longitudinal incision is useful if repeated operations on the wrist are necessary. The extensor retinaculum is entered through the third compartment, and retinacular flaps are raised radially and ulnarly by dividing the septae between extensor compartments. If the dorsal capsule is torn, the arthrotomy simply can be extended. If possible, the preferred capsulotomy is the ligament sparing approach described by Berger and coworkers [42]. This allows sparing of the dorsal intercarpal and the dorsal radiocarpal ligaments.

If a closed reduction was not achieved, an open reduction is performed at this time. It is often

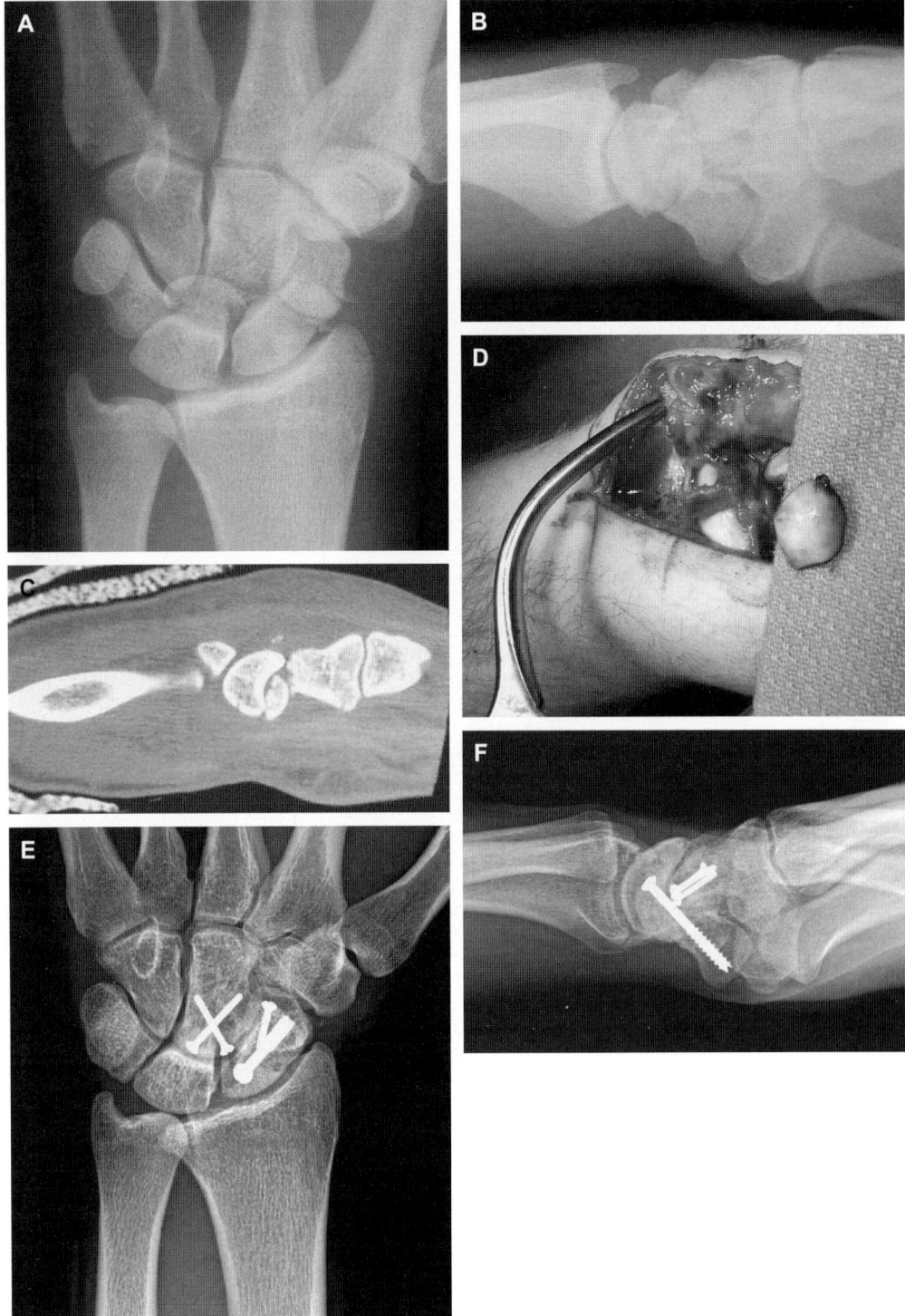

Fig. 7. A clinical case of scaphocapitate syndrome. Posteroanterior (*A*) and lateral (*B*) radiographs, and a sagittal reformat of a CT scan (*C*) show the scaphoid fracture and the head of the capitate which is rotated 180°. An intraoperative photo of the completely detached head of the capitate (*D*). Final follow up radiographs (*E*, *F*) show screw fixation and both fractures healing. (*Courtesy of* Graham J. King, MD, FRCSC, London, Ontario, Canada.)

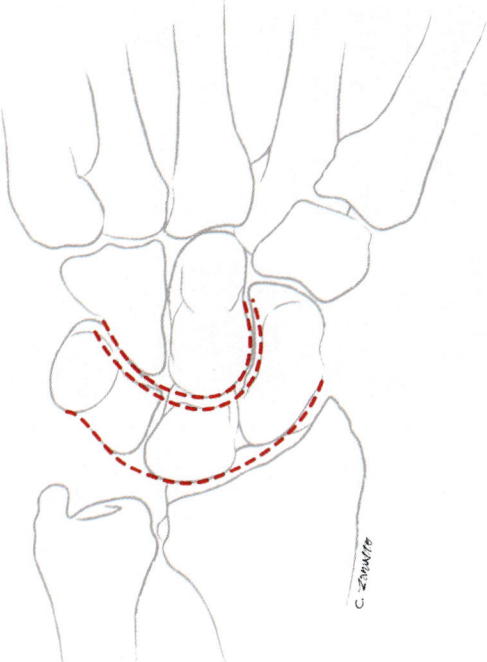

Fig. 8. An illustration of Gilula's lines. Three smooth arcs should be present on a posteroanterior radiograph of the wrist.

helpful to place 1.6 mm Kirschner wire (K wire) pins transversely into the scaphoid and the triquetrum using an inside-out technique prior to performing the initial reduction maneuver. These K wires are advanced until they reach the articular surface. Traction and downward pressure on the perilunate carpus with volar stabilization of the lunate should accomplish a gentle reduction. A flat, blunt instrument can be used to shoehorn the capitate head onto the distal lunate.

Fractures are identified and reduced. The scaphoid is most often fractured through the waist [1]. It is commonly comminuted and can be difficult to reduce [3]. Once reduced and stabilized by a K wire, a single headless compression screw is introduced antegrade to achieve rigid internal fixation. K wires can be used as the definitive fixation and are preferred by the senior author (KJF). The capitate or triquetrum may be reduced and fixed in a similar manner.

After fractures are stabilized, the carpus can be anatomically reduced with the help of K wires as joysticks. The lunate is flexed and the scaphoid is extended. This maneuver is used to obtain an anatomic scapholunate angle and avoid the tendency for DISI deformity. After carpal realignment, the transverse pins that had been placed previously into the scaphoid and the triquetrum are reversed into the lunate to stabilize the proximal carpal row.

The dorsal portion of the scapholunate ligament usually pulls off of the scaphoid and is left attached to the lunate. The ligament can be grasped with suture and repaired to the scaphoid with minisuture anchors buried in the scaphoid. Alternatively, drill holes can be used in the scaphoid to pass suture and tie over a button. The lunotriquetral ligament is then repaired in a similar fashion. Fluoroscopy is used to confirm reduction and adequate placement of fixation devices. K wires may be left percutaneous; however, the authors prefer to bury the wire beneath the skin then apply a bulky splint (Fig. 9).

Postoperative management

Patients are maintained in a splint for 1–2 weeks. They are then converted to a thumb spica fiberglass cast for 10 weeks. Interosseous pin removal is accomplished at 10 weeks when the fiberglass cast is removed. The scaphoid takes an average of 16 weeks to heal [29]. Range of motion and strength are gained with rehabilitation after immobilization is removed. There is some suggestion that a dart-throwing motion may be ideal for rehabilitation because it would limit scapholunate motion [43].

Results

The most common scoring system in the literature is the Mayo score described by Cooney and colleagues and modified from Green and O'Brien [20,23]. This rating instrument gives a maximum score of 100 with a higher score demonstrating a better outcome. The four parameters assessed are pain, functional status (ability to work), range of motion, and grip strength; each area is worth 25 points. A score of 90–100 points is excellent, 80–90 points is good, 65–80 points is fair, and less than 65 points is poor.

The results following nonoperative treatment are poor. Aspergis and coworkers [27] treated eight people who had closed reduction under anesthesia and casting, and compared them with an operative group. The nonoperative group had 100% (6/6) scaphoid nonunion rate. The patients had three fair and five poor results at an average follow-up

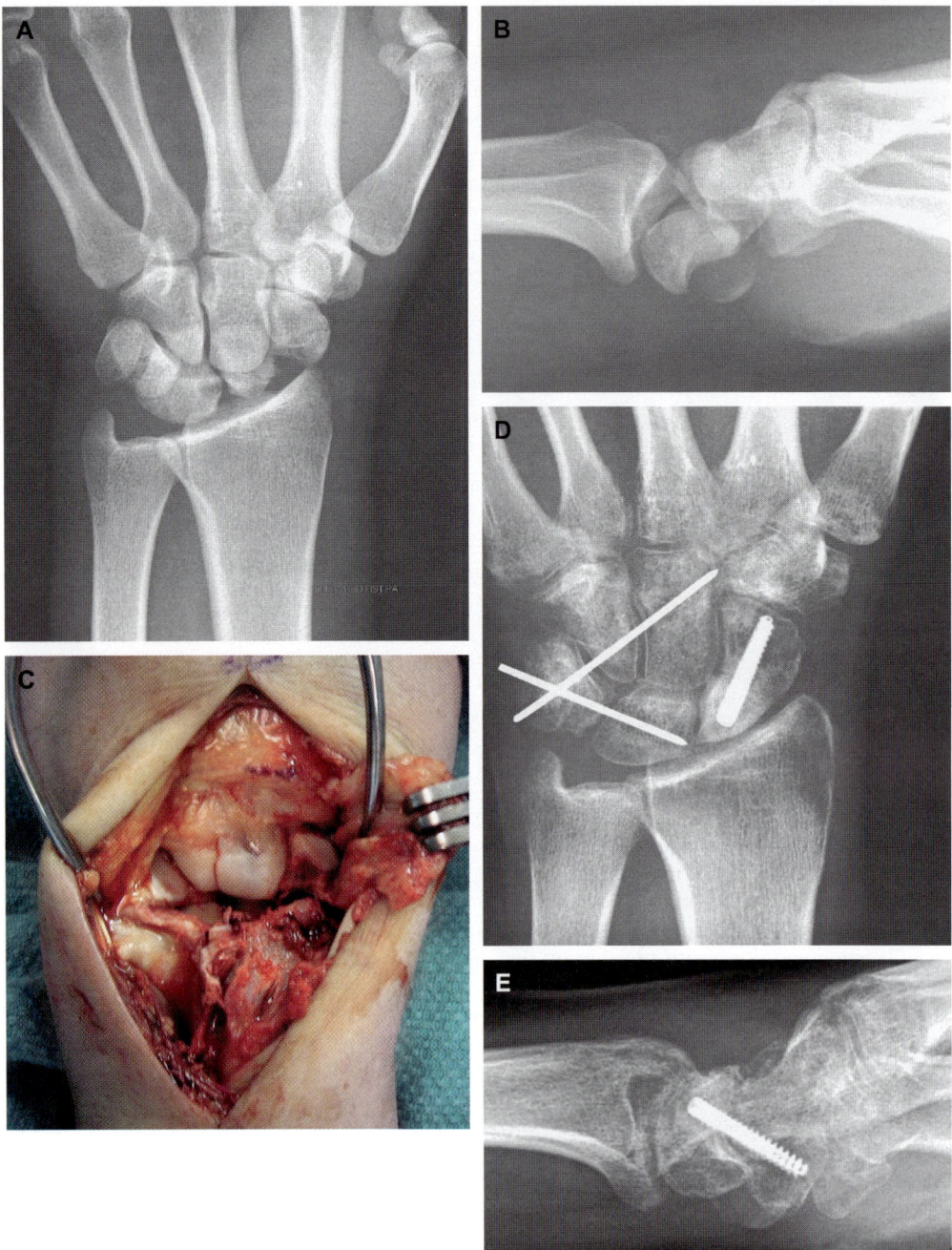

Fig. 9. A clinical case of a transscaphoid dorsal perilunate fracture dislocation of the wrist. Posteroanterior (*A*) and lateral (*B*) radiographs show the head of the capitate dislocated dorsally relative to the lunate. The scaphoid has a comminuted fracture through the waist. An intraoperative photograph (*C*) was taken before the reduction, which shows the capitate, hamate, and distal pole of the scaphoid dislocated dorsally. Two-month follow-up radiographs (*D, E*) after open reduction and internal fixation of the carpus with headless screw fixation and bonegrafting of the scaphoid demonstrate restoration of carpal alignment. The radiodensity of the proximal scaphoid suggests avascular necrosis.

of 6 years. Adkison and Chapman [19] demonstrated a 59% loss of reduction overall with closed treatment. In the TSPLD population, they reported a 68% loss of reduction and a 75% rate of avascular necrosis or nonunion in their scaphoids.

Much better results occur with operative management. Outcomes from PLD and TSPLD do not differ significantly [1,3,29,33]. For most series of operatively stabilized scaphoids, the rate of union is 100% [3,29,44]. The average time to union using a headless compression screw is 16 weeks [29]. A gradual loss of alignment after surgical intervention is observed often [3]. However, Trumble and Verheyden [18] found no loss of alignment after an average 4-year follow-up in perilunate injuries treated with interosseous cerclage wiring.

Clinical outcomes are often significantly better than the radiographic outcomes. Herzberg and Forissier [44] reported an 8-year follow-up for TSPLD. All patients maintained anatomic wrist alignment and 57% had a good or excellent Mayo score, despite 86% of patients who had radiographic evidence of arthritis at the radiocarpal or midcarpal joints. Hildebrand and colleagues [3] found a 50% rate of arthritis at an average follow-up period of 3 years. Yet, 73% of patients were engaged in full regular activities. This prevalence of midcarpal arthritis despite normal alignment may be explained by the common finding of capitate cartilage damage found at the time of surgery. Compared with the contralateral side, range of motion varies between 69% and 91% [3,28,29]. Most of the authors immobilize the wrist for 6 to 10 weeks. Inoue and Imaeda [32] advocate for 4 weeks of immobilization to prevent loss of range of motion. They found an increased range of motion when they immobilized for 4 weeks as opposed to an average of 7.6 weeks (114° versus 96°). Grip strength varies between 73% and 80% [3,28,29]. Most people are able to resume previous levels of activities (72%–92%) [3,28,29,44]. This usually entails a return to their previous occupation. Some patients can return to work, but only with modified duties. Very few are severely disabled in short- and medium-term follow up.

Missed diagnosis

Patients who have PLI often go undiagnosed. Herzberg and colleagues [1] had a rate of 25% in their series. Untreated patients do poorly; they develop degenerative arthritis and pain and often have accompanying median nerve compression.

Inoue and Shionova [45] reviewed 34 patients who had chronic, unreduced perilunate injuries. With injuries less than 2 months old, the patients showed good outcomes of open reduction and internal fixation. For patients who presented after 2 months, Inoue and Shionova recommended proximal row carpectomy for patients in whom cartilage on the capitate was preserved. These acceptable results for proximal row carpectomy have been confirmed by others [46].

Summary

PLDs are complex injuries of the bony and ligamentous anatomy of the wrist. They require operative management with careful restoration of carpal alignment and internal fixation. Even with optimal treatment, mild to moderate dysfunction affects most patients.

References

[1] Herzberg G, Comtet JJ, Linschied RL, et al. Perilunate dislocations and fracture-dislocations: a multicenter study. J Hand Surg [Am] 1993;18:768–79.
[2] Destot E. The classic: injuries of the wrist: a radiologic study. Clin Orthop 2006;445:8–14.
[3] Hildebrand KA, Ross DC, Patterson SD, et al. Dorsal perilunate dislocations and fracture-dislocations: questionnaire, clinical, and radiographic evaluation. J Hand Surg [Am] 2000;25:1069–79.
[4] Garcia-Elias M, Geissler WB. Carpal instability. In: Green's operative hand surgery. 5th edition. Philadelphia: Elsevier Churchill Livingstone; 2005. p. 535–604.
[5] Berger RA. The gross and histologic anatomy of the scapholunate interosseous ligament. J Hand Surg [Am] 1996;21:170–8.
[6] Berger RA. The anatomy of the ligaments of the wrist and distal radioulnar joints. Clin Orthop 2001;383:32–40.
[7] Berger RA. The ligaments of the wrist; a current overview of anatomy with considerations of their potential functions. Hand Clin 1997;13(1):63–82.
[8] Walsh JJ, Berger RA, Cooney WP. Current status of scapholunate interosseous ligament injuries. J Am Acad Orthop Surg 2002;10:32–42.
[9] Mayfield JK. Patterns of injury to carpal ligaments: a spectrum. Clin Orthop 1984;187:36–42.
[10] Mayfield JK, Johnson RP, Kilcoyne RK. Carpal dislocations: pathomechanics and progressive perilunar instability. J Hand Surg [Am] 1980;5:1199–201.
[11] Mayfield JK. Wrist ligamentous anatomy and pathogenesis of carpal instability. Orthop Clin North Am 1984;15(2):209–16.

[12] Mayfield JK, Johnson RP, Kilcoyne RF. The ligaments of the human wrist and their functional significance. Anat Rec 1976;186:417–28.

[13] Johnson RP. The acutely injured wrist and its residuals. Clin Orthop 1980;149:33–44.

[14] Fenton RL. The naviculo-capitate fracture syndrome. J Bone Joint Surg Am 1956;12:335–47.

[15] Raemisch ME, Rothman MB. Palmar dislocation of the scaphoid and lunate as a unit. Orthopedics 2004;27(11):1199–201.

[16] Kamano M, Honda Y, Kazuki K. Palmar lunate transscaphoid fracture-dislocation caused by a palmar flexion injury. J Orthop Trauma 2001;15:225–7.

[17] Cheng C-Y, Hsu K-Y, Tseng I-C, et al. Concurrent scaphoid fracture with scapholunate ligament rupture. Acta Orthop Belg 2004;70:485–91 [in French].

[18] Trumble T, Verheyden J. Treatment of isolated perilunate and lunate dislocations with combined dorsal and volar approach and intraosseous cerclage wire. J Hand Surg [Am] 2004;29:412–7.

[19] Adkison JW, Chapman MW. Treatment of acute lunate and perilunate dislocations. Clin Orthop 1982;164:199–207.

[20] Green DP, O'Brien ET. Classification and management of carpal dislocations. Clin Orthop 1980;149:55–72.

[21] Gilula LA. Carpal injuries: analytical approach and case exercises. AJR Am J Roentgenol 1979;133:503–17.

[22] Gilula LA, Destouet JM, Weeks PM, et al. Roentgenographic diagnosis of the painful wrist. Clin Orthop 1984;187:52–64.

[23] Cooney WP, Bussey R, Dobyns JH, et al. Difficult wrist fractures: perilunate fracture-dislocations of the wrist. Clin Orthop 1987;214:136–47.

[24] Watson-Jones R. Fractures and joint injuries. 3rd edition. Edinburgh (Scotland): E & S Livingstone; 1943. p. 568–77.

[25] DioGiovanni B, Shaffer J. Treatment of perilunate and transscaphoid perilunate dislocations of the wrist. Am J Orthop 1995;24(11):818–26.

[26] Jasmine MS, Packer JW, Edwards GS. Irreducible trans-scaphoid perilunate dislocation. J Hand Surg [Am] 1988;13:212–5.

[27] Aspergis E, Maris J, Theodoratos G, et al. Perilunate dislocations and fracture-dislocations: closed and early open reduction compared in 28 cases. Acta Orthop Scand 1997;68(Suppl 275):55–9.

[28] Linscheid RL, Dobyns JH, Beaubout HW, et al. Traumatic instability of the wrist. J Bone Joint Surg Am 1972;54:1612–32.

[29] Knoll VD, Allan C, Trumble TE. Trans-scaphoid perilunate fracture dislocations: results of screw fixation of the scaphoid and lunotriquetral repair with a dorsal approach. J Hand Surg [Am] 2005;30:1145–52.

[30] Herzberg G. Acute dorsal trans-scaphoid perilunate dislocations: open reduction and internal fixation. Tech Hand Up Extrem Surg 2000;4:2–13.

[31] Inoue G, Kuwahta Y. Management of acute perilunate dislocations without fracture of the scaphoid. J Hand Surg [Br] 1997;22:647–52.

[32] Inoue G, Imaeda T. Management of trans-scaphoid perilunate dislocations: Herbert screw fixation, ligamentous repair and early wrist mobilization. Arch Orthop Trauma Surg 1997;116:338–40.

[33] Hee HT, Wong HP, Low YP. Transscaphoid perilunate fracture/dislocations—results of surgical treatment. Ann Acad Med Singapore 1999;28:791–4.

[34] Minami A, Kaneda K. Repair and/or reconstruction of scapholunate interosseous ligament in lunate and perilunate dislocations. J Hand Surg [Am] 1993;18:1099–106.

[35] Melone CP Jr, Murphy MS, Raskin KB. Perilunate injuries: repair by dual dorsal and volar approaches. Hand Clin 2000;16:439–48.

[36] Blazar PE, Murray P. Treatment of perilunate dislocations by combined dorsal and palmar approaches. Tech Hand Up Extrem Surg 2001;5:2–7.

[37] Sotreanos DG, Mitsionis GJ, Giannakopoulos PN, et al. Perilunate dislocation and fracture dislocation: a critical analysis of the volar-dorsal approach. J Hand Surg [Am] 1997;22:49–56.

[38] Pourgiezis N, Bain G, Roth J, et al. Volar ulnar approach to the distal radius and carpus. Canadian Journal of Plastic Surgery 1999;7:273–8.

[39] Slade JF III, Jaskwhich D. Percutaneous fixation of scaphoid fractures. Hand Clin 2001;17:553–74.

[40] Slade JF III. Percutaneous treatment of trans-scaphoid trans-capitate fracture dislocations with arthroscopic assistance. Atlas of the Hand Clinics 2003;8:77–94.

[41] Weil WM, Slade JF, Trumble TE. Open and arthroscopic treatment of perilunate injuries. Clin Orthop 2006;445:120–32.

[42] Berger RA, Bishop AT, Bettinger PC. New dorsal capsulotomy for the surgical exposure of the wrist. Ann Plast Surg 1995;35(1):54–9.

[43] Werner FW, Green JK, Short WH, et al. Scaphoid and lunate motion during a wrist dart throw motion. J Hand Surg [Am] 2004;29:418–22.

[44] Herzberg G, Forissier D. Acute dorsal trans-scaphoid perilunate fracture-dislocations: medium-term results. J Hand Surg [Br] 2002;27:498–502.

[45] Inoue G, Shionova K. Late treatment of unreduced perilunate dislocations. J Hand Surg [Br] 1999;24:221–5.

[46] Rettig ME, Raskin KB. Long-term assessment of proximal row carpectomy for chronic perilunate dislocations. J Hand Surg [Am] 1999;24:1231–6.

Traumatic Injuries of the Distal Radioulnar Joint

Jonathan S. Mulford, BMedSc, MBBS, FRACS[a],
Terry S. Axelrod, MD, MSc, FRCS(C)[a,b,*]

[a]Division of Orthopaedic Surgery, Sunnybrook Health Sciences Centre, University of Toronto, MG301,
2075 Bayview Avenue, Toronto, Ontario, Canada M4N 3M5
[b]Department of Surgery, Sunnybrook Health Sciences Centre, University of Toronto,
2075 Bayview Avenue, Ontario, Canada M4N 3M5

Traumatic injuries of the distal radioulnar joint (DRUJ) give rise to wrist pathologies that require special consideration for management. There may be substantial ongoing disability arising from failure to recognize, treat, and rehabilitate individuals with injuries to the DRUJ. These may occur as isolated injuries without associated fractures, but occur more commonly with fractures of the radius. These challenging DRUJ injuries may be simple or complex (irreducible or severe instability). They also may be acute or become a chronic problem. An adequate knowledge of the stabilizers of the DRUJ is essential in understanding treatment options. Traumatic instability of the DRUJ, its anatomy, and its stabilizing factors are reviewed, followed by an algorithm to guide selection of treatment options in complex cases.

The anatomy and stabilizers of the distal radioulnar joint

The DRUJ is stabilized by way of a complex arrangement involving bony congruence and soft tissue constraints.

The gross anatomy of the DRUJ is illustrated in Figs. 1 and 2. The DRUJ consists of a complex articulation between the bony elements of the ulnar head and the sigmoid notch of the distal radius. This articulation is shallow and relies on soft tissue stabilizers to maintain joint integrity. The triangular fibrocartilage complex (TFCC) is the most essential soft tissue stabilizer of the DRUJ.

Bony stabilizers

The ulnar head articulates with the sigmoid notch of the distal radius. The congruence between the two bones provides some stability to the DRUJ [1,2]. The sigmoid notch and the ulnar head have different arcs of curvature. The sigmoid notch arc of curvature is larger and so with forearm rotation, translation also occurs at the DRUJ. There is volar translation of the ulnar head with supination and dorsal translation with pronation.

Soft tissue stabilizers

There are primary and secondary soft tissue stabilizers of the DRUJ. The degree of instability may occur in definable stages, depending on the magnitude of injury to the soft tissue stabilizers of this joint [3].

Primary stabilizer

The TFCC is an essential stabilizer of the DRUJ. It encompasses the sheath of the extensor carpi ulnaris tendon, the ulnocarpal ligaments, the radioulnar ligaments, and the triangular fibrocartilage. The dorsal and volar radioulnar ligaments are the major stabilizers [2,4,5]. The foveal insertion of the TFCC is the most important [6] attachment for stability.

* Corresponding author. Division of Orthopaedic Surgery, Sunnybrook Health Sciences Centre, University of Toronto, MG301, 2075 Bayview Avenue, Toronto, Ontario, Canada M4N 3M5.
E-mail address: Terry.Axelrod@sunnybrook.ca (T.S. Axelrod).

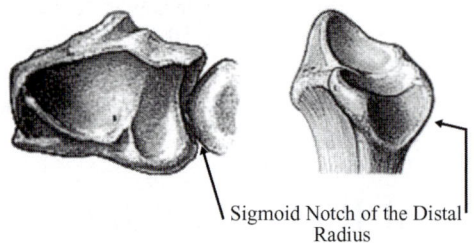

Fig. 1. Bony anatomy of the DRUJ. Note the sigmoid notch of the distal radius and the conical shape of the ulnar head.

Secondary stabilizers

There are static and dynamic stabilizers of the DRUJ [2,7,8]. Static secondary stabilizers include the joint capsule and the interosseous membrane. Dynamic stabilizers include the extensor carpi ulnaris (ECU) and pronator quadratus.

Isolated distal radioulnar joint dislocation

Isolated DRUJ dislocation involves trauma to the joint that is not associated with a fracture of the radius. It is neither a Galeazzi injury nor one with injury to the distal radius articular segments of the DRUJ.

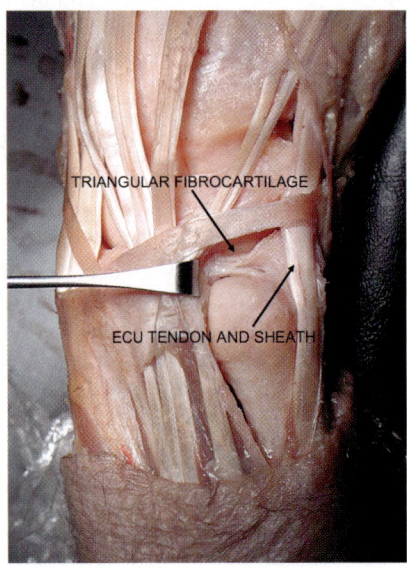

Fig. 2. Soft tissue anatomy of the DRUJ, specifically the TFCC. Note the ulnar sheath of the extensor carpi ulnaris tendon, the ulnocarpal and radiocarpal ligaments, and the triangular fibrocartilage itself. (*Courtesy of* Amit Gupta, MD, and Makoto Tamai, MD, Louisville, KY.)

Typically, these injuries are traumatic dislocations of the distal ulnar, either dorsal or volar. Soft tissue injuries, including TFCC injuries, causing instability are included in this group.

Volar

Isolated volar dislocation of the DRUJ is uncommon. Typically, the mechanism of injury is the classic fall on the outstretched arm, usually with a rotational supination force to the impact. The physical examination is notable for the absence of the typical dorsal prominence of the ulnar head and the lack of forearm rotation. Radiographs illustrate an overlap of the distal ulnar to the distal radius on the posteroanterior (PA) film (Fig. 3).

A review of the literature identified 23 cases of isolated volar DRUJ dislocation since 1960 [9]. Fifteen of the 23 cases were misdiagnosed initially. If the injury was diagnosed acutely, most (9 of 11) were reduced successfully by closed reduction. Only 1 out of 12 chronic cases was treated successfully with closed reduction. Reasons to account for the irreducible dislocations included block from the TFCC [10] or the pronator quadratus [11], interposition of the extensor tendons and extensor retinaculum [12], and impaction ulnar head fracture resulting in locking on the sigmoid notch [9].

Only one chronic dislocation was treated successfully with closed reduction [13]. Most required salvage surgery (five Darrach procedures [14], three Suave Kapanji procedures [12], and one hemiresection of the ulnar head [13]). It has been suggested that a forceful closed reduction should be attempted in a chronic dislocation. This may lead to fracture if there is locked dislocation. The authors advocate the use of a CT scan of the DRUJ to exclude any impacted fracture before any attempt at a closed reduction (Fig. 4). If there is a locked dislocation with bony impaction, the authors advise open reduction of the dislocation.

Dorsal

Dorsal dislocation is more common than volar dislocation of the DRUJ. Dorsal dislocations also occur with a similar mechanism to the volar dislocation as described above. The rotational moment usually is in pronation. The physical examination usually indicates excessive prominence of the ulnar head and the similar lack of forearm rotation.

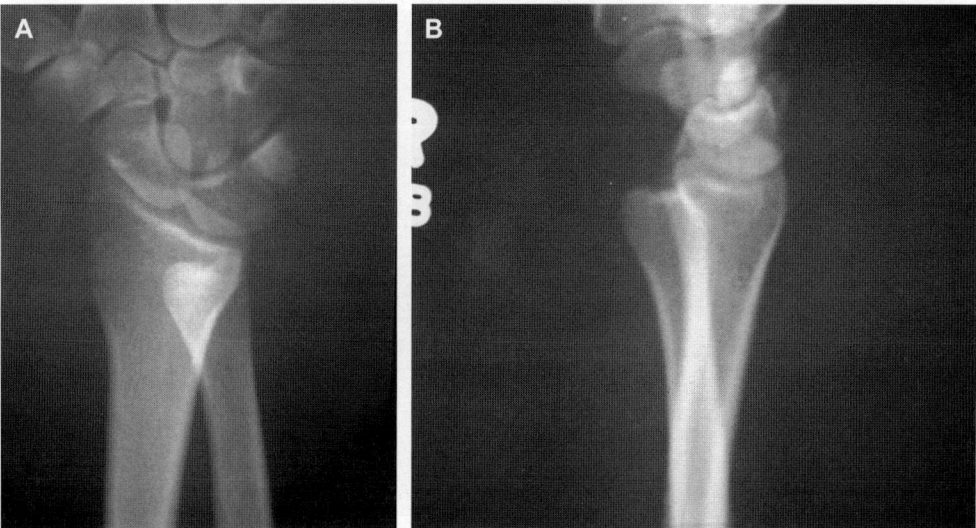

Fig. 3. PA (*A*) and lateral (*B*) radiographs of an acute DRUJ dislocation. There is overlap of the ulnar head with the distal radius, whereas a normal joint space should be seen. Note the volar position of the ulnar head on the lateral projection.

Radiographs show findings similar to those for volar dislocations, except that the ulnar head is displaced in the dorsal direction on the lateral projection.

Usually, closed reduction is successful using digital pressure over the ulnar head and supination. The dislocation may be complicated by irreducibility or ongoing instability (complex dislocation). In these cases, the patient can be managed as described below for patients with combined injuries. Underlying factors that may block reduction are similar to those described above for isolated volar dislocation.

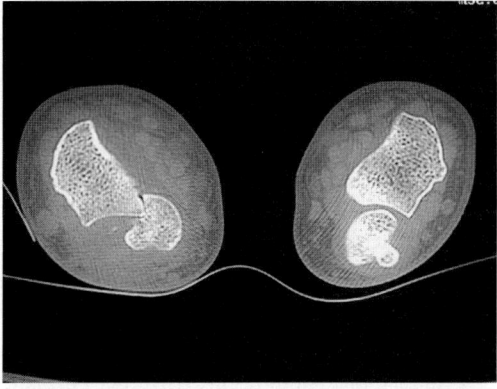

Fig. 4. CT axial cut of a locked volar dislocation of the DRUJ, comparison with the normal contralateral wrist is provided.

Combined injury with fractured radius

Combined injuries include Galeazzi injuries or distal radial fractures with DRUJ injury.

A Galeazzi injury is characterized by a displaced distal radius fracture with a dislocation of the DRUJ. Usually, the diagnosis is straightforward, owing to the often dramatic appearance of the disruption of the DRUJ with the displaced radius (Fig. 5). Typically, the dislocation is dorsal, but it can occur in any direction depending on the displacement of the distal segment of the radius.

Frequently, fractures of the distal radius associated with displacement result in an injury to the ulnar side of the wrist. This may involve the ulnar shaft, neck, or head fracture. More typically, there is some disruption of the soft tissue supporting structures of the DRUJ, resulting in varying degrees of instability, subluxation, or dislocation.

Traditionally, DRUJ instability was believed to occur rarely in combined injuries [15–17]. Sixty percent [15] of patients with a distal radius fracture have an ulnar styloid fracture, but most do not have instability. Recent outcome reviews found that ulnar-sided wrist problems occur in 3% to 37% of distal radial fractures [18–23] and often are due to DRUJ instability. A large-sized ulnar styloid fragment (type II fractures [19]) with displacement is more likely to result in DRUJ instability [19,21,24]. Many patients with a distal radius fracture have accompanying

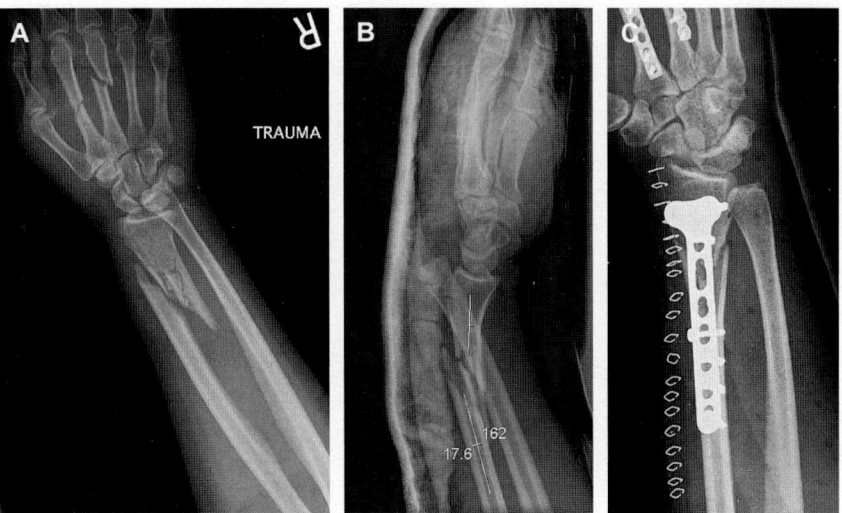

Fig. 5. Galeazzi fracture-dislocation of the wrist. Preoperative initial radiographs reveal the gross displacement of the radius fracture with the dislocation of the distal radioulnar joint. Preoperative initial lateral radiograph with dorsal dislocation of the ulnar head. Postoperative radiographs indicate anatomic reduction of the radius and the DRUJ.

TFCC tears; however, they are likely to remain asymptomatic if the joint is stable [25]. Reduced outcome scores have been well documented in radial fractures complicated by instability [23,26–28]. If the clinician has an awareness of the possibility of these associated DRUJ injuries, clinical and radiological testing can be directed toward recognizing and effectively treating these injuries and improving their outcome.

The instability of the DRUJ in association with radial fractures can be addressed acutely or chronically.

Acute injury

Early treatment of acute injury gives rise to better results than does surgical management of chronic instability [18,21,29]. An algorithm is described for the management of acute DRUJ instability (Fig. 6) associated with radial fracture. This is based on a series of difficult cases [30] that was managed by the senior author and a review of the literature.

The risk for DRUJ instability can be assessed according to the mechanism of injury (eg, high-energy trauma with rotational component) and initial radiographs. Radiological indicators of potential DRUJ instability include (1) an ulnar styloid fracture involving the base with more than 2 mm displacement [18,21,31], (2) an irreducible dislocation of the DRUJ, (3) fractures involving the sigmoid notch of the radius, (4) a wide displacement of the DRUJ, and (5) radial shortening.

In the operating room, the initial goal is anatomic reduction of the radius. Following reduction of the radius, the DRUJ can be assessed for stability in different positions of forearm rotation using the piano key sign [32]. The presence of this sign can be subtle and comparison to the contralateral DRUJ may be required. If the joint is stable, no further operative intervention is required, whereas any ongoing instability must be addressed.

If instability is detected, the quality of the radius fracture reduction should be reassessed to ensure restoration of the anatomy. If the reduction in nonanatomic, it must be revised, and the status of the DRUJ must be reevaluated.

Instability that occurs in some positions of forearm rotation may be considered for casting in a position of stability. Typically, dorsal dislocations are stable in supination, whereas the unusual volar dislocations are stable in pronation. The limb can be immobilized in the stable position with an above-elbow splint or brace for a period of 4 to 6 weeks until the soft tissue structures stabilize.

Complex instability occurs when the DRUJ is irreducible or unstable in all positions. Fig. 7 illustrates the typical pathology noted with a complex injury of the DRUJ.

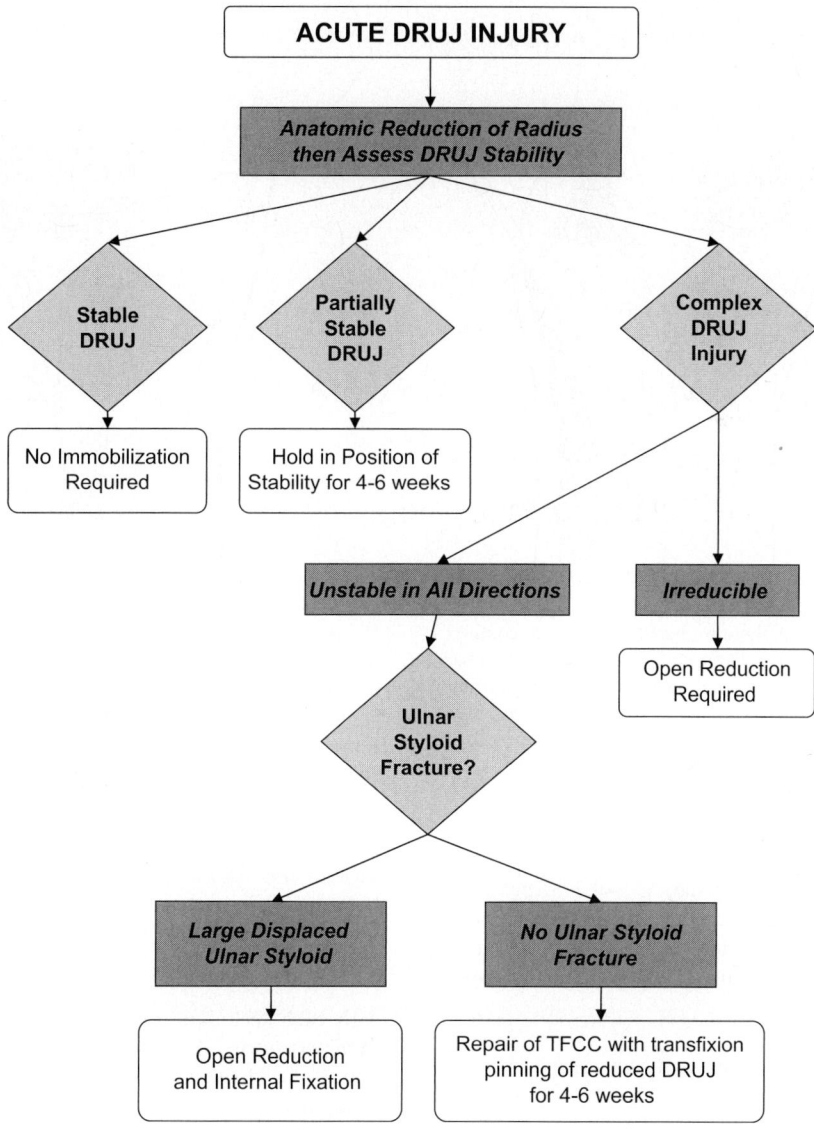

Fig. 6. Algorithm for the management of acute injuries of the DRUJ.

Irreducible distal radioulnar joint

An irreducible DRUJ has a block to reduction. This is characterized by soft tissue, or less often, bone interposition within the joint. Complete joint reduction may be blocked by (1) the ulnar head incarceration through a rent in the capsule of the DRUJ, (2) tendons, such as the ECU or flexor carpi ulnaris, (3) a bone fragment from the ulnar or sigmoid notch of the radius.

If the joint cannot be reduced, an arthrotomy is performed, and the offending obstacle to reduction is removed. The approach is dictated by the pattern of displacement of the dislocation. Often, the simplest approach is to expose the DRUJ by way of the ECU subsheath. This involves mobilizing the ECU with a dorsal ulnar linear incision. The skin incision is made, and the dorsal sensory branch of the ulnar nerve is identified and protected. The ECU tendon is retracted, and the subsheath is incised longitudinally. This brings the surgeon directly onto the ulnar styloid. This exposure allows reconstruction of the TFCC and the ulnar styloid, should it be indicated (Fig. 8). If the ulnar head is trapped

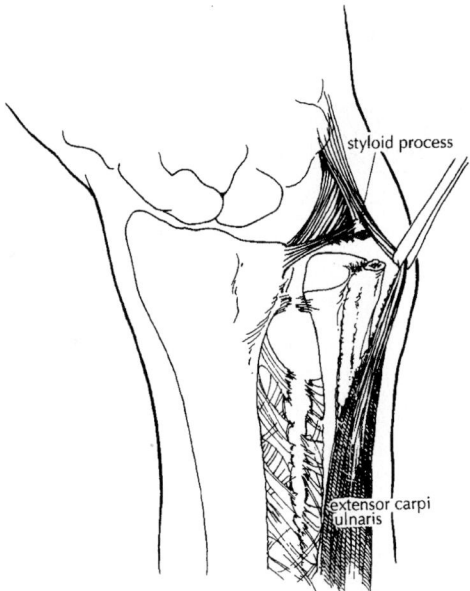

Fig. 7. Typical pathology associated with a complex dislocation, showing disruption of the distal radioulnar joint ligaments, a portion of the interosseous membrane, the floor of the ECU tendon sheath, and an avulsion fracture of the ulnar styloid process. (*From* Cheng SL, Axelrod TS. Management of complex dislocations of the distal radioulnar joint. Clin Orthop Relat Res 1997;341:186; with permission.)

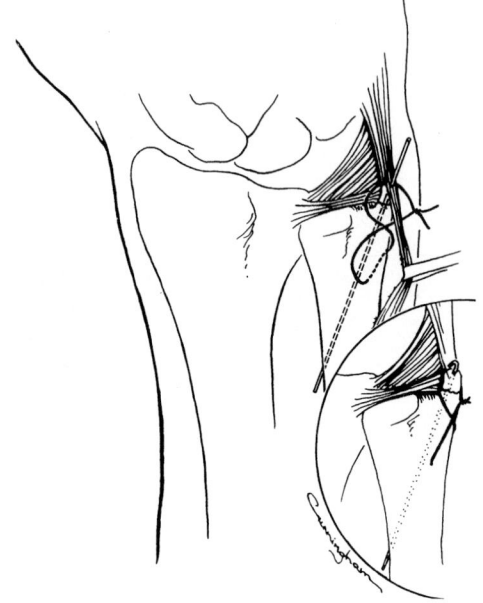

Fig. 8. The technique of tension band wire fixation of the ulnar styloid process. A 1.6-mm K-wire is used to fix the styloid process to the ulnar shaft, and a 22-gauge wire is passed around the ulnar collateral ligament complex and the ulnar styloid. It is then passed through a drill hole in the ulnar shaft and tied in a figure-of-eight fashion. The inset shows completed fixation with the K-wire bent over and cut short to prevent irritation of the adjacent soft tissues. (*From* Cheng SL, Axelrod TS. Management of complex dislocations of the distal radioulnar joint. Clin Orthop Relat Res 1997;341:187; with permission.)

within the volar capsule, a volar exposure—between the long flexors and the ulnar neurovascular structures—allows adequate visualization of the joint and capsule to perform an open reduction.

Reducible but unstable distal radioulnar joint

Usually, instability in all positions is associated with a large, displaced ulnar styloid fracture and is managed by way of internal fixation. Often, this also addresses the stability of the DRUJ because the TFCC is attached to the fragment (see Fig. 8) [24,33].

If the ulnar is not fractured, the TFCC is likely to have a peripheral tear. Closed treatment of an unstable DRUJ results in a high incidence of recurrent subluxation or dislocation and residual pain [34]. Surgical options in this situation include reduction of the DRUJ with ulno-radial transfixion pins [35–38], repair of the TFCC (open [18], mini-open [39], or arthroscopically [40–46]), or an external fixateur of the radius with an outrigger to the ulnar [47]. There are few studies to guide which of these techniques has the best outcome, with each technique having reported success in small case series. The authors favor mini-open repair of the TFCC with short-term transfixion pins in supination. The suture repair of the TFCC with a grossly unstable DRUJ dislocation is not strong enough with current techniques to hold the reduction until healing is complete. Transfixion pinning gives initial protection to the repair.

Chronic instability following fracture of the distal radius

Chronic instability of the DRUJ can undergo a trial of nonoperative management, including bracing [48]. These cases can have other causes of ulnar-sided wrist pain that may mimic or coexist with DRUJ instability. These include DRUJ arthritis, ECU tendonitis, ulnar abutment, central TFCC tear, and ulnar carpal instability. These

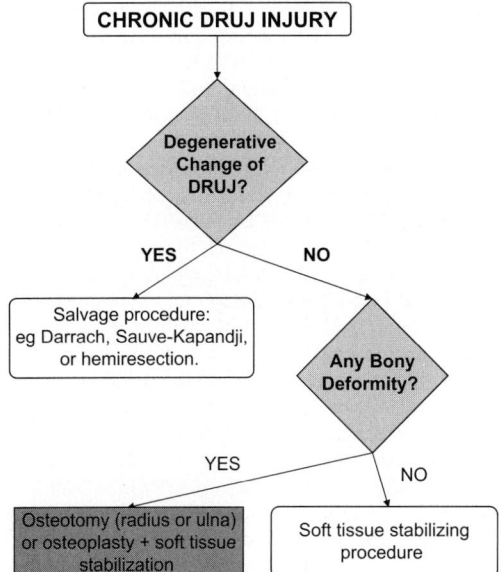

Fig. 9. Algorithm for the management of chronic post-trauma instability of the DRUJ.

conditions should be considered in the clinical and radiological assessment.

If nonoperative treatment is unsuccessful, the goals of surgical treatment are to restore stability and obtain a functional painless arc of forearm rotation. To achieve this, one must identify any bony deformity or ligament injuries. An algorithm is described for the management of chronic DRUJ instability (Fig. 9).

Bony abnormalities causing instability include radial or ulnar malunion or loss of the curve of the radius on the sigmoid notch. Osteotomies of the radius [49,50] or ulnar [51] or an osteoplasty of the sigmoid notch [52] can improve stability in these situations.

Once the bony anatomy is restored, the soft tissue can be addressed. Late repair of the TFCC complex can be considered [53], although attenuated tissues may preclude primary repair. Reconstructive procedures can be used if there is no DRUJ arthritis and the sigmoid notch is competent. Possible reconstructions include indirect radioulnar link by way of an ulnar carpal sling or tenodesis [54–57] or reconstruction of the distal radioulnar ligaments [58,59]. These techniques were reported to give improvement in small series. Cadaveric studies, however, showed that tenodesis procedures do not restore DRUJ mechanics [60], whereas intra-articular reconstructive procedures restore stability without limitations on forearm rotation [61].

Finally, if repair or reconstructive procedures are unsuccessful or not indicated (eg, DRUJ degenerative changes), salvage surgery can be considered. These include Darrach [62], Sauve-Kapandji [63], ulnar head arthroplasty, and hemiresection [64] procedures.

Summary

A knowledge and awareness of the stabilizing factors of the DRUJ are important in managing DRUJ instability. An algorithm for management options presented here allows the clinician to make sound clinical decisions for the management of complex instability of the DRUJ in trauma.

References

[1] Cole DW, Elsaidi GA, Kuzma KR, et al. Distal radioulnar joint instability in distal radius fractures: the role of sigmoid notch and triangular fibrocartilage complex revisited. Injury 2006;37:252–8.

[2] Garcia-Elias M. Soft-tissue anatomy and relationships about the distal ulna. Hand Clin 1998;14:165–76.

[3] Moore TM, Lester DK, Sarmiento A. The stabilizing effect of soft-tissue constraints in artificial Galeazzi fractures. Clin Orthop Relat Res 1985;194:189–94.

[4] Palmer AK, Werner FW. The triangular fibrocartilage complex of the wrist–anatomy and function. J Hand Surg [Am] 1981;6:153–62.

[5] Ward LD, Ambrose CG, Masson MV, et al. The role of the distal radioulnar ligaments, interosseous membrane, and joint capsule in distal radioulnar joint stability. J Hand Surg [Am] 2000;25:341–51.

[6] Haugstvedt JR, Berger RA, Nakamura T, et al. Relative contributions of the ulnar attachments of the triangular fibrocartilage complex to the dynamic stability of the distal radioulnar joint. J Hand Surg [Am] 2006;31:445–51.

[7] Gofton WT, Gordon KD, Dunning CE, et al. Soft-tissue stabilizers of the distal radioulnar joint: an in vitro kinematic study. J Hand Surg [Am] 2004;29:423–31.

[8] Johnson RK, Shrewsbury MM. The pronator quadratus in motions and in stabilization of the radius and ulna at the distal radioulnar joint. J Hand Surg [Am] 1976;1:205–9.

[9] Mulford JS, Jansen S, Axelrod TS. A review of isolated volar distal radioulnar joint dislocation and case report. Submitted to Journal of Orthopaedic Trauma under review. References available from authors on request. 2007.

[10] Dameron TB Jr. Traumatic dislocation of the distal radio-ulnar joint. Clin Orthop Relat Res 1972;83:55–63.

[11] Kikuchi Y, Nakamura T. Irreducible Galeazzi fracture-dislocation due to an avulsion fracture of the fovea of the ulna. J Hand Surg [Br] 1999;24:379–81.

[12] Kikuchi Y, Nakamura T, Horiuchi Y. Irreducible chronic palmar dislocation of the distal radioulnar joint–a case report. Hand Surg 2005;10:319–22.

[13] Schiller MG, af Ekenstam F, Kirsch PT. Volar dislocation of the distal radio-ulnar joint. A case report. J Bone Joint Surg Am 1991;73:617–9.

[14] Saito J, Sakai A, Okimoto N, et al. [Three cases of chronic volar dislocation of the distal radioulnar joint that were treated with the Sauve-Kapandji procedure]. J Uoeh 2003;25:249–57.

[15] Frykman G. Fracture of the distal radius including sequelae–shoulder-hand-finger syndrome, disturbance in the distal radio-ulnar joint and impairment of nerve function. A clinical and experimental study. Acta Orthop Scand 1967;(Suppl 108):3+.

[16] Solgaard S. Function after distal radius fracture. Acta Orthop Scand 1988;59:39–42.

[17] Stewart HD, Innes AR, Burke FD. Factors affecting the outcome of Colles' fracture: an anatomical and functional study. Injury 1985;16:289–95.

[18] Geissler WB, Fernandez DL, Lamey DM. Distal radioulnar joint injuries associated with fractures of the distal radius. Clin Orthop Relat Res 1996;327:135–46.

[19] Hauck RM, Skahen J 3rd, Palmer AK. Classification and treatment of ulnar styloid nonunion. J Hand Surg [Am] 1996;21:418–22.

[20] Lindau T, Adlercreutz C, Aspenberg P. Peripheral tears of the triangular fibrocartilage complex cause distal radioulnar joint instability after distal radial fractures. J Hand Surg [Am] 2000;25:464–8.

[21] May MM, Lawton JN, Blazar PE. Ulnar styloid fractures associated with distal radius fractures: incidence and implications for distal radioulnar joint instability. J Hand Surg [Am] 2002;27:965–71.

[22] Oskarsson GV, Aaser P, Hjall A. Do we underestimate the predictive value of the ulnar styloid affection in Colles fractures? Arch Orthop Trauma Surg 1997;116:341–4.

[23] Stoffelen D, De Smet L, Broos P. The importance of the distal radioulnar joint in distal radial fractures. J Hand Surg [Br] 1998;23:507–11.

[24] Mikic ZD. Treatment of acute injuries of the triangular fibrocartilage complex associated with distal radioulnar joint instability. J Hand Surg [Am] 1995;20:319–23.

[25] af Ekenstam F, Jakobsson OP, Wadin K. Repair of the triangular ligament in Colles' fracture. No effect in a prospective randomized study. Acta Orthop Scand 1989;60:393–6.

[26] Lindau T. Treatment of injuries to the ulnar side of the wrist occurring with distal radial fractures. Hand Clin 2005;21:417–25.

[27] Melone CP Jr, Nathan R. Traumatic disruption of the triangular fibrocartilage complex. Pathoanatomy. Clin Orthop Relat Res 1992;65–73.

[28] Morrissy RT, Nalebuff EA. Dislocation of the distal radioulnar joint: anatomy and clues to prompt diagnosis. Clin Orthop Relat Res 1979;154–8.

[29] Fernandez DL. Fractures of the distal radius: operative treatment. Instr Course Lect 1993;42:73–88.

[30] Cheng SL, Axelrod TS. Management of complex dislocations of the distal radioulnar joint. Clin Orthop Relat Res 1997;341:183–91.

[31] Bruckner JD, Alexander AH, Lichtman DM. Acute dislocations of the distal radioulnar joint. Instr Course Lect 1996;45:27–36.

[32] Darrow JC Jr, Linscheid RL, Dobyns JH, et al. Distal ulnar recession for disorders of the distal radioulnar joint. J Hand Surg [Am] 1985;10:482–91.

[33] Shaw JA, Bruno A, Paul EM. Ulnar styloid fixation in the treatment of posttraumatic instability of the radioulnar joint: a biomechanical study with clinical correlation. J Hand Surg [Am] 1990;15:712–20.

[34] Strehle J, Gerber C. Distal radioulnar joint function after Galeazzi fracture-dislocations treated by open reduction and internal plate fixation. Clin Orthop Relat Res 1993;240–5.

[35] Bhan S, Rath S. Management of the Galeazzi fracture. Int Orthop 1991;15:193–6.

[36] Macule Beneyto F, Arandes Renu JM, Ferreres Claramunt A, et al. Treatment of Galeazzi fracture-dislocations. J Trauma 1994;36:352–5.

[37] Mikic ZD. Galeazzi fracture-dislocations. J Bone Joint Surg Am 1975;57:1071–80.

[38] Moore TM, Klein JP, Patzakis MJ, et al. Results of compression-plating of closed Galeazzi fractures. J Bone Joint Surg Am 1985;67:1015–21.

[39] Chou KH, Sarris IK, Sotereanos DG. Suture anchor repair of ulnar-sided triangular fibrocartilage complex tears. J Hand Surg [Br] 2003;28:546–50.

[40] Chen AC, Hsu KY, Chang CH, et al. Arthroscopic suture repair of peripheral tears of triangular fibrocartilage complex using a volar portal. Arthroscopy 2005;21:1406.

[41] de Araujo W, Poehling GG, Kuzma GR. New Tuohy needle technique for triangular fibrocartilage complex repair: preliminary studies. Arthroscopy 1996;12:699–703.

[42] Fellinger M, Peicha G, Seibert FJ, et al. Radial avulsion of the triangular fibrocartilage complex in acute wrist trauma: a new technique for arthroscopic repair. Arthroscopy 1997;13:370–4.

[43] Haugstvedt JR, Husby T. Results of repair of peripheral tears in the triangular fibrocartilage complex using an arthroscopic suture technique. Scand J Plast Reconstr Surg Hand Surg 1999;33:439–47.

[44] Ruch DS, Papadonikolakis A. Arthroscopically assisted repair of peripheral triangular fibrocartilage complex tears: factors affecting outcome. Arthroscopy 2005;21:1126–30.

[45] Skie MC, Mekhail AO, Deitrich DR, et al. Operative technique for inside-out repair of the triangular fibrocartilage complex. J Hand Surg [Am] 1997;22:814–7.

[46] Zachee B, De Smet L, Fabry G. Arthroscopic suturing of TFCC lesions. Arthroscopy 1993;9: 242–3.
[47] Ruch DS, Lumsden BC, Papadonikolakis A. Distal radius fractures: a comparison of tension band wiring versus ulnar outrigger external fixation for the management of distal radioulnar instability. J Hand Surg [Am] 2005;30:969–77.
[48] Millard GM, Budoff JE, Paravic V, et al. Functional bracing for distal radioulnar joint instability. J Hand Surg [Am] 2002;27:972–7.
[49] Adams BD. Effects of radial deformity on distal radioulnar joint mechanics. J Hand Surg [Am] 1993;18:492–8.
[50] Kihara H, Palmer AK, Werner FW, et al. The effect of dorsally angulated distal radius fractures on distal radioulnar joint congruency and forearm rotation. J Hand Surg [Am] 1996;21:40–7.
[51] Chidgey LK. Treatment of acute and chronic instability of the distal radio-ulnar joint. Hand Clin 1998; 14:297–303.
[52] Wallwork NA, Bain GI. Sigmoid notch osteoplasty for chronic volar instability of the distal radioulnar joint: a case report. J Hand Surg [Am] 2001;26: 454–9.
[53] Hermansdorfer JD, Kleinman WB. Management of chronic peripheral tears of the triangular fibrocartilage complex. J Hand Surg [Am] 1991;16: 340–6.
[54] Breen TF, Jupiter JB. Extensor carpi ulnaris and flexor carpi ulnaris tenodesis of the unstable distal ulna. J Hand Surg [Am] 1989;14:612–7.
[55] Fulkerson JP, Watson HK. Congenital anterior subluxation of the distal ulna. A case report. Clin Orthop Relat Res 1978;131:179–82.

[56] Hui FC, Linscheid RL. Ulnotriquetral augmentation tenodesis: a reconstructive procedure for dorsal subluxation of the distal radioulnar joint. J Hand Surg [Am] 1982;7:230–6.
[57] Tsai TM, Stilwell JH. Repair of chronic subluxation of the distal radioulnar joint (ulnar dorsal) using flexor carpi ulnaris tendon. J Hand Surg [Br] 1984; 9:289–94.
[58] Adams BD, Berger RA. An anatomic reconstruction of the distal radioulnar ligaments for posttraumatic distal radioulnar joint instability. J Hand Surg [Am] 2002;27:243–51.
[59] Scheker LR, Belliappa PP, Acosta R, et al. Reconstruction of the dorsal ligament of the triangular fibrocartilage complex. J Hand Surg [Br] 1994;19: 310–8.
[60] Petersen MS, Adams BD. Biomechanical evaluation of distal radioulnar reconstructions. J Hand Surg [Am] 1993;18:328–34.
[61] Martineau PA, Bergeron S, Beckman L, et al. Reconstructive procedure for unstable radial-sided triangular fibrocartilage complex avulsions. J Hand Surg [Am] 2005;30:727–32.
[62] Gaebler C, McQueen MM. Ulnar procedures for post-traumatic disorders of the distal radioulnar joint. Injury 2003;34:47–59.
[63] Lamey DM, Fernandez DL. Results of the modified Sauve-Kapandji procedure in the treatment of chronic posttraumatic derangement of the distal radioulnar joint. J Bone Joint Surg Am 1998;80: 1758–69.
[64] Imbriglia JE, Matthews D. Treatment of chronic post-traumatic dorsal subluxation of the distal ulna by hemiresection-interposition arthroplasty. J Hand Surg [Am] 1993;18:899–907.

Index

Note: Page numbers of article titles are in **boldface** type.

A

Acute scaphoid fractures, **229–235**
  causes of, 229
  classification of, 231
  diagnosis of, 229–231
  treatment of, 231–233
    authors' preferred approach in, 232
    scaphoid nonunions after, 232–233

Arthrography, in scapholunate instability diagnosis, 266

Arthroscopic debridement, for scapholunate instability, 269

Arthroscopy, in scapholunate instability diagnosis, 266–267

Arthrosis, distal radius fractures and, 223

Association for the Study of Internal Fixation, 169

B

Body fractures, 253

Bone fractures, carpal, **251–260**. See also *Carpal bone fractures.*

Bone graft(s), for post-traumatic malunion of distal radius fractures, 212

Bone scintigraphy, in scapholunate instability diagnosis, 266

Bone–retinaculum–bone/bone ligament–bone, for scapholunate instability, 271

C

Capitate fractures, 255–256

Capitolunate instability, provocative tests of, 163–164

Capsulodesis, dorsal, for scapholunate instability, 270–271

Carpal bone fractures, **251–260**
  body fractures, 253
  capitate fractures, 255–256
  hamate fractures, 251–253
  hook fractures, 251–253
  lunate fractures, 256
  pisiform fractures, 255
  prevalence of, 251
  trapezium fractures, 256–258
  trapezoid fractures, 258
  triquetral fractures, 253–255

Carpal fusion, limited, for scapholunate instability, 272–273

Carpal instability, provocative tests of, 160–164
  capitolunate instability, 163–164
  lunotriquestral instability, 161–162
  midcarpal instability, 162–163
  radiocarpal instability, 162
  scapholunate instability, 160–161

Carpectomy, proximal row, for scapholunate instability, 273

Carpometacarpal (CMC) joints, physical examination of, 157

Cast issues, distal radius fractures and, 219

Casting, for scapholunate instability, 269

Closed reduction, Kirschner wire fixation and, for scapholunate instability, 269

CMC joints. See *Carpometacarpal (CMC) joints.*

Compartment syndrome, distal radius fractures and, 218–219

Complex regional pain syndrome (CRPS), distal radius fractures and, 223

CRPS. See *Complex regional pain syndrome (CRPS).*

D

de Quervain's tenosynovitis, physical examination of, 154

Differential lidocaine injection, in physical examination of wrist, 164

Distal radioulnar joint (DRUJ)
  anatomy of, 289, 290
  dislocation of, isolated, 290–291
  physical examination of, 159
  stabilizers of, 289–290
  traumatic injuries of, **289–297**
    chronic instability following fracture of distal radius, 294–295
    combined injury with fractured radius, 291–294
    isolated DRUJ dislocation, 290–291

Distal radius fractures
  chronic instability of DRUJ after, 294–295
  classification of, 167–169
  complications of, **217–228**
    arthrosis, 223
    cast issues, 219
    compartment syndrome, 218–219
    CRPS, 223
    infection, 219–221
    loss of reduction, 219
    malunion, 224–226
    missed associated injury, 219
    nerve injuries, 217
    nerve-related, 223
    neurologic, 221–222
    nonunion/delayed union, 223–224
    open injuries, 218
    skin injury during manipulation, 218
    tendon rupture, 222
    tendon-related, 226
  post-traumatic malunion of, management of, **203–216**
    bone graft alternatives in, 212
    computer-assisted techniques in, 209–211
    evolving trends in, 209–212
    extra-articular malunion, 203–108
      anatomy of, 203
      disorders of distal radioulnar joint associated with distal radius malunion, 206–208
      goals of, 205
      indications for, 205
      kinematics of, 203–205
      surgical techniques, 205–206
    intra-articular malunion, 208–209
    volar fixed-angle plate osteosynthesis, 211–212
  traumatic injuries of DRUJ with, 291–294
  treatment of, **167–173**
    classification of, 167–169
    external fixation in, **187–192**
      algorithm for, 188
      case example, 190
      discussion of, 192
      operative technique, 188–190
      patient evaluation in, 187–188
      postoperative care, 190–191
      results of, 191–192
    nonoperative, **175–180**
      complications of, 179
      follow-up and aftercare, 177
      indications for, 175–176
      outcomes of, 179–180
      reduction techniques, 176–177
      successful, predicting of, 177–179
    percutaneous pinning options in, **180–182**
    plating in, **193–201**
      discussion of, 193
      techniques, 193–200
        fragment-specific fixation, 195–196
        locking vs. nonlocking plates, 196–197
        special plates, 197–199
        titanium vs. stainless plates, 199–200
        volar plates vs. dorsal plates, 193–195
    surgical
      associated injuries and, 171
      fracture pattern and, 169–170
      fracture stability and, 170–171
      indications for, 169–171
      patient factors in, 169

Dorsal capsulodesis, for scapholunate instability, 270–271

Dorsal wrist, physical examination of, 157

DRUJ. See *Distal radioulnar joint (DRUJ)*.

E

Electrothermal collagen shrinkage, for scapholunate instability, 269–270

External fixation, of distal radius fractures, **187–192**. See also *Distal radius fractures, treatment of, external fixation in.*

F

Fifth extensor compartment, physical examination of, 157

First CMC joint, physical examination of, 155

First dorsal compartment, of wrist, physical examination of, 153–154

Flexor carpi radialis, physical examination of, 152–153

Fourth extensor compartment, physical examination of, 157

Fracture(s)
  acute scaphoid, **229–235.** See also *Acute scaphoid fractures.*
  body, 253
  bone, carpal, **251–260**
  capitate, 255–256
  carpal bone, **251–260.** See also *Carpal bone fractures.*
  distal radius, **167–173.** See also *Distal radius fractures.*
  hamate, 251–253
  hook, 251–253
  lunate, 256
  pisiform, 255
  trapezium, 256–258
  trapezoid, 258
  triquetral, 253–255

H

Hamate fractures, 251–253

Hook fractures, 251–253

I

Immobilization, for scapholunate instability, 269

Infection(s), distal radius fractures and, 219–221

Instability
  capitolunate, provocative tests of, 163–164
  carpal, provocative tests of, 160–164. See also *Carpal instability, provocative tests of.*
  lunotriquetral, provocative tests of, 161–162
  midcarpal, provocative tests of, 162–163
  radiocarpal, provocative tests of, 162
  scapholunate, **261–277.** See also *Scapholunate instability.*

Intersection syndrome, physical examination in, 154

J

Joint(s). See also specific types, e.g., *Scaphotrapezial joint.*

K

Kirschner wire fixation, closed reduction and, for scapholunate instability, 269

L

Lidocaine injection, differential, in physical examination of wrist, 164

Lunate fractures, 256

Lunotriquetral instability, provocative tests of, 161–162

M

Magnetic resonance imaging (MRI), in scapholunate instability diagnosis, 266

Malunion
  distal radius fractures and, 224–226
  post-traumatic, of fractures of distal radius, management of, **203–216.** See also *Distal radius fractures, post-traumatic malunion of, management of.*

Midcarpal instability, provocative tests of, 162–163

Missed associated injury, distal radius fractures and, 219

MRI. See *Magnetic resonance imaging (MRI).*

N

Nerve(s), distal radius fractures effects on, 223

Nerve injuries, distal radius fractures and, 217

Nonunion(s), scaphoid, management of, **237–249.** See also *Scaphoid nonunions, management of.*

Nonunion/delayed union, distal radius fractures and, 223–224

O

Open injuries, distal radius fractures and, 218

Open reduction, internal fixation with repair of ligaments and, for scapholunate instability, 270

Osteology, of wrist, 127–128

P

Palmar scaphoid, physical examination of, 150–152

Palmar ulnar structures, physical examination of, 159–160

Palmar wrist, physical examination of, 160

Percutaneous pinning, in distal radius fracture management, **180–182**

Perilunate injuries, **279–288**
  anatomy in, 279–280
  classification of, 281
  diagnosis of, 280–282
    missed, 287
  management of
    initial, 281–283
    operative, 283–285
    postoperative, 285
    results of, 285–287
  pathomechanics of, 280

Pisiform fractures, 255

Plating, for distal radius fractures, **193–201.** See also *Distal radius fractures, treatment of, plating in.*

Post-traumatic malunion, of fractures of distal radius, management of, **203–216.** See also *Distal radius fractures, post-traumatic malunion of, management of.*

Proximal row carpectomy, for scapholunate instability, 273

R

Radial artery, physical examination of, 153

Radial nerve, superficial branch of, physical examination of, 154

Radial wrist, physical examination of, 150–157. See also *Wrist, radial, physical examination of.*

Radiocarpal instability, provocative tests of, 162

Radiography, in scapholunate instability diagnosis, 264–266

Radius, distal, fractures of. See *Distal radius fractures.*

Range of motion, in wrist examination, 149

Reduction, loss of, distal radius fractures and, 219

S

Scaphoid
  fractures of, acute, **229–235.** See also *Acute scaphoid fractures.*
  nonunion of, after acute scaphoid fracture management, 232–233
  palmar, physical examination of, 150–152
  radial approach to, 140–144
  volar approach to, 135–137

Scaphoid excision with four-corner fusion (SLAC procedure), for scapholunate instability, 273

Scaphoid nonunions, management of, **237–249**
  approach to, 237–238
  complications of, 247–248
  dorsal approach in, 241–243
  dorsal-radial approach with vascularized graft in, 243–245
  palmar approach in, 238–241
  volar-radial approach with vascularized graft in, 245–246

Scapholunate dissociation, natural history of, 268

Scapholunate instability, **261–277**
  clinical stages of, 267–268
  diagnosis of, 263–267
    arthrography in, 266
    arthroscopy in, 266–267
    bone scintigraphy in, 266
    MRI in, 266
    radiographic examination in, 264–266
  history of, 261
  mechanism of, 263
  pathophysiology of, 261–263
  provocative tests of, 160–161
  treatment of, 268–273
    arthroscopic debridement in, 269
    bone–retinaculum–bone/bone ligament–bone in, 271
    casting/immobilization in, 269
    closed reduction and Kirschner wire fixation in, 269
    dorsal capsulodesis in, 270–271
    electrothermal collagen shrinkage in, 269–270
    limited carpal fusion in, 272–273
    open reduction, internal fixation with repair of ligaments in, 270
    proximal row carpectomy in, 273
    reduction and association of scaphoid and lunate in, 272
    SLAC procedure in, 273
    tenodesis in, 271–272

Scapholunate interval, physical examination of, 157

Scaphotrapezial joint, physical examination of, 153

Scintigraphy, bone, in scapholunate instability diagnosis, 266

Skin injury during manipulation, distal radius fractures and, 218

SLAC procedure, for scapholunate instability, 273

Snuffbox, physical examination of, 155–157

Stabilizer(s), of distal radioulnar joint, 289–290

T

Tendon(s)
    distal radius fractures effects on, 226
    rupture of, distal radius fractures and, 222

Tenodesis, for scapholunate instability, 271–272

Tenosynovitis, de Quervain's, physical examination of, 154

Trapezium fractures, 256–258

Trapezoid fractures, 258

Traumatic injuries, of distal radioulnar joint, **289–297**. See also *Distal radioulnar joint, traumatic injuries of.*

Triquetral fractures, 253–255

U

Ulnar wrist, physical examination of, 157–160

V

Volar fixed-angle plate osteosynthesis, for post-traumatic malunion of distal radius fractures, 211–212

W

Wrist
    anatomy of, **127–148**
        joint, 127–128
        ligament, 128–130
        retinacular, 130–131
        surface landmarks, 127
        vascular, 131–134
    dorsal, physical examination of, 157
    osteology of, 127–128
    physical examination of, **149–165**
        carpal instability, 160–164. See also *Carpal instability, provocative tests of.*
        differential lidocaine injection in, 164
        distal, 157–160
        dorsal, 157
        DRUJ, 159
        observation in, 149
        palmar, 160
        palmar ulnar structures, 159–160
        palpation in, 149
        radial, 150–157
        range of motion in, 149
        special tests in, 149–150
        ulnar, 157–160
    radial, physical examination of, 150–157
        de Quervain's tenosynovitis, 154
        first carpometacarpal joint, 155
        first dorsal compartment, 153–154
        flexor carpi radialis, 152–153
        intersection syndrome, 154
        palmar scaphoid, 150–152
        radial artery, 153
        scaphotrapezial joint, 153
        snuffbox, 155–157
        superficial branch of radial nerve, 154
    surgical approaches to, **127–148**
        application of external fixator, 146–148
        approach to Guyon's canal, 139–140
        carpal tunnel approach, 137–138
        central palmar approach, 138–139
        direct ulnar approach, 145–146
        dorsal approach to distal radioulnar joint, 145
        extended flexor carpi radialis approach, 130
        longitudinal dorsal approach, 144–145
        radial approach to scaphoid, 140–144
        volar approach to scaphoid, 135–137
        volar radial approach, 134–135
    ulnar, physical examination of, 157–160

Moving?

Make sure your subscription moves with you!

To notify us of your new address, find your **Clinics Account Number** (located on your mailing label above your name), and contact customer service at:

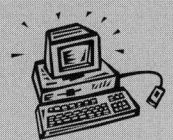

E-mail: elspcs@elsevier.com

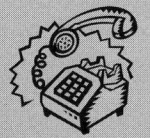

800-654-2452 (subscribers in the U.S. & Canada)
407-345-4000 (subscribers outside of the U.S. & Canada)

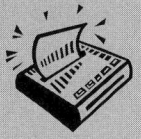

Fax number: 407-363-9661

Elsevier Periodicals Customer Service
6277 Sea Harbor Drive
Orlando, FL 32887-4800

*To ensure uninterrupted delivery of your subscription, please notify us at least 4 weeks in advance of move.

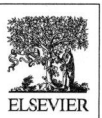

Monito?

Make sure your audience moves with you.